Allergy & Candida Cooking— Rotational Style

God Bless You!
Matthew 19:26
Sondra

Sondra K. Lewis

with Lonnett Dietrich Blakley
illustrations by Christine Hicks

Published by
Canary Connect Publications
Coralville, Iowa

Allergy & *Candida* Cooking—Rotational Style

First Printing, December 1994

Information contained in this book is intended to be useful and educational. It is not intended to replace medical diagnosis or treatment, but rather to provide recipes and information that may be of assistance in implementing a food allergy, *Candida* control, and/or rotational diet prescribed by your health-care provider. Please consult your nutritionally oriented health-care provider for medical advice before changing your diet.

The publisher and authors declare that to the best of their knowledge all material in this book is accurate. We shall have neither liability nor responsibility to any person with respect to any loss or damage caused, or alleged to be caused, directly or indirectly by the information contained in this book.

There are no warranties with the education of this book. We shall have neither liability nor responsibility to any person with respect to any loss or damage alleged to be caused, directly or indirectly, by the information contained in this book.

ISBN: 0-9643462-0-6
Library of Congress Catalog Number 94-92451

Printed in the United States of America

Published by Canary Connect Publications, P.O. Box 5317, Coralville, IA 52241-0317

Reviews of Allergy and *Candida* Cooking—Rotational Style

A superb book written by a person who's been there! This book should serve as an invaluable resource for any person with yeast-related health problems. I especially recommend it for those who continue to experience problems even though they take antifungal medication, avoid chemical pollutants, and take nutritional supplements.

—William G. Crook, M.D., author of The Yeast Connection, Chronic Fatigue Syndrome and the Yeast Connection, and Help for the Hyperactive Child

* * * * *

Congratulations on a job well done! The comprehensive information in Allergy and *Candida* Cooking—Rotational Style will help many people with food allergies and *Candida* yeast infections, especially those recently diagnosed and just getting into treatment. I especially like the care you have taken in suggesting appropriate treats and snacks for each of the four days. In my experience, people just won't stick with a diet that forbids all forms of fun foods. Yours appears to be a very livable plan for eating one's way to recovery—and it's already rotated. Thank you!

—Marjorie Hurt Jones, R.N., Editor, Mastering Food Allergies Newsletter

* * * * *

Sondra Lewis' knowledge of *Candidiasis* and the treatments for it is very impressive. In Allergy and *Candida* Cooking—Rotational Style she gives the medical background for problems related to *Candidasis* and food allergies as well as providing useful techniques to help individuals affected by them feel better. I highly recommend this book to anyone with *Candidiasis* and/or food allergies who is eager to actually get well by putting some much-needed effort into improving their diet while enjoying what they eat.

—Nicolette M. Dumke, author of Allergy Cooking with Ease and More Allergy Cooking with Ease #1

* * * * *

If you were to gather a few books together for a library covering natural foods preparation, this book by Sondra Lewis would be one of the best to add to your shelf. Many books have been written covering the field, however this book occupies a unique place because of its ease of use, helpfulness and applicability, and good basic coverage over a wide range of topics. It is especially valuable because it was developed through the personal needs and hands-on experience of the author. The thoughts and concepts were gathered and developed from a wide range of references, with the references fully documented. Highly recommended from beginner to expert!

—Larry Hendershot, Director of Technical Services, Arrowhead Mills, Inc.

* * * * *

Finally, I'll have a complete guide for my patients who are willing to go this route. What a wealth of information for me as a nutritionist! It should sit on all nutritionists' reference shelf.

—Barbara Schiltz, Nutritionist, New York

Reviews of <u>Allergy and *Candida* Cooking—Rotational Style</u> (continued)

* * * * *

I wish to congratulate you on an excellent book.

—George F. Kroker, M.D., FACAI, Allergy Associates of La Crosse, Ltd., Wisconsin

* * * * *

It was nice to get a cookbook I didn't need to outgas before reading. The "Helpful Hints" section is full of ideas to make the special diet easier to follow. I will often use the substitution tables for grains, thickeners, and eggs to adapt family recipes. Sondra gives detailed instructions on making tortillas and crackers from many types of grains and grain alternatives. The "Specialty Foods" section has fun stories of where different grains come from and explains how to use them. We will enjoy the wild game recipes. And I look forward to using the Resources section to order organic foods I cannot purchase locally.

—Judy J., Iowa

* * * * *

This is the best cookbook I have seen on the subject of Allergy and *Candida*. Compared to other cookbooks, it is much more detailed and has a larger variety of foods and recipes. I like the idea of the four day meal planning and recipes with a wide variety of foods. It makes meal planning much easier to follow. The spiral binding allows the book to lay flat so that it is easier to read when following the recipes. Thank you for a much needed book on Allergy and *Candida*.

—Ross R., Wisconsin

* * * * *

This is the most fantastic cookbook for EI (Environmental Illness) people I have ever seen. It is most exceptional! Sondra has done a great deal of testing and retesting in the process of developing her recipes as well as incorporating many different grains, nongrains, and alternative sweeteners. I have had the opportunity to be a tasting "guinea pig" for her recipes in addition to preparing them for my husband and myself. This is the type of book I needed when I was diagnosed with food allergies and MCS/EI (Multiple Chemical Sensitivities/Environmental Illness). It would have been a Godsend to be able to bring a book of this caliber home to read and use in learning more about food allergies, rotational diet, food families, and cooking with alternative foods.

—Elva W., Iowa

* * * * *

I found this cookbook to be just what I needed for planning meals for my family to keep our food allergies from increasing. Problems with *Candida* have affected five generations of my family, down to my 7-year-old daughter, and being able to prepare meals that help deal with this condition is important to me.

—Jo Ellyn O., Texas

ACKNOWLEDGMENTS

I wish to thank so many for their direct and/or indirect help in making this book a reality.

◊ Almighty God and His Son Jesus Christ, my Lord and Savior, for without their presence and guidance in my life this book would not have been conceived.

◊ Jedn and Iowa Vocational Rehabilitation for their belief in me and the beginning funds that brought Lonnett and I together in the Fall of 1991.

◊ Lonnett for her writing skills in taking my thoughts and words and turning them into understandable sentences.

◊ My great appreciation to all those who came before me in the study of food allergy, rotational diet, and *Candida* Related Complex for their knowledge, inspiring recipes, guidance, and examples through their writings as well as through many kind words of assistance. Just to mention a few—

William G. Crook, M.D. Marjorie Hunt Jones, R.N. Nicolette M. Dumke Sally Rockwell
Charlene Grimmett Pat Connolly Natalie Golos Frances Golos Golbitz
Gail Burton Stephanie Hayes Barbara Maynard

◊ Many thanks to Drs. Crook and Kroker for all their assistance with technical information—especially with Chapter 1.

◊ For the positive comments and constructive suggestions, a special thank you to those who reviewed my book

William G. Crook, M.D. George F. Kroker, M. D. Marjorie Hunt Jones, R.N.
Nicolette M. Dumke Larry Hendershot Barbara Schiltz
Elva Judy Ross Jo Ellyn

◊ Lonnett, Bob, Elva, and others for recipe ideas.

◊ Family and friends for their patience, encouragement, prayers, and being part of my quality control and assurance team as "official tasters."

◊ Special Friends—Betty, Elva, Judy, and Lonnett.

◊ Chris for graphic illustrations that add life and fun to my words.

◊ Members of the Caring Connection Writing Circles for their encouragement, patience, and prayers.

◊ My health-care team—Dr. Kroker, Sorrel, Dr. Kauffman, Kay, Dr. Kammeyer, Dr. Zdrazil, Dr. Carr, Betty, and James.

◊ Betty for her artistic flare with photography.

◊ Thanks for the encouragement from fellow food allergy and *Candida* warriors that I have met by phone and mail through my FOS sales.

◊ Thanks for all the encouragement, information, guidance, and support from all of the "beautiful" people I have met and/or talked with through gathering the information provided in this book.

◊ Business Systems International, Inc.—David and Koreen for their assistance in automating my office with computer equipment/software and education.

PREFACE

My goal and purpose in developing the rotational diet, recipes, and supplementary materials contained in this cookbook is to reach those persons who are searching for a healthier lifestyle and/or are seeking help with current health problems. My hope is to reach as many people as possible to encourage them to "wake up and smell the roses." This could involve making changes now to prevent the possibility of developing disabling conditions which could drastically affect their lives. Or it could involve implementing special methods to counter conditions already present. Changes in dietary habits, as well as in home, work, and other environments, can be essential steps in preventing the development of or in dealing with the presence of such conditions as *Candida* Related Complex (CRC), food allergies, and/or Multiple Chemical Sensitivities/Environmental Illness (MCS/EI)

As a symbol of my goal and purpose, I chose the name **Canary Connect** to illustrate the focus of my endeavors. Canaries were used in coal mine tunnels to warn miners of dangerous coal gases. Since canaries are more sensitive to coal gases than humans, they would stop singing (or even die) when the dangerous gases were present in the mine shafts. Coal miners would then know to leave immediately.

Those of us who are affected by Multiple Chemical Sensitivities/Environmental Illness (MCS/EI) have come to regard ourselves as warning canaries for today's world. Since we are more sensitive to chemicals and other dangerous substances present in today's world, we, as human "canaries," are singing out the message of danger to any and all who will hear and respond. We "sing" not only to reach those around us, but to connect with other human "canaries" to share information and techniques that may assist us in our daily lives.

This cookbook was developed from the wealth of available information regarding treatments for, as well as from personal experience in dealing with, *Candida* Related Complex (CRC) and food allergies. It presents an eating program which can assist in the treatment of these conditions. Based on those foods allowed on a *Candida* control diet, it uses a rotational format. Using a rotational eating program can help treat food allergies, prevent development of new food allergies, and maintain current food tolerances. The rotational format can also be used as a technique for uncovering and diagnosing food allergies. It is designed so that it can be used for the rest of your life, as well as for shorter time periods.

Although many cookbooks which address the areas of CRC and/or food allergies recommend the rotation of foods, only a few of them actually provide a complete rotational format to use. This cookbook not only provides a complete 4-day rotational diet, but it includes meal planning techniques and over 350 recipes to aid you in incorporating it into your daily life.

I wish I could write a rotational diet complete with recipes that everyone could use without modifications. But because of the circumstances and requirements involved for each individual, the specific rotational diet found in this cookbook will not be a "perfect fit" for everyone. However, it can be adjusted and tailored to provide a personalized plan to meet individual needs using the rules and techniques contained in this cookbook. The basic information and techniques; the specialty food information and resources; the helpful hints for planning and cooking; and the delicious, “healthy” recipes can be of great assistance for persons working to control *Candida* Related Complex (CRC) and/or food allergies through dietary means. It is an accomplishable goal and this cookbook may just provide the help, encouragement, hope, and support needed to achieve success.

YOU *CAN* DO IT—AND *ENJOY* THE PROCESS!

Best wishes to you as you begin the adventure of incorporating a rotational diet into your life. Remember, you are not alone and there are many resources available to you in this endeavor. It is my hope that this cookbook will be a useful and important part of your journey.

Read . . . Cook . . . Eat . . . Enjoy!

Sondra

TABLE OF CONTENTS

If you have a problem you must know that it simply is not going to go away—you might as well face it, tackle it, do something about it.

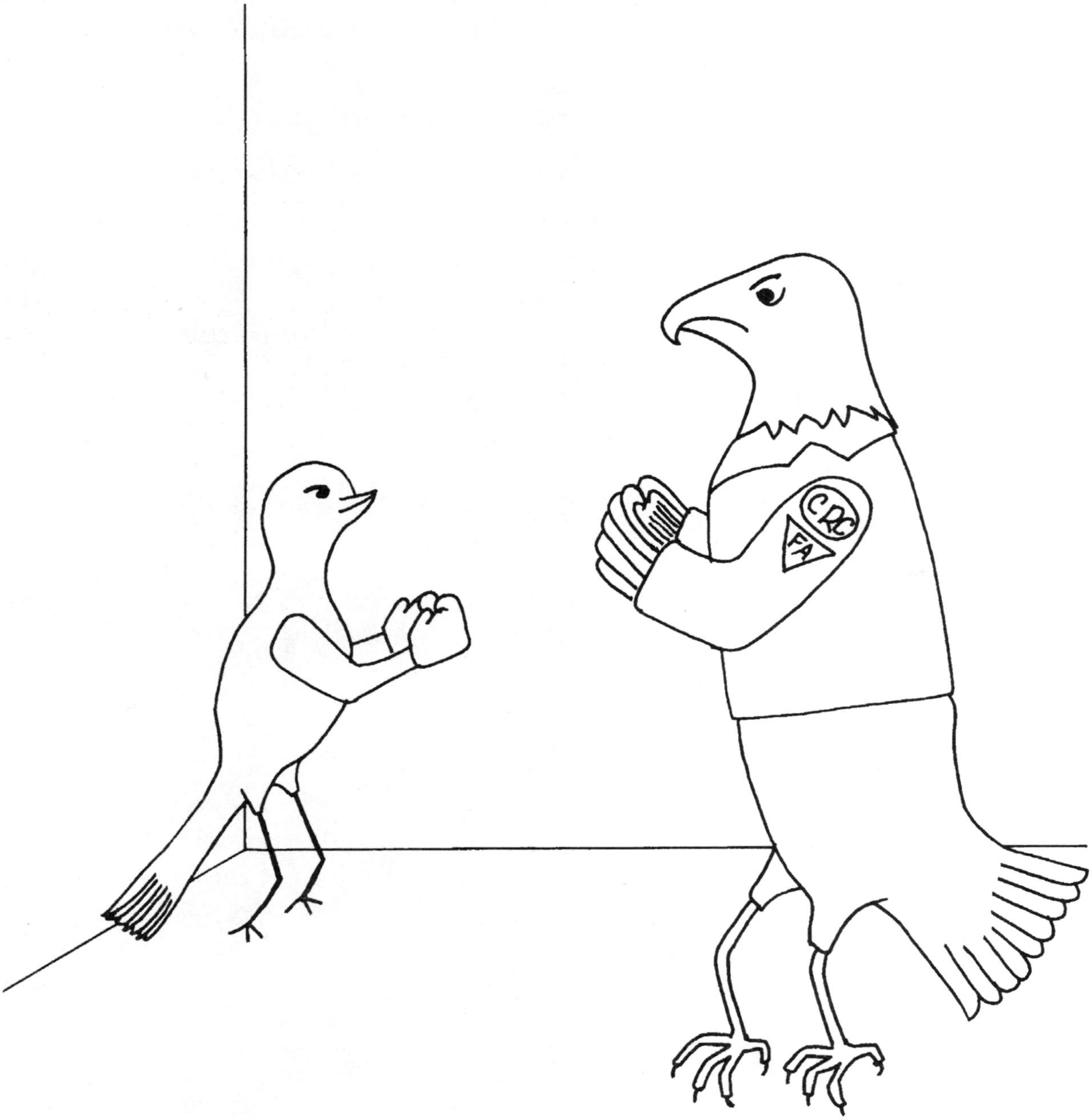

HOW TO USE THIS COOKBOOK

To receive the full benefit from this cookbook, I strongly recommend that you read it in its entirety before starting a food allergy, *Candida* control, and/or rotational diet. However, if you have a good knowledge base regarding *Candida* Related Complex, food allergies, and the rotary diversified diet, you can begin by scanning Chapters 4–6. Then read and study Chapter 7—Meal Planning before beginning the rotational diet set forth in this cookbook. *Meal planning is the* ***core*** *of beginning and remaining on a food allergy, Candida control, and/or rotational diet.*

The most important tool that you need to be able to use the information and recipes in this cookbook is a level of ***commitment*** which grows with experience. The recipes follow the *Candida* control diet as well as a 4-day rotational food plan. The cookbook's format was developed to be user friendly to help the reader avoid the long trial-and-error process often experienced when beginning a food allergy, *Candida* control, and/or rotational diet. Through the helpful information and delicious recipes in this cookbook, and with commitment on your part, success can be achieved quickly with this diet plan.

The recipes and 4-day rotational diet in this cookbook were developed from my first-hand experience with *Candida* Related Complex and food allergies. I did not have all the information and recipes in this cookbook when I first started. It took about 1 1/2 years before I was eating almost all organic foods. My use of specialty foods gradually grew over a five year time period, as did my number of recipes, and the rotational diet was under constant revision over a three year time period. Recently (past 1 1/2 years), through the use of this diet and other techniques incorporated into my health care plan, I have experienced enough healing to give me the energy needed to complete this cookbook. Now the rotation and the recipes are available to you just waiting for the addition of your commitment to use them.

About the Recipes

Many of the recipes emphasize taste and variety, but they also emphasize "traditional" foods with slight changes. The recipes may have different ingredients than those to which you are accustomed, but there are only slight changes in flavor and texture. Before you know it your taste buds will not crave or need the original version. In addition, the similarities will help other family members become accustomed to eating the same foods as you do, which will save you meal preparation time.

A low percentage of my recipes contains common food allergens such as egg, dairy, soy, and corn. Wheat is totally omitted unless you count the wheat alternatives such as spelt and Kamut® (see Chapter 4—Specialty Foods for more information on these two grains).

Before beginning a recipe, read through it first to be sure you have all the ingredients. Set out the ingredients and organize them in the order they are listed, which is the order that you will most likely need them in the recipe. Also, set up your mixing and/or cooking area.

Chicken Cabbage Rolls
(from This Cookbook)

1/2 pound	ground chicken
1 cup	celery, diced
1/4 teaspoon	sea salt
1 cup	cooked brown rice
2 cups	Chicken Broth
2 tablespoons	hulled sesame seeds
1/4 cup	brown rice flour
1/4 teaspoon	sea salt
4–6	medium-size cabbage leaves

Chicken Cabbage Rolls
(As It May Appear in Other Cookbooks)

1/2 pound ground chicken
1 cup celery, diced
1/4 teaspoon sea salt
1 cup cooked brown rice
2 cups Chicken Broth
2 tablespoons hulled sesame seeds
1/4 cup brown rice flour
1/4 teaspoon sea salt
4–6 medium-size cabbage leaves

The ingredient and amount sections of the recipes are formatted with the amount column on the left and the ingredient column on the right with a small space in between. This allows you to move your finger down the list of ingredients very quickly to see if you have all of them before you start. If you do not usually keep a specific food product on hand or know you have a limited amount of an ingredient, a quick glance to the left will let you check the amount needed for the recipe. This format allows you to check the list quickly without constantly moving your eyes back and forth (see comparison).

The recipe instructions are written in great detail using a numbered, step-by-step outline. At first glance, many of the recipes may appear very long and complicated and as though they will take a great deal of time to prepare. Please take the time to read through the directions to discover that in reality they are an easy step-by-step guide to preparation. The numbered outline helps you refer back to each step as you are completing it. Once you complete a step you can then review the next step before beginning it.

There are not a great number of recipes in this cookbook that describe how to cook vegetables plain. If you need assistance in this area, as many people do—especially with the unfamiliar vegetables, I highly recommend that you acquire The Yeast Connection Cookbook by William G. Crook and Marjorie Hurt Jones. Marge has written an excellent forty page chapter on vegetable cookery (see pages 229-269). She gives you an introduction to unfamiliar vegetables as well as pointers about selection, storage, and simple preparation. This information will assist you in adding more vegetables and diversity to your diet.

If you begin your journey with the attitude shown by the canary on page xiv—"I may be backed into a corner, but I'm not giving up!"—you can achieve more than you may have imagined. The canary shown just inside the back cover (page 370) has used the tools of commitment and knowledge (in the form of this cookbook) to fight the battle against *Candida* Related Complex and/or food allergies and is doing well in his/her search for better health. Many persons facing these challenges feel discouraged and as though they are "cornered." But it is important to remember that in some ways this is not a bad position to start from. The walls at your back protect you from that direction and the only way you can go is forward. Gather your resources and begin the fight!

Ready to start on your culinary adventure? Give yourself a hug and be proud of yourself for each accomplishment—minor or major. You will be in my prayers as I ask for success and encouragement for you in this endeavor.

Sandra

1. *CANDIDA* RELATED COMPLEX (CRC)

Following is a review of the literature available on *Candida* Related Complex (CRC) and should not be substituted for medical advice from a nutritionally oriented, health-care professional.

What is *Candida Albicans*?

Yeasts are members of the Fungi Family, which is part of the vegetable kingdom. These single-cell, opportunistic organisms, like their "cousins" the molds, can be found everywhere—in the air, soil, and water as well as in our food and bodies. One family of yeasts that lives in the warm, moist mucous membranes of our bodies, particularly in the digestive and genitourinary regions, is *Candida albicans*. *Candida albicans* is a part of the body's normal flora.

Another part of the body's normal flora is friendly bacteria. In a healthy body, there is a correct balance of *Candida albicans* and friendly bacteria. However, in a weakened body a reduction of friendly bacteria allows the normally harmless *Candida albicans* to multiply out of control. This results in an overgrowth of this organism, which is a major cause of chronic illness. The medical term for this overgrowth of *Candida albicans* is *Candidiasis* (pronounced can-di-DIE-ah-sis).

A graphic illustration of *Candida albicans* overgrowth, may be found on pages 10–11 of Dr. William G. Crook's book The Yeast Connection where drawings and symbols are used to demonstrate a normal balance of friendly bacteria and *Candida* compared to the imbalance of these factors found in persons with *Candidiasis*.[1]

So What is the *Candidia* Related Complex (CRC)?

Until the late 1970's, the common yeast *Candida albicans* was thought to cause health problems in only two categories—minor infection of the mucous membrane, skin, or nails in the average person and blood-borne infections in individuals with severely weakened immune systems.

By contrast, this often-misdiagnosed illness also can manifest itself as a severe chronic systemic infection which can cause extensive tissue damage throughout the body. Several factors may be involved in this systemic infection.

First, when the *Candida albicans* (yeast) in the body multiplies severely out of balance it throws off toxins. These toxins are chemical compounds that are picked up and absorbed into the bloodstream and body tissues causing an allergic reaction to the toxins.

Second, an allergic reaction to the *Candida albicans* organism can cause a release of chemicals such as histamines. These chemicals react with different parts of the body resulting in various symptoms.

Third, an overgrowth of *Candida albicans* in the gut (as well as other possible factors)[2,3] can cause the intestinal mucosa (the gut lining) to become inflamed which

---

[1] William G. Crook, M.D. The Yeast Connection (New York, NY: Vintage Books, A Division of Ramdom House, 1986), 10-11.

[2] Marjorie Hurt Jones. "Candida—A Different Approach," Mastering Food Allergies (Vol. IV, No. 7, Issue No. 37, July-August 1989), 3.

[3] Marjorie Hurt Jones. "Leaky Gut: A Common Problem with Food Allergies," Mastering Food Allergies (Vol. VIII, No. 5, Issue No. 75, September-October, 1993), 1.

weakens the gut wall and allows it to become more permeable. Undigested food particles are then able to leak into the blood stream. The food particles are identified as foreign "invaders" and are attacked by the immune system resulting in allergic reactions (food allergies) and the development of various symptoms. This condition is referred to as "leaky gut syndrome."[4]

Because the symptoms of *Candidiasis* are numerous and complex, we will discuss them later in the section called "What Are the Symptoms of *Candida* Related Complex (CRC)?"

Over the years many different names have been used to label the condition suffered by individuals with *Candida*-related health problems. These names include "*Candida* Toxicity Syndrome,"[5] Chronic *Candidiasis*, Chronic Polysystemic *Candidiasis*, *Candidiasis*-Hypersensitivity Syndrome, "The Yeast Connection," the Yeast Syndrome, and "*Candida*." However, George F. Kroker, M.D., of LaCrosse, Wisconsin, suggested a new name, *Candida* Related Complex or CRC.[6] For simplicity, in this cookbook the term *Candida* Related Complex (CRC) is used to describe any or all health problems attributed to the overgrowth of *Candida albicans*.

What Causes *Candida* Related Complex (CRC)?

What Causes CRC

- Diet rich in sugar and yeast
- Antibiotic use
- Steroids (cortisone, prednisone)
- Pregnancy hormonal changes
- Menstrual cycle hormonal changes
- Birth control pills
- Chemical, physical, and emotional stress
- "Leaky gut syndrome"

There are several factors that cause the normally harmless *Candida albicans* (yeast) to grow out of control. Interestingly, our twentieth-century American diet, rich in sugar and yeast, encourages yeast growth. In addition, because of the effectiveness of antibiotics in alleviating bacterial infections, the medical profession has come to rely heavily on them in their treatment programs. This extensive use of antibiotics, while effective in the short term, can cause complications resulting in yeast overgrowth. Also, in women the hormonal changes caused by taking birth control pills or the hormonal changes that occur during pregnancy and the menstrual cycle encourage yeast growth.

"Leaky gut syndrome," a condition which results from a breakdown of the gut mucosa[7] (the gut lining), can also contribute to an overgrowth of *Candida albicans* since it can result in a weakened immune system and an imbalance in the intestinal flora.

When *Candida* yeast overmultiplies, it releases toxins that weaken the body's immune system. The immune system can also be weakened by physical, chemical, and emotional stress as well as by allergies. In addition, steroids (cortisone, prednisone) suppress the immune system's ability to fight the overgrowth of *Candida albicans*. A weakened immune system allows germs that cause nose, throat, sinus, ear, bronchial, bladder, and other infections to invade our bodies.

These infections make us sick, and often we take antibiotics, especially "broad spectrum" antibiotics, to get well. Also, extended antibiotic cycles of tetracycline are often used to treat teenagers and others with severe acne problems. Unfortunately, antibiotics, including tetracyclines, cannot discriminate between friendly bacteria and the disease-causing

---

[4] Ibid.

[5] Gail Burton. The *Candida* Control Cookbook (New York, NY: New American Library Books, a Division of Penguin Books USA, Inc., 1989), 1.

[6] William G. Crook, M.D., and Marjorie Hurt Jones, R.N. The Yeast Connection Cookbook (Jackson, TN: Professional Books, 1989), 25.

[7] Marjorie Hurt Jones. "Leaky Gut: A Common Problem with Food Allergies," Mastering Food Allergies (Vol. VIII, No. 5, Issue No. 75, September-October, 1993), 1.

bacteria. Thus the antibiotics destroy both, leaving the *Candida albicans* (yeast) a proper environment for overgrowth because there are not enough friendly bacteria in the body to keep the yeast growth under control.

Since the yeast is not harmed by the antibiotics, it begins to multiply and to throw off toxins. It adheres to the cell membranes by sending out projections that penetrate the cell lining.[8] To further complicate the situation, even after the antibiotics are stopped the yeast continues to multiply at a higher rate releasing more toxins into the body. Again, this is due to the fact that the controlling friendly bacteria population has been reduced by the antibiotics.

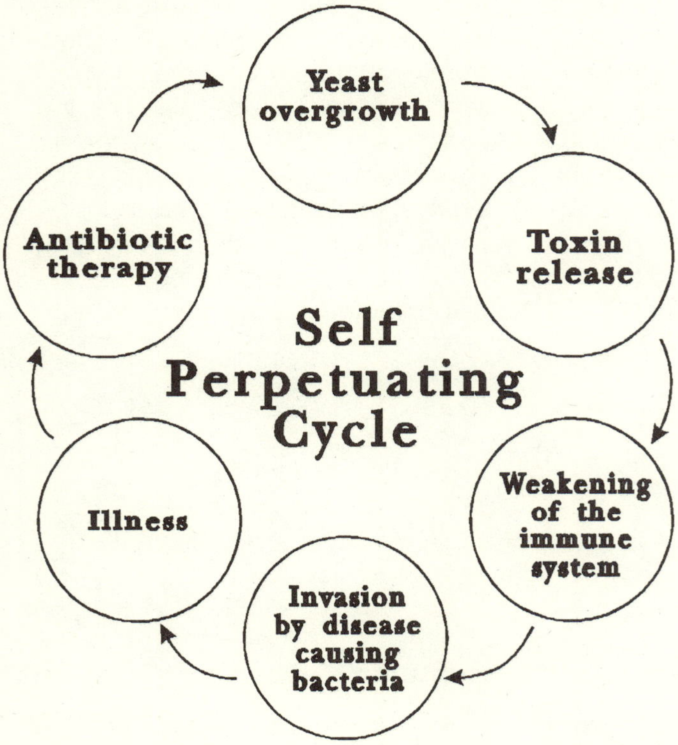

This pattern of yeast overgrowth, toxin release, weakening of the immune system, invasion by disease-causing bacteria, illness, antibiotic therapy, and resulting additional yeast overgrowth is a self-perpetuating cycle. The overgrowth of yeast causes more and more health problems as the cycle repeats again and again. As an additional contributing factor, when people get sick often they lose their taste for healthy foods. Instead they desire "junk" foods, particularly sugar-laden desserts, which add to the problem.

The continued use or overuse of antibiotics, birth control pills, and steroids is often a major contributing factor in the development of CRC. Too few modern health-care professionals have realized the dangers involved in the extensive use of these substances and the resulting physical changes they initiate.

An analogy used by Dr. George F. Kroker of LaCrosse, Wisconsin, to help patients understand what is happening to them involves the comparison of a heart attack to *Candida* Related Complex and the underlying causes for both.

When a person has a heart attack, the illness itself really does not involve just the heart—it involves the entire cardiovascular system. Heart attacks do not just "occur." They often are the result of many years of wear and tear on the cardiovascular system from things such as high blood pressure, elevated cholesterol levels, smoking history, etc. Therefore, a good cardiovascular physician not only focuses on the heart attack, but also on the underlying causes of the attack. Treatment includes eliminating or lessening as many of these factors as possible to help prevent a further heart attack.

Dr. Kroker views CRC as a "heart attack of the immune system" with the immune system weakness and the underlying causes for it as the key factors. In 85% of CRC patients, this immune system weakness is caused by allergic illness preceding the yeast-related problems. A very common scenario is one where the CRC patient had recurrent infections as a result of untreated allergies earlier in life. Then the antibiotics used in treating these infections set the patient up to have more yeast-related problems. Simply treating CRC directly with a sugar-free diet and antifungal medication may be inadequate if underlying

[8] Gail Burton. The Candida Control Cookbook, 1.

issues such as mold allergy, chemical sensitivity, malnutrition, and immune system weakness are not directly addressed.

To better understand what happens in your body when there is an overgrowth of *Candida albicans*, try this experiment using active dry yeast (bread yeast). Bread yeast and *Candida albicans* yeast are different, but they both desire the same environment and have similar growth patterns. In a clear, two-cup measure, add one package of active dry yeast to one-half cup of lukewarm water (approximately 100–110° F.). Do not stir. Watch what happens over a three-minute period. Now add one tablespoon of granulated sugar (again, do not stir) and watch what happens. What you have just seen was yeast in its inactive state and its reaction when you gave it a warm, moist place to live and it started to slowly grow. Then you fed it sugar and it grew faster. In fact, within three minutes you created a population explosion. After ten minutes you will find a thick layer of rapidly growing yeast colony on top of the water. If the yeast is allowed to grow with further nourishment but the water becomes cold, the yeast will stop reproducing. However, your digestive tract is always a dark, moist, warm place. So to control the yeast's growth in a weakened system where the friendly bacteria are reduced, you need to omit foods on which *Candida albicans* feeds (sweets and other simple carbohydrates). Then you need to include friendly bacteria-enhancing substances in your diet. (See sections on friendly bacteria supplements, pages 18–19, and on FOS probiotic enhancer, pages 19 and 50–52.)

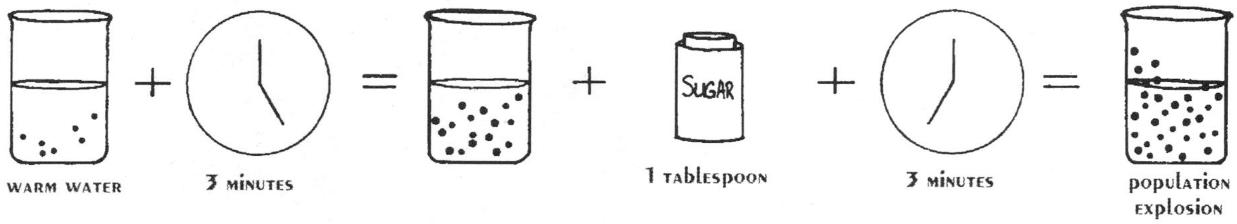

Who Discovered *Candida* Related Complex (CRC)?

C. Orian Truss, M.D., an allergist and internist, first pioneered the awareness of *Candida* Related Complex, which he called Chronic *Candidiasis*. He has studied the connection between human illness and the yeast, *Candida albicans*, for over twenty years. Many who have benefited from his studies say that he deserves recognition from organized medicine for his work, but this will probably not happen in his lifetime.

Only a few in the medical professions have accepted the idea that yeast can cause so many health problems. This is partly due to the fact that the toxic substances produced by the overgrowth of *Candida albicans* have not been specifically isolated or characterized. Nonacceptance or nonrecognition of this condition by many health-care professionals and the resulting lack of treatment or mistreatment greatly contributes to the continuance and worsening of its symptoms.

Often the health-care professional who does recognize CRC and is working to aid those with the condition has firsthand experience of the devastating effects of the overgrowth of *Candida albicans*. Whether because of personal health problems or those of a family member, he/she has learned of the underlying causes of the condition and the available treatments to alleviate its effects.

The discovery of CRC is a major medical breakthrough that brings hope to thousands of desperate and distraught people. This is particularly important to women who are not crazy as they have been led to believe by many in the medical field. Since Dr. Truss's discovery, many others in the health-care professions have added additional research and information to the study of CRC and have greatly improved understanding of the condition and treatment options.

What Are the Symptoms of *Candida* Related Complex (CRC)?

The symptoms of CRC are numerous and complex. This may be the most prevalent reason why physicians either ignore CRC as a real condition or misdiagnose it as some type of emotional disorder.

Often people say that they are "sick and tired of being sick and tired." You may feel almost like a hypochondriac or people may label you a hypochondriac if you talk about all your aches and pains. This feeling is perpetuated because the symptoms may come and go as your body and mind adapt to feeling ill. Or your immune system may wax and wane as it struggles to deal with the demands placed upon it causing your symptoms to appear and disappear. Often so many things are bothering you that the symptoms become masked like some food allergy reactions (see discussion of masked food allergies starting on page 24).

Following is a list of the most common symptoms of CRC, which are divided into four categories. You should be aware that if you have CRC you do not necessarily exhibit all of these symptoms.

Allergic reactions include:

- acne
- asthma
- bronchitis
- dizziness
- earaches and itchy ears
- food allergies and/or food cravings
- hay fever
- headaches
- hives
- itchy and/or burning eyes
- mold allergies, symptoms flare up on damp days or in moldy places
- severe chemical sensitivities
- sore throat

Emotional and mental problems include:

- confusion, fretfulness
- extreme irritability and anxiety
- insomnia
- lethargy, fatigue, a "drained" feeling
- loss of libido (loss of sexual drive)
- memory lapses, poor memory, inability to concentrate
- severe depression

Intestinal and urinary tract symptoms are:

- bowel problems, diarrhea and/or constipation
- gas, abdominal pain, bloating, indigestion
- inflammations of the stomach lining and/or colon
- menstrual complaints, especially PMS
- nausea
- prostate problems
- urinary tract infections
- yeast vaginitis

Other physical manifestations include:

- appetite changes*
- athlete's foot, jock itch, nail fungus, oral thrush
- blurred vision
- myalgias, muscular flu-like symptoms
- numbness, tingling, muscle weakness
- tightness in chest
- weight gain or loss

*Many CRC patients lose their taste for vegetables and animal protein, foods on which *Candida* does not thrive. Cravings for foods on which *Candida* thrives often appear and compulsive overeating of these foods is common. Women often experience these cravings a week prior to their menstrual period. For the health-conscious person, food cravings may include honey, granola bars, whole-grain bread, cheese, dried fruit, nut mixes, or peanut butter. Persons who follow an all-American "junk" food diet may crave chocolate chip cookies, milk, pizza, alcoholic beverages, or other refined carbohydrates such as white sugar or bleached flour.

Diagnosis of *Candida* Related Complex (CRC)

Patient history and an evaluation of symptoms are keys to making a correct diagnosis of CRC. The health-care professional pays careful attention to the patient's history of medications that destroy the delicate balance between *Candida albicans* and the friendly bacteria in the body. These medications include antibiotics, steroids, and birth control pills, especially if used over extended periods. Symptoms that the health-care professional would be listening for include any from the above list, especially chronic vaginitis or urinary tract infection. Also, yeast and mold allergies occur commonly in people with CRC. The patient's own positive response to the treatment for CRC will help to confirm a correct diagnosis.

If you would like to do a self-evaluation to help determine if you are affected by a *Candida albicans* overgrowth, the *Candida* Questionnaire and Score Sheet developed by William G. Crook, M.D., can be found in Appendix B. Filling out and scoring this questionnaire should help you and your nutritionally oriented, health-care professional evaluate how *Candida albicans* may be contributing to your health problems.

Who Treats *Candida* Related Complex (CRC)?

Finding a caring, nutritionally oriented, health-care professional who treats CRC is sometimes difficult. First, ask around your community for possible referrals for a physician, chiropractor, and/or certified nutritionist. Another good source of information could be employees at an organic grocery or health-food store.

If needed, several sources that you can contact for more information on physicians who treat CRC in your geographical area can be found in Section 4: Resources for Locating a Physician of Appendix C: Resources. These organizations may require a small monetary donation for their list. Also, for the fastest service, I would suggest you include a #10, self-addressed, stamped envelope with your request.

Because of the nature of CRC and the many facets involved in its treatment, I feel it is essential for your health-care professionals to be very nutritionally and naturally, as well as medically, oriented in their treatment program. They should have a thorough understanding of all immune factors that can weaken the system and promote CRC. Also, your health-care professionals need to have a very caring attitude as they work with you. Therefore, when I refer to your health-care professional in the following sections, please keep in mind the importance of these factors in your treatment program.

> *The world is round,*
> *and the place which may*
> *seem like the end may also*
> *be only the beginning.*
> *Ivy Baker Priest*

2. TREATMENTS FOR *CANDIDA* RELATED COMPLEX (CRC)

Because of the multifaceted nature of CRC symptoms and causes and the very individual-oriented factors involved, not all health-care professionals will use identical treatment programs for all their patients. Each treatment program works best if specifically tailored for the patient's needs. Because of these factors, this book should not be substituted for medical advice from a nutritionally oriented, health-care professional.

The dietary and additional treatment methods which follow are one facet of treatment that may be recommended by your health-care professional.

Dietary Treatment for CRC

A special sugar-free, yeast-free, mold-free, and diversified diet is the single most important yet most difficult part of the treatment for CRC. When you omit sweets from the diet, which is difficult, the yeast seems to yell for more sweets, creating a craving. You crave, dream of, and salivate for sweets while just thinking or talking about food. You may respond favorably to the diet in as few as ten days to two weeks. However, it is important to remember that although your major symptoms may disappear rather quickly, the *Candida* overgrowth was probably well established before it was identified. You must be persistent in the treatment and adhere to the diet for months and perhaps years to attain and maintain good health.

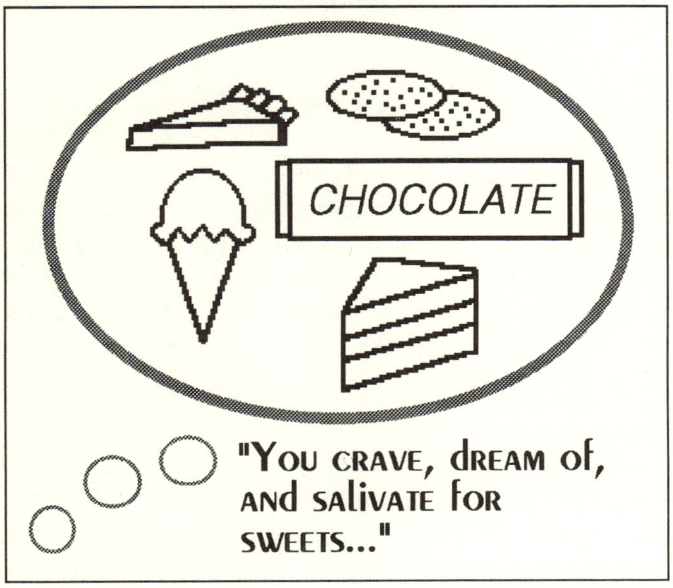

Even though you may not believe it, especially when you first start, the diet is manageable and can be incorporated into your lifestyle easily with support and guidance. (See more information about support on page 33.)

Your health-care professional may also suggest a low-carbohydrate diet, ranging from 60–100 grams per day. These carbohydrates should be consumed evenly throughout the day and can be gradually increased in amount as you improve. However, a prolonged high-protein/low-carbohydrate diet may cause problems for individuals with CRC in the form of persistent fatigue and weakness or excessive weight loss and malnutrition.

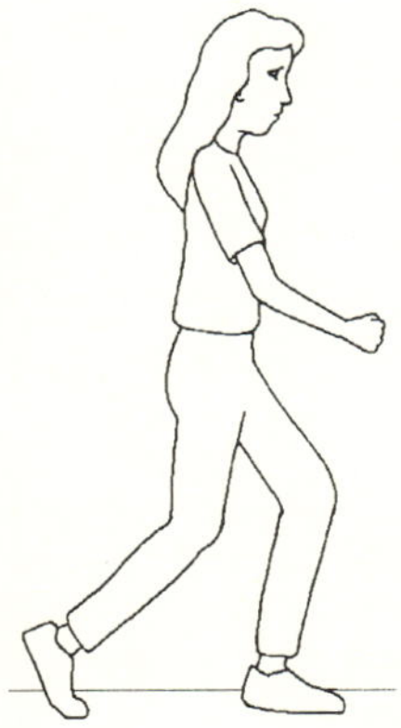

Many health-care professionals recommend regular exercise to aid in toxin elimination during the treatment. However, they feel that if carbohydrate intake is limited, the patient's energy level for exercise will also be limited. These professionals usually recommend eating complex carbohydrates freely (unless you are allergic to them). Instead they will only limit simple carbohydrates such as fruits.

You will probably need to eliminate simple carbohydrates for at least the first two weeks and often longer. Then gradually add individual fruits to discover which ones you can tolerate and in what amount. After doing this fruit challenge described in "Foods Partially Restricted" (page 13), you can gradually add sweeteners such as pure maple syrup, brown rice syrup, and honey to your diet.

The gluten in gluten grains such as wheat, rye, barley, oat, spelt, and Kamut® converts readily to glucose in the body which feeds the *Candida* yeast.[9] In addition, some of these grains are common food allergens so you may desire to test them carefully and watch for immediate and delayed reactions.

Remember, everyone is different and only you can listen to your body and make the best decision for you. Since *Candida* Related Complex (CRC) often clouds your ability to concentrate and make decisions, keep a notebook to record all the food you are eating. You will want to record date, time, food eaten, amount eaten, and any noticeable reactions you experienced as well as any possible other causes such as environmental factors.

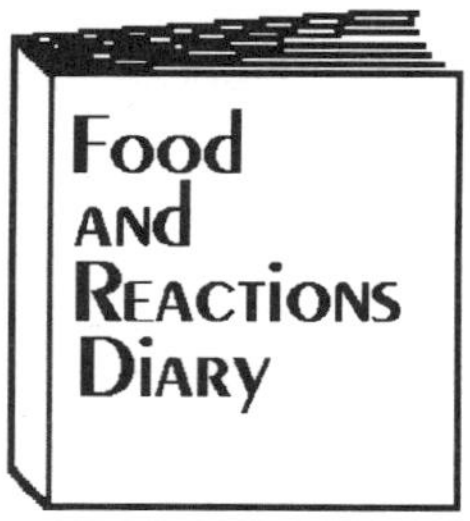

Day/Date	Time	Food & Form Eaten	Amount Eaten	Reaction & Possible Cause
8/25/94	*6 pm*	*Shrimp* *Corn on Cob with margarine* *Sliced Tomatoes*	*6 jumbo fried* *2 large ears* *1 large*	*developed a headache approximately 30 minutes after meal that lasted for 2 days—suspect corn*

Take this notebook and discuss it with your health-care professional for advice on customizing your diet. Also, sometimes a friend experienced with dealing with CRC and its treatment in his/her own life may be able to help you understand what is happening to you and help you adjust your diet. In addition, you may need to adjust your diet with the seasons. For example, because of the way my body reacts it is important for me to eat fewer fruits and other simple carbohydrates when it is rainy, damp, and moldy outside for long periods of time. During these times I crave something sweet, but I am much better off if I control these cravings.

Another word on complex carbohydrates—they are good for everyone. In fact, the old basic four food groups chart has been recently changed to a pyramid with complex carbohydrates consisting of whole grains at the base.[10] Your diet should contain 6–11 servings of complex carbohydrates per day,[11] around 55% of your total daily caloric intake.[12] Complex carbohydrates aid in the prevention and treatment of high blood pressure and heart disease, osteoporosis, and digestive disorders. As quoted in The Yeast Connection Cookbook, in a lecture given in January 1987, Sidney M. Baker, M.D., said that "eating a diet rich in complex carbohydrates is the best way to promote normal bowel flora in the person who has some immune dysfunction."[13]

Food cravings are part of the reason why the diet is the most difficult aspect of CRC treatment to follow. These cravings add to feelings of denial and lead to low self-esteem when you eat foods that are not on your diet plan. In addition, many CRC patients may temporarily

---

[9] Gail Burton. The *Candida* Control Cookbook (New York, NY: New American Library Books, a Division of Penguin Books USA, Inc., 1989), 4.
[10] Department of Agriculture. Food Guide Pyramid: A Guide to Daily Food Choices (Washington, DC: Government Printing Office, 1992).
[11] Ibid.
[12] Marjorie Hurt Jones, R.N. Mastering Food Allergies Newsletter (Vol. V, No. 9, Issue No. 49, October 1990).
[13] William G. Crook, M.D., and Marjorie Hurt Jones, R.N. The Yeast Connection Cookbook (Jackson, TN: Professional Books, 1989), 24.

lose their taste for vegetables and animal protein. Retraining your taste buds is difficult but possible. Soon you will be able to satisfy your sweet tooth by enjoying the desserts as well as other recipes I have developed for this cookbook. Also, the very different whole-grain and nongrain entrees, tortillas, crackers, breads, biscuits, and muffins will satisfy your desire for yeast breads.

Some health-care professionals say mold and yeast foods do not promote *Candida* growth, but they are removed from the diet because many people are actually allergic to yeast products. After your symptoms have cleared, you can do a challenge by trying a yeast food such as Brewer's yeast or vinegar. Watch closely for immediate and delayed reactions. Also, chemical reactions in your body involving yeast foods may cause hormonal changes which encourage the overgrowth of *Candida albicans* as mentioned in Chapter 1—*Candida* Related Complex (CRC) under the section entitled "What Causes CRC?" (page 4). You need to avoid yeast foods as one effort to stop the cycle of *Candida albicans*' overgrowth.

Another interesting factor to consider is that "recent research indicates that antibiotic-resistant strains of microorganisms can be spread by eating meats raised on steroids and antibiotics."[14] Choose meats and poultry raised without the use of antibiotics and growth hormones. Also, many times these meats have another plus because the animals are often fed organically raised grains. In addition, organically raised foods are recommended since the chemicals (herbicides and pesticides) in nonorganic foods can possibly weaken your immune system. (For more information on organic foods read Chapter 12—Organics—The Only Way to Go.)

It is important to drink 6–8 glasses (approximately 2 quarts) of water throughout each day. It is equally important for you to consider using some type of "purified" water: reverse osmosis, distilled, or bottled water. All brands of bottled water are not the same and some can have pesticides or other contaminants in them such as can be found in regular tap water. Also, city tap water contains chlorine and possibly fluoride which may weaken your immune system. In addition, consider using a natural toothpaste without fluoride. (See Appendix C: Resources for help in making an informed decision about purchasing "purified" water and/or a home water-purification unit.)

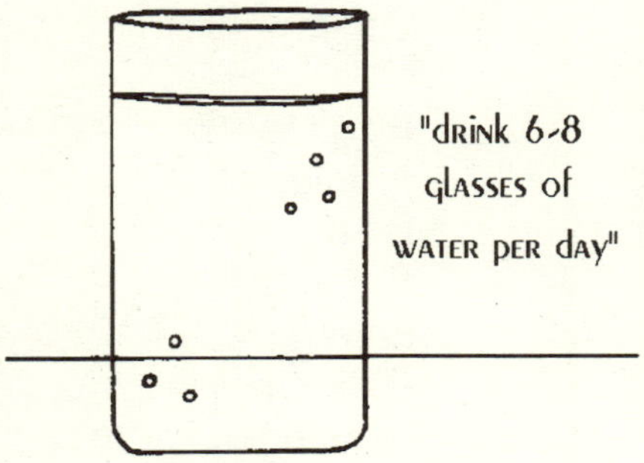

The time to relax is
when you don't
have time for it.
Sydney J. Harris

[14] Gail Burton. The *Candida* Control Cookbook, 5.

Candida Control Diet

The diet for treatment of *Candida* Related Complex (CRC) is unique to the individual. Therefore, since each person differs, what works for one may not work for another. The following diet guidelines may need to be modified for each individual.

Foods You Can Eat Freely (unless you are allergic to them)

Vegetables and Legumes

Artichoke
Asparagus
Beans, all kinds
Beet
Broccoli
Brussels Sprout
Cabbage
Carrot
Cauliflower
Celery
Chard
Cucumber
Eggplant
Garlic
Green Bean
Greens: Beet
Collard
Kale
Mustard
Kohlrabi
Leek
Lettuce, all kinds
Okra
Onion
Parsley
Parsnip
Peppers, all kinds
Pimento
Radish
Peas, all kinds
Potatoes, white & sweet
Rutabaga
Soybean
Spinach
Sprouts, all kinds
Squash, all kinds
Tofu
Tomato
Turnip
Yam

Nuts

Almond
Brazil Nut
Filbert
Macadamia Nut
Pecan
Pine Nut
Walnut

Seeds

Pumpkin
Sesame
Sunflower

Butters

Almond
Sesame
Sunflower

Fats

Butter
Oils, all kinds
except peanut

Whole Grains

Barley
Brown Rice
Corn
Job's Tears
Kamut®
Millet
Oat
Rye
Spelt
Teff
Wheat

Nongrains

Amaranth
Buckwheat
Quinoa

Fish/Shellfish

Cod
Crab
Halibut
Orange Roughy
Salmon
Shrimp
Trout
Tuna
Other fish/shellfish

Poultry

Chicken
Cornish Hen
Duck
Eggs
Goose
Pheasant
Turkey
Other poultry

Red Meats

Antelope
Beef
Buffalo
Lamb
Pork, uncured &
unsmoked only
Rabbit
Squirrel
Veal
Venison
Other red meat

Dairy

Yogurt, plain only

Starches

Arrowroot
Kudzu/Kuzu
Tapioca

Beverages

Water, "purified" is preferred
Sparkling Water
Lemon or Lime in Water
Pau D'Arco Tea (See Coffee and tea listing on page 14 and the paragraph in the section on "Other Treatments for CRC" on page 20)

Foods Partially Restricted

As with many CRC patients, you may need to omit the following fruits and sweeteners for the first two or more weeks. Depending upon your response to a food challenge of these individual fruits and sweeteners, you may not be able to add them to your diet.

Fresh Fruits

2–3 servings of the following may be eaten per day

1 medium apple
1/2 avocado
1/2 banana
1 cup blackberries
1 cup blueberries
1/2 cantaloupe
1 wedge Casaba melon
1 cup cherries
1 cup fresh shredded coconut
1/2 large grapefruit
1 cup grapes
1 medium lemon
1 medium orange
1 cup papaya cubes
1 medium peach
1 medium pear
1 wedge Persian melon
1 cup fresh diced pineapple
1 medium plum

Sweeteners

Limit the following to 1–2 teaspoons per day

Brown Rice Syrup
Honey
Pure Maple Syrup

After your major symptoms have cleared, you can do a food challenge. You can do this by gradually adding individual foods, in this case fruits, to discover which ones you can tolerate and in what amount.

To do a food challenge, select a food that you have not eaten in at least two or more weeks. As an example, we will select apple. To eliminate one more factor, we will peel the apple and only eat a very small apple or one-half of a medium-size apple. For the next 48 hours do not try any other fruits or foods that you are wanting to "challenge." This allows you to check for immediate and delayed reactions because you could have either or both of them for this one particular food.

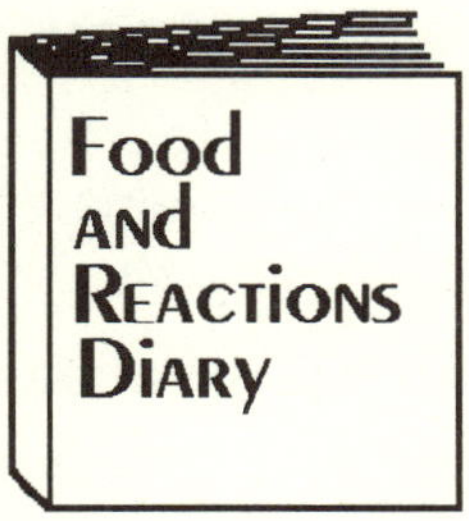

Keep a notebook to record the food you are trying. You will want to record date, time, food eaten, amount eaten, and any noticeable reactions you experience as well as any other possible causes such as environmental factors.

Day/Date	Time	Food & Form Eaten	Amount Eaten	Reaction & Possible Cause
8/25/94	*10 am*	*peeled apple*	*small size*	*no reaction for up to 2 days*

If you are very sensitive, it is always better to try your food challenges in a very controlled environment (such as home) where you are not going to be chemically challenged also.

After this approximate two-day period, if you have not noticed any reactions, you can add apple (or your selected food) to your list of foods that you can eat. In addition, the next time you try apple you may want to expand the challenge by eating the peeling and again waiting 48 hours to check for immediate and/or delayed reactions.

Now that you are continuing to stay well, select another food or fruit that you would like to try to add to your diet. This time you may wish to select a peach, a grape, or some other fruit that you would not peel to add that additional factor to your challenge.

Later you can try the sweeteners listed. When experimenting with fruits and other sweeteners, **I cannot emphasize enough** trying only a small amount of one at a time and being sure to wait for both immediate and delayed reactions (48 hours) before trying an additional amount or another food.

Foods You Must Avoid

Sugars and Sugar-containing Foods: Brown, granulated, and powdered sugar, and other sugars such as dextrose, fructose, galactose, glucose, glycogen, lactose (milk sugar), maltose, mannitol, monosaccharides, polysaccharides, sorbitol, and sucrose. Also avoid Sucanat (organic raw sugar), molasses, maple sugar, date sugar, and turbinado sugar. Read all labels of packaged foods to make sure there are no hidden sugars.

Artificial Sweeteners: NutraSweet and Equal (aspartame) often cause allergic reactions. Some can tolerate them in moderation, but be aware that they contain milk sugar or corn sugar which are also common allergens.

Common Table Salt: Most table salts contain dextrose and other chemicals. Instead use sea salt that may be free of these substances. Be sure to read the ingredient list on the label.

Milk and Milk-containing Products: Milk contains lactose, a simple carbohydrate which feeds the yeast, and should be avoided at least until you improve. Also, many persons are allergic to milk. Some can tolerate plain yogurt which is free of fruit, sugar or other sweeteners, preservatives, and additives.

Black Pepper: Black pepper is hard to digest so it is not recommended. However, in contrast, cayenne (red) pepper seems to promote digestion.

Caffeine and Caffeine-containing Products: Avoid coffee, tea, and other beverages that contain caffeine and chocolate. Instead drink water or sparkling mineral water and substitute naturally sweet-tasting carob for chocolate.

Yeast and Moldy Foods:

* Alcoholic beverages, beer, and wine are fermented and/or brewed with yeast.
* Breads, pastries, and other yeast-leavened bakery products.
* Cheeses: Aged, processed, cheese-containing foods are made from mold-fermentation methods and some also contain additives. Avoid foods containing whey, which is a by-product of the cheese-making process.
* Coffee and tea: Includes all varieties either caffeinated or decaffeinated, except Pau D'Arco tea. Mold collects on the beans and leaves during the drying process for coffee and tea. Even though herbal teas do contain molds, some are able to tolerate them. To start, try no more than one cup of herbal tea per day. As an exception, Pau D'Arco tea is beneficial in combating yeast and comes from the bark of trees resistant to fungi.
* Condiments, sauces, and other vinegar-containing foods are fermented. This includes mustard and catsup, barbecue, chili, shrimp, soy, steak, and tamari sauces. This also includes vinegar-containing foods such as green olives, horseradish, mayonnaise, pickles, pickled vegetables, relishes, salad dressings, and sauerkraut.

* Cream of tartar is made from the fermented residue in wine barrels and may aggravate your symptoms.
* Dried herbs: Mold collects on the leaves during the drying process. When possible, use fresh herbs. One teaspoon of dry herbs equals one tablespoon of fresh herbs. Note: Garlic is really not an herb and garlic in any form is beneficial in combating yeast. Cloves also kill yeast.
* Edible fungi: Includes citric acid, morels, mushrooms, and truffles.
* Fermented beverages such as cider and root beer.
* Fruit juices of all kinds except freshly prepared juices and unsweetened cranberry juice. Packaged juice is usually made from seconds, fruit that drops off the tree and bruises. Bruised fruit develops more mold growth that is often not cut away before processing. If you prepare your own juices, you can wash the fruit more thoroughly and avoid using fruits of second quality.
* Fruits that are moldy and dried fruits: This may include strawberries and other berries and melons. Dried fruits collect mold during the drying process. Also, avoid canned fruit.
* Malted products such as barley malt found in many cereals, candies, and malted milk drinks.
* Peanuts and pistachios harbor fungus. Also, avoid peanut oil.
* Processed and smoked meats such as pickled and smoked meat and fish: This includes beef jerky, corned beef, hot dogs, luncheon meats, pastrami, pickled meat, and sausages.
* Skins of fruits and vegetables accumulate mold during growth. Grapes and tomatoes especially have a particular fungus which grows on them. Scrub the skins of all vegetables and fruits before peeling or cutting to avoid spreading the mold.
* Tempeh and Miso: Tempeh is a cake of cooked split soybeans held together by a dense, white cultured mold closely related to mushrooms. Miso is a fermented soybean product.

General Tips to Follow in the *Candida* Control Diet

1. Avoid eating any foods that you are craving, even if they are listed as acceptable foods in the above diet. Chances are that you are allergic to that food or that the particular food (e.g., fruit, honey) will promote yeast growth and the yeast is yelling for that food.
2. Buy fresh or frozen vegetables, fruits, fish, poultry, and meats. Purchase only whole grains, whole-grain flours, raw nuts, and cold-pressed, unrefined oils. Organic and/or natural foods are the best alternatives.

3. Read all labels when buying foods to check for ingredients that need to be eliminated from your diet. For instance, most canned tomato products contain citric acid.
4. Food begins to collect bacteria, which can be harmful to your health, within 24 hours. To prevent mold growth, freeze leftovers soon after preparation. You may store them in the refrigerator for a while, but the freezer is better.

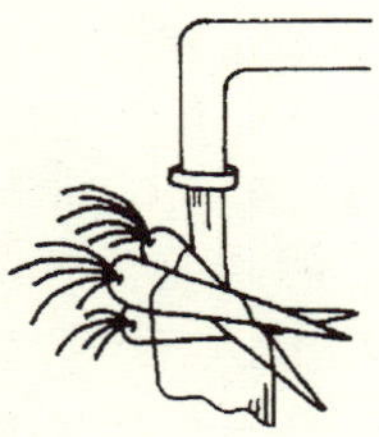

5. Rinse fresh vegetables and fruits thoroughly before using. Also, dispose of any fruit or vegetable with evidence of mold.
6. You may need to omit nuts and seeds in the beginning stages of the diet if you have a sensitive digestive system. However, ground nuts and seeds are easier to digest.

7. Choose alcohol-free flavorings and extracts but read the labels for other ingredients that may not be allowed.
8. Read and reread a variety of different materials on *Candida* Related Complex (CRC) so you can fully understand, visualize, and conquer it. (See Appendix D: Recommended Reading.)
9. Here are some tips for when you are eating at a restaurant or banquet:

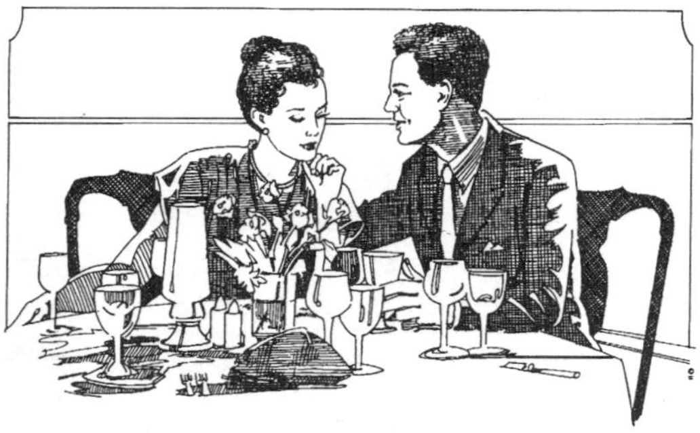

   - Plan ahead. Call ahead for the menu, particularly if you are attending a banquet.
   - Skip the appetizer or order a shrimp cocktail without the sauce. Eat the shrimp with just a squeeze of lemon or take your own Picante Sauce (page 196).
   - Order unflavored mineral water instead of wine or a mixed drink.
   - Use oil and a squeeze of lemon on the salad for dressing. Ask what is on the salad before ordering so you do not get foods that you need to avoid, e.g., bacon bits, croutons, etc.
   - Order animal protein without sauce—broiled dry is the best choice. We have a steak house restaurant in our town which offers a grilled shrimp dinner. They normally grill it in vegetable shortening. However, I take my own Clarified Butter (page 195) and have them use it instead of their vegetable shortening in preparing my dinner. I even ask them to scrape the grill to remove most of any leftover beef juices and vegetable shortening.
   - Order steamed vegetables instead of bread. Skip the bread, crackers, and dessert or take your own muffin or bread.
   - Order your baked potato dry and take your own Clarified Butter or flaxseed oil. If you usually enjoy your baked potato with sour cream, try substituting Sunflower Mayo or Creamy Italian Dressing (page 180). Also, do not eat the skin of the potato.
   - If you can tolerate herbal tea, sip that while others are eating dessert. However, my best suggestion is to eat slowly, more slowly than the others at your table, so you are still enjoying your meal while they are having dessert.
10. One of the most important tips that I can share with you is to enjoy your meals and make them attractive on the plate or in the serving bowls. Also, relax before, during, and after your meals to aid digestion. Eating slowly and chewing every bite aids in digestion. In order to relax before a meal, try to plan and prepare some things in advance. I will often wash and prepare my fresh vegetables ahead of time to avoid being rushed when it is time to prepare a meal.

Other Treatments for *Candida* Related Complex (CRC)

Treatment for CRC starts with a simple, effective goal of getting the yeast and toxins out of the body tissues and building up the body's ability to keep them out. In addition to diet, treatment can include several facets with the ultimate goal of building up the weakened immune system and moving toward a healthy lifestyle.

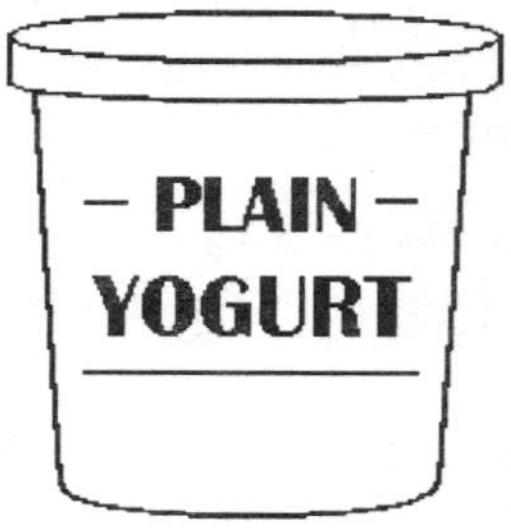

Because birth control pills encourage *Candida* growth, you should seriously consider a natural alternative method of birth control. Another important step is to avoid the use of all antibiotics and steroids unless absolutely necessary.

To help remedy chronic vaginal yeast infections, use a yogurt intravaginal treatment at night. The yogurt should be plain and sweetener-free with live active cultures. Over-the-counter vaginal yeast creams can help to eliminate the symptoms of the yeast infection, but they do not attack the cause of chronic infections. The yogurt treatment reintroduces good bacteria into the vaginal system to provide a natural check on the overgrowth of *Candida albicans*. Generally speaking, this has a better and longer-lasting effect on the yeast infection than the over-the-counter antifungal creams.

Also, since allergies weaken the immune system, you should be tested to discover any allergies you may have. Allergies are a serious factor and should not be treated lightly. Seek treatment for allergies, especially for those to yeast and mold. These allergies fight against the body's immune system and ability to resist infection. Allergies to mold are a major problem for persons with CRC. This is because a symptom (such as itchy or burning eyes) can result from an allergic reaction to airborne mold OR from an overgrowth of *Candida* making it difficult to determine the symptom's cause.

If you have food allergies, it is best to entirely avoid eating the foods to which you are allergic. Your second choice is to eat them only occasionally on a rotational basis. Eating the foods to which you are allergic on a rotational basis involves eating the food at least four days apart and usually **more** than four days apart. This time spread needs to be long enough that you do not notice any allergic reactions after consuming the food. This will lighten the load on your immune system. (More information about eating foods on rotation can be found in Chapter 3—Rotational Diet.)

Other Treatments for CRC

- Natural birth control methods
- Avoidance of antibiotics and steroids
- Yogurt intravaginal treatment
- Allergy testing and desensitization treatments
- Regular exercise
- Stress reduction
- Attitude adjustment
- Regular chiropractic care
- Therapeutic massage
- Avoidance of antacids
- *Acidophilus* supplements
- Natural probiotic enhancer (FOS)
- Vitamin and mineral supplements
- EFAs (essential fatty acids)
- Antifungal medications or supplements

If you are seeing a physician who is an allergist or a clinical ecologist, you may be tested for an allergy to *Candida*. Sublingual drops or shots may be prescribed to build your body's natural defense system and to lower your allergic reactions to *Candida albicans*.

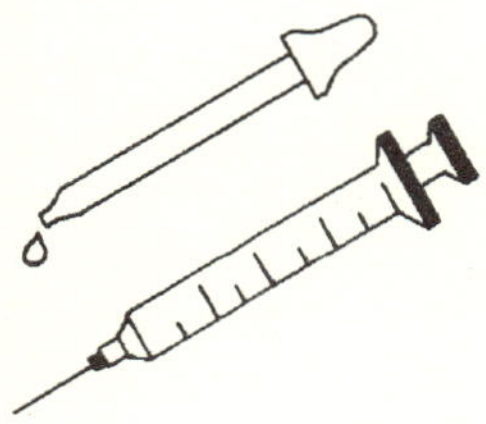

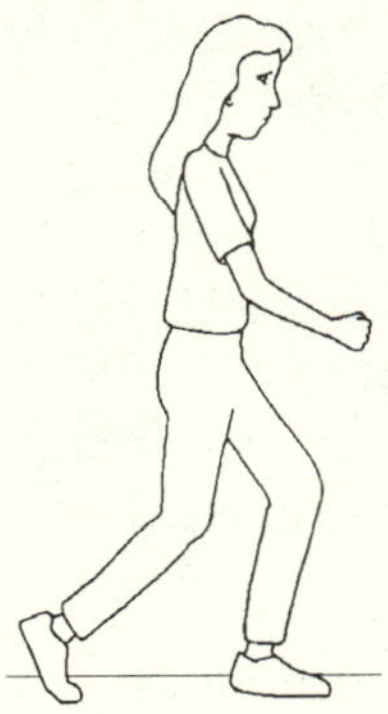

Regular exercise is important because it increases circulation, improves digestion, relieves stress, and helps release toxins that have become lodged in the muscles. Sweat created through exercise is a good avenue for toxin removal. Remember to breathe deeply during exercise. Those of us who are adversely affected by many odors may have developed a habit of shallow breathing. We need to make it a point to learn to breathe normally and also to take deep breaths when we know our air is of good quality.

Stress puts your body into an "alarm mode" that does not allow your immune system to heal. Even though exercise relieves stress, you need to regularly practice other methods for handling stress. I suggest prayer, personal Bible study, laughter, deep breathing coupled with progressive relaxation, talks with an understanding friend, and balancing your time indoors and outdoors, especially getting plenty of sunlight and enough restful sleep each day.

A positive mental attitude about your health is very important to your recovery. A healthy mind and a religious attitude are effective in determining how you deal with your situation and how you work mentally to heal your body and adopt a healthy life style. Strive for warm fuzzies in your life and reject the cold pricklies that could bring you down. A warm fuzzy is a warm, cozy, comforting hug (mental or physical) that lifts your outlook and attitude. A cold prickly is that person whom you have heard say to you "It's all in your head. There's nothing wrong with you." Cherish those warm fuzzies and seek them out at every opportunity.

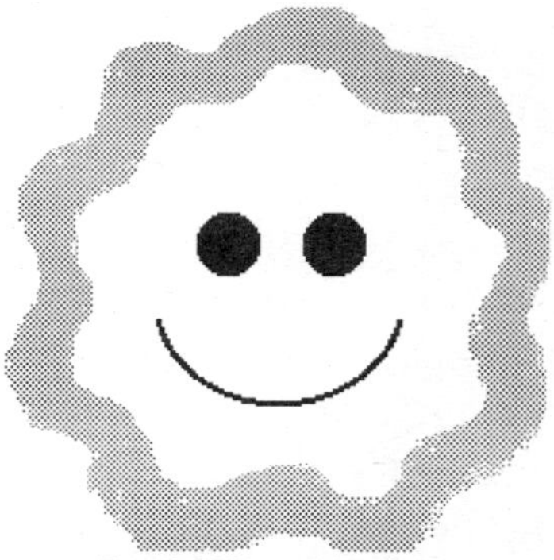

Seek Warm Fuzzies

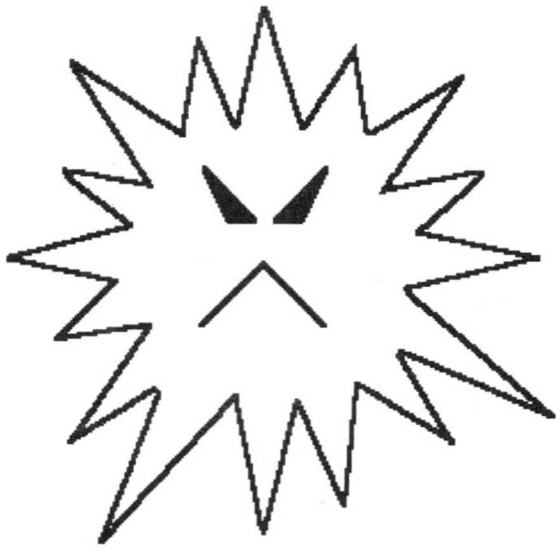

Reject Cold Pricklies

Consider seeking regular chiropractic care so structural stress is not weighing on your immune system. Skeletal misalignment can cause nerve interference, which blocks the energy flow and may slow down your healing. Nerves control all body functions and are responsible for the proper functioning of the immune system. Because of this, regular chiropractic care to naturally correct inefficient nerve and energy patterns is an important part of the healing process. This allows the immune system to fight back and attack the overgrowth of *Candida albicans* which is at the root of your health problems.

> A hug is a great gift.... One size fits all, and its easy to exchange.
>
> Lilly Biles

Likewise, therapeutic massage enhances energy flow and the release of toxins by keeping the muscles relaxed and loosened. This encourages increased and more complete blood circulation throughout the entire body. Since the circulatory system delivers nutrients to all parts of the body and removes toxins and waste, the increased efficiency resulting from therapeutic massage can greatly aid the body's healing process.

Avoid antacids since they promote an acid-free environment in your digestive system which encourages yeast growth. Instead, your health-care professional may suggest charcoal capsules or tablets for stomach distress. However, your stomach distress may be caused by just the opposite condition—too alkaline an environment. An alkaline stomach does not have the proper environment for food digestion and therefore may allow undigested food particles to appear in your stool. Repeated occurrences of this situation can lead to constipation, diarrhea, and nutrient deficiency. Hydrochloric acid capsules or tablets may be recommended by your health-care professional to aid in digestion as well as to combat yeast growth by returning your stomach to a proper acidic nature.[15]

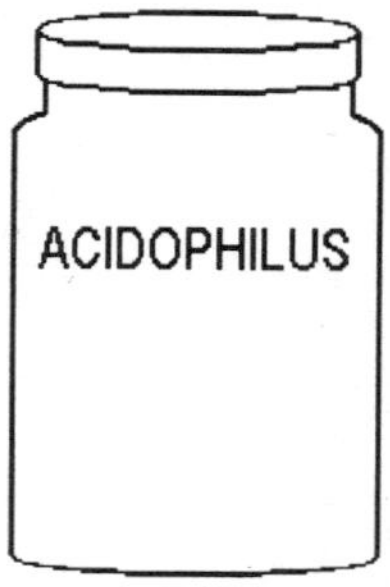

To help reestablish the normal flora in your digestive tract, take a good quality friendly bacteria supplement, commonly referred to as *acidophilus*. This supplement may contain *Lactobacillus acidophilus* (*L. acidophilus* or *L. dophilus*), *Bifidobacterium bifidum* (*B. bididum* or *L. bifidus*), *Streptococcus faecium*, and/or *Lactobacillus bulgaricus* (*L. bulgaricus*). To evaluate the quality of different brands, read the product label for a listing of ingredients included. Also look for substances specifically avoided in their production, such as common allergens—dairy, yeast, grains, soy, etc. Depending upon what bacterial culture medium is

[15] Gardiner Harris. "Low Stomach Acidity," Medical Nutrition (Spring 1989).

used, you may need to rotate your friendly bacteria supplement along with other supplements and foods. (See more information about rotation of foods in Chapter 3.) Also, compare different products for concentrations of *Lactobacillus* per gram. More specific information and research about *Lactobacillus* supplements can be obtained from several companies who market the product. Each company's research supports their product and often differs widely from what another manufacturer's research supports. Individual experimentation may be the best solution when choosing this **VERY IMPORTANT SUPPLEMENT** for your own use. Check with your health-care professional to see if he/she has a specific product to recommend. The *acidophilus* supplement that is right for one person may not be right for another.

Two factors are especially important when using an *acidophilus* supplement. First, be sure to choose a good quality supplement that displays an expiration date. Since good quality products contain live active cultures, they have a limited "shelf life" after which they lose much of their effectiveness. Inexpensive *acidophilus* products can be found in the supplement sections of grocery or discount stores. However, they may not contain the more effective active cultures and would therefore not be very effective in replacing the beneficial intestinal flora. Good quality supplements can be purchased from some health-care professionals, at health-food stores, through food-buying cooperatives, and from mail-order sources such as N.E.E.D.S. (see Appendix C: Resources).

Second, many of the individual *acidophilus* floras (especially *Bifidobacteria*) are acid sensitive and may have trouble surviving through the upper gastrointestinal tract. Because of this, it is important to support the existing beneficial flora in the gut by "feeding" it with a probiotic enhancer such as FOS to help it multiply naturally.

NATURAL PROBIOTIC ENHANCER

100% NUTRAFLORA™

FOS

FRUCTOOLIGOSACCHARIDES CONCENTRATE

FOS (fructo-oligo-saccharides) is a natural probiotic enhancer that "feeds" the beneficial bacteria in the gut, but which cannot be used by *Candida* and other yeast or by certain other harmful bacteria. Since the FOS molecule is too large to be broken down and used by the body, it reaches the intestines intact where it can be broken down and used by the beneficial bacteria. FOS is a relatively fine white powder with a clean taste. It is about half as sweet as sugar with no aftertaste or bitterness and is very simple to use. (For more information on FOS, see the section on Sugar Substitutes in Chapter 4—Specialty Foods.)

Your health-care professional will probably prescribe multivitamin and mineral supplements that do not have yeast as a base. Some companies which carry supplements that are yeast-free are Freeda Vitamins, Nutricology/Allergy Research Group, Twin Labs, Standard Process (except vitamin B supplements), and Metagenics. Again, just as when choosing an *acidophilus* supplement, read the labels to make sure the supplement is not made from any common allergens or from any food which causes you allergic reactions. If the supplement does not say yeast-free, there is an almost 100% chance that the B vitamins are grown on yeast. In any case, your wisest choice is to purchase a quality brand rather than the inexpensive supplements often found in discount stores or supermarkets.

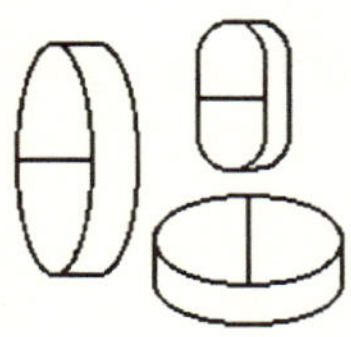

In addition to multivitamin and mineral supplements, your health-care professional may suggest a supplement such as chlorophyll or Nutricology/Allergy Research Group's AntiOx to help eliminate toxins from the blood and gastrointestinal tract. An antioxidant is a "substance that scours the body for unstable oxygen molecules call free radicals, which can cause cell damage."[16] It may include beta carotene, dimethylglycine (also called DMG or vitamin B_{15}), selenium, vitamin A, vitamin C, and/or vitamin E. Keeping your colon moving (elimination of solid body waste) every day is also important in the removal of toxins from your body.

Another recommended supplement may be essential fatty acids, commonly referred to as EFAs. These essential fatty acids help in balancing the body systems, including the immune system. EFAs include Omega-3 (EPA) and Omega-6 or gamma linolenic acid (GLA) and are available in vegetable forms (flaxseed oil, evening primrose oil, or borage oil) or an animal form (fish oil supplements). Instead of taking flaxseed oil by the spoonful, I prefer to pour this buttery-tasting oil on pancakes, muffins, potatoes, vegetables, or other foods each day. However, when using flaxseed oil for its nutritional properties, you should not add it to foods before cooking them because the oil looses its beneficial factor when heated.

Your treatment for *Candida* Related Complex (CRC) may need to include one or more antifungal medications or supplements. Antifungal medications that must be prescribed by a physician are Nystatin (a powder taken by mouth or a cream for vaginal use), Nizoral, Diflucan, and, most recently introduced, Sporanox. Nystatin is poorly absorbed by the body so that while it is effective in reducing the *Candida albicans* in the large bowel it causes no side effects except for a little nausea. The newer antifungal medications, such as Difucan and Sporanox, are easily absorbed by the body, which enhances their effectiveness in reducing *Candida albicans* in all body tissues.

Paramicocidin is an antifungal supplement derived from extracts of grapefruit seeds and does not need a prescription, but it is usually not readily available over-the-counter. It is often available from health-care professionals such as chiropractors or certified nutritionists who treat CRC or in health-food stores.

As mentioned earlier, garlic and cloves are beneficial in combating yeast. Taking yeast-free odorless Kyolic garlic tablets or capsules is an easy way to benefit from garlic's antifungal properties.

Large amounts of biotin, a B vitamin available in capsules or tablets, is beneficial because a deficiency of biotin allows for yeast overgrowth. Biotin is produced by your normal bowel flora. When this delicate balance is disturbed, so is the biotin production that would help to keep *Candida albicans* in check.

Pau D'Arco tea is very helpful in discouraging yeast growth. It is a nutritional tea that is derived from the inner bark of the Pau D'Arco tree in the rain forests of Argentina. These trees are resistant to fungi. I recommend the bulk tea rather than the tea bags because the bag may be made from allergenic materials. To prepare, boil 4 cups of water in a large stainless steel saucepan. Add 1 heaping tablespoon of the bulk tea. Remove from heat, cover, and allow to steep for 20 minutes or longer. Pour the steeped tea through a fine mesh strainer to remove the leaves and store in the refrigerator. Drink 3–6 cups of unsweetened tea evenly and slowly throughout each day, either warm or cold on an empty stomach. If you need a sweeter flavor, add a teaspoon of fresh basil when preparing 4 cups of tea.

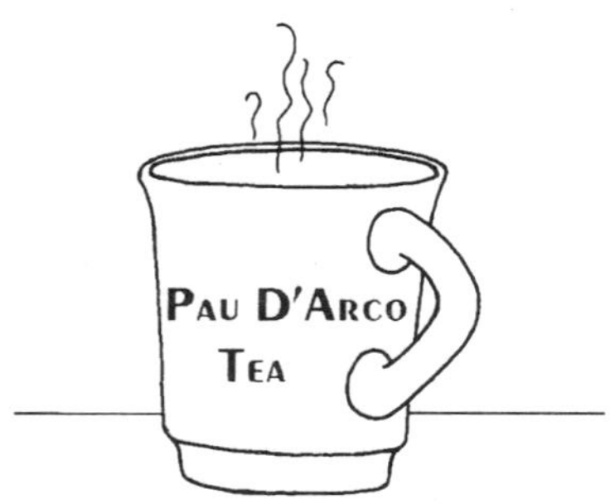

Caprylic acid, a short-chain fatty acid, has been found to be antifungal. This is available in capsules, liquid, or tablets and is derived from coconut.

Other nonprescription antifungal supplements may be suggested by your health-care professional. These may include Nature's Herb Myrrh liquid or Tea Tree Oil from Australia.

[16] Beth Ann Meehan. "Linus Pauling's Rehabilitation," Discover Magazine (Vol. 14, No. 1, January, 1993), 54.

Treatment using antifungal medications and supplements most often causes a worsening of symptoms at first, usually during the first two weeks. This temporary increase in symptoms is called "yeast die-off." Also, as with food, you can develop an allergy (sensitivity) to anything you ingest each day. You may need to consider rotating some or all of your vitamin, mineral, antifungal, and *acidophilus* supplements because of the food source from which they are derived.

In Conclusion

Since I am not a physician, a chiropractor, or a certified nutritionist, I am not making any medical claims or recommendations for the diet, treatments, or supplements discussed in this chapter. The information is based on literature that I have read, lectures I have heard, and personal experience. Each individual is different and any treatment initiated or medication taken needs to be determined by you and your nutritionally oriented health-care professional. However, it is important for you to read and reread materials about *Candida* Related Complex (CRC) to become as knowledgeable as possible. You need to understand which treatments can be beneficial as well as which may be detrimental to your recovery. Also, you may by chance read some material and, by taking it to your physician, open his/her eyes to your recovery. No one has all the answers to the complex problem of *Candida* Related Complex. Whichever treatment(s) you choose, I cannot emphasize enough that you need an understanding health-care professional to supervise your recovery.

It is astonishing
how short a time it takes
for very wonderful things
to happen.

Frances Burnett

Reflect upon your present blessings,
of which every man has many,
not on your past misfortunes,
of which all men have some.

Charles Dickens

The real art of living is
beginning where you are.

Martin Vanbee

3. ROTATIONAL DIET

Rotation of foods accomplishes three main goals:

1. Helps you to maintain your tolerance to the foods you can eat now, greatly lessening your chances of becoming allergic to other foods.
2. Helps in the treatment of current food allergies.
3. Aids you in identifying foods that could be causing you problems.

If you have *Candida* Related Complex (CRC), frequently you will also be sensitive to individual foods, additives, and preservatives. Also, due to the interrelationship of causes and effects, CRC, food allergies, and "leaky gut" syndrome often go hand-in-hand.[17] Because of this it is very important to rotate your foods. It is especially advantageous to rotate and diversify your foods during the early weeks and months of the CRC treatment program. This is when your body is the weakest, so there is a good chance of your weakened body becoming allergic to foods. In addition, if you are already allergic to some foods but not aware of it, a rotational diet can help you identify these allergies and therefore aid in your recovery from CRC. The whole point of rotation is to let your body recover from the effects of a food before you eat it again.

When you first start a CRC treatment diet, you may feel deprived because there are foods that you can no longer eat. More than likely this will lead you to overeat a substitute for the foods lacking in your diet. When you abuse a food by eating it too often, it increases your chances of developing an allergy to it. For example, when I had to avoid eating wheat (my first known food allergen), I substituted rye crackers and popcorn. Because I ate these foods too often, within two months I had developed allergies to rye and corn. So I substituted rice cakes. Again, because I ate them too often, an allergy to rice developed.

Certain events have triggered the onset of CRC and/or food allergies in your system so you now need to minimize your chances of developing additional food allergies.

Rotary Diversified Diet

Rotary diversified diet was first developed in 1934 by Dr. Herbert J. Rinkel. It is used by people who (1) have multiple food sensitivities, (2) are diagnosed chemically susceptible, (3) are healthy members of a family prone to food allergies, or (4) are health-conscious individuals.[18] The rotational diet is more enjoyable and less limiting than other diets to which you may be accustomed. The diet calls for you to eat in a controlled, rational way while allowing for flexibility. The whole point of a rotational diet is to allow time for your body to recover from the effects of a food before eating the food again.

Foods eaten frequently are the most common food allergens. For example, the diet of most Americans includes one or more servings of wheat, milk or other dairy products, egg, corn, and/or soy each day. You may say, "I do not eat egg, corn, or soy each day." However, if you glance at the labels of prepared foods, you will find these ingredients in common foods eaten daily. These include salad

<u>Common Food Allergens</u>

- wheat
- milk/dairy products
- eggs
- corn
- soy

---

[17] Marjorie Hurt Jones. "Leaky Gut: A Common Problem with Food Allergies," <u>Mastering Food Allergies</u> (Vol. VIII, No. 5, Issue No. 75, September-October, 1993), 1.

[18] Natalie Golos and Frances Golos Golbitz. <u>Coping with Your Allergies</u> (New York, NY: A Fireside Book, Published by Simon and Schuster, Inc., 1986), 85.

dressing, catsup, pancake syrup, breakfast cereal, bread, English muffins, snack cakes, chips, "healthy" granola bars, etc. The list goes on and on. To reduce the symptoms of food sensitivities, the offending food or class of food needs to be identified and eliminated or consumed less often by the sensitive person. Avoiding foods to which you are allergic allows your immune system to rest. In addition, eating foods on a rotational basis may help prevent the development of new food sensitivities.

What Is a Food Allergy?

An allergy is an individual's adverse response to a substance such as dust, pollen, food, or a chemical that normally does not cause a problem for an individual who is not allergic to the substance. Through repeated exposure to the substance eventually the immune system reaches a state where it just cannot handle the problem exposure any longer and an allergic reaction develops. Allergic reactions can be as varied in form as there are individuals. Because they are often inherited, you may have a predisposition to allergies. They sometimes appear relatively late in life, but you may be able to think back and remember the subtle effects of allergies throughout your life.

When you eat foods to which you are allergic, the food causes the lymphocytes (white blood cells) to release certain proteins called immunoglobulins. These immunoglobulins then react with other cells in your body (tissues of your nose, lungs, skin, digestive tract, etc.) to release chemicals such as histamine. The symptoms (allergic reactions) that you perceive are caused by the histamine reacting with parts of your body.

Food allergies have either fixed or cyclical reactions. Fixed food allergies are the type that you have every time you eat or even breathe the fumes of a small amount of a particular food. A fixed reaction will usually have appeared earlier in your life and at the first time you consumed the food. The reactions are very strong, often potentially dangerous, and appear rather soon after contact with the food. They have a lifelong pattern, are very unlikely to disappear, and the food causing the reaction always needs to be eliminated from the diet. Fish and nuts are two common fixed food allergens. Often, people who react to fish and/or nuts need to avoid all fish and/or nuts but have no other allergies.

Cyclical reactions are much different in that you may or may not notice a reaction or may not notice the reaction every time you eat the food. The level of reaction may range from quite weak to severe, but is seldom dangerous and may depend on how much of a particular food you eat or how often you eat it. For example, eating one cup of popcorn once a week may not cause you any noticeable reaction. But if you eat an increased amount (let's say four cups of popcorn once a week) or if you increase the frequency (one cup of popcorn every night while enjoying your favorite TV show), an immediate or a delayed reaction may occur. Also, constant consumption of a food allergen may cause acute symptoms to temporarily disappear or become chronic as your body tries to adapt to the exposure. Corn is a good example because it is a hidden ingredient in several foods you may consume daily.

Cyclical food allergies usually depend upon exposure so any food can be an allergen. However, in the Western diet, common food allergens are beef, chocolate, citrus, corn, egg, milk, peanut, shellfish, soy, tomato, wheat, and yeast.

A cyclical food reaction can be either masked or unmasked. An unmasked reaction is when you have a reaction soon after eating a food or you know which food causes the reaction. However, the most common reaction is a masked cyclical reaction, which occurs many hours after eating the food. Many times you do not make any connection between your health problems and the foods you eat. Repeated consumption of a food to which you are allergic causes symptoms that become chronic and do not necessarily occur or worsen at the time you eat the food. Instead, symptoms vary from feeling slightly stimulated (which may be a good feeling) to actually craving the allergic food or feeling worse if you avoid eating it for a couple of days. Often you feel that the food may be needed by your body to maintain good health. This pattern is called a "food addiction." The craving leads to over-consumption of the reactive food.

To unmask a food allergy it is necessary to completely avoid eating the suspected food(s) for approximately two weeks. Also, read all labels on the foods you eat to be sure you are omitting all sources of the suspected food(s). After your chronic symptoms have cleared, you can eat a small amount of one of the suspected foods.

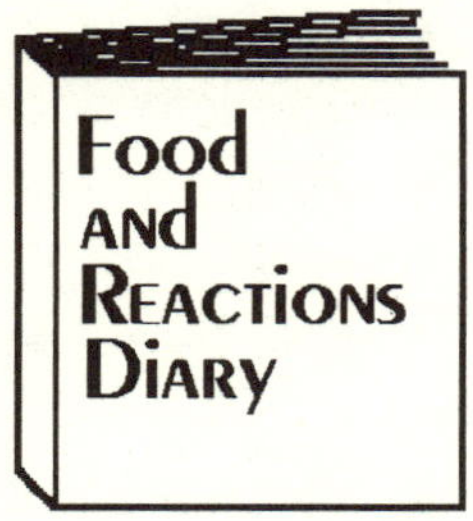

Keep a notebook to record the food you are trying. You will want to record date, time, food eaten, amount eaten, and any noticeable reactions you experienced as well as any other possible causes such as environmental factors.

Day/Date	Time	Food & Form Eaten	Amount Eaten	Reaction & Possible Cause
8/25/94	*8 am*	*egg, scrambled with butter*	*2 large size*	*Mild headache 2 hours following breakfast lasting until midafternoon* *Itchy rectum around noon on 8/26* *Suspect the butter as well as the egg. Next time try using Clarified Butter.*

Your body's response may appear as a noticeable and/or unexpected reaction. However, if you do not notice an immediate reaction, wait for a delayed reaction before eating more or eating another suspected food. (A delayed reaction can occur relative soon [as little as 30 minutes] after eating the food or as long as up to 48 hours later.)[19] This delayed reaction is caused by the fact that it takes time for the allergens to travel through the blood stream and encounter the sensitized cells in your body.[20] If you have an immediate or delayed reaction, you should avoid eating the food for three to six months before trying it again. Your list of suspected foods should include the common food allergens as well as foods you normally eat more than two times a week.

An example of how a food allergy becomes masked is described in Coping with Your Allergies.[21] An allergy to peanuts is used as an example. For instance, you would begin by avoiding peanuts for at least 10 days. This would also include being careful to avoid foods which may include other forms of peanuts such as peanut oil (e.g., granola bars). After the 10 days when you reintroduce peanuts into your diet, you have a definite immediate or delayed reaction. If you continue to eat peanuts every day, your reaction still continues, but it occurs at a lesser level of severity. Soon you do not notice the reaction you are having—the symptoms have become masked or hidden. You no longer associate any reaction with eating this food. The masked symptoms become chronic ailments. If you have many food allergies that are masked, you end up having a lot of chronic ailments. When you reach this acute stage you often feel better when you eat the foods you are allergic to or you begin to crave them.

---

[19] Alan Scott Levin, M.D., and Merla Zellerbach. The Type 1/Type 2 Allergy Relief Program (Los Angeles, CA: Jeremy P. Tarcher, Inc., 1983), 96.
[20] Alan Scott Levin, M.D., and Merla Zellerbach. The Type 1/Type 2 Allergy Relief Program, 96.
[21] Natalie Golos and Frances Golos Golbitz. Coping with Your Allergies, 85.

Typical Allergic Reactions to Food[22,23]

Respiratory

- Dry mouth
- Ear infections
- Ringing in ears
- Rubbing nose all the time
- Sensitivity to odors

Gastrointestinal

- Gain in weight
- Craving for food, alcohol, or tobacco
- Constipation
- Colic
- Diarrhea

Genitourinary

- Chronic bladder irritation
- Bedwetting
- Premenstrual tension
- Menstrual cramps

Skin

- Sweating
- Flushing
- Outer ears hurt
- Bright red ear lobes

Systemic

- Fluid retention in any part of body
- Unexplained fluctuation of weight
- Muscle and joint swelling, redness, and pain
- Backache
- Fatigue
- Hyperactive
- Dark circles under eyes
- Leg aches
- Muscle aches

Cardiovascular

- Abnormal heart rhythms
- Severe chest pain
- Heart palpitations

Cerebral

- Migraine headaches or chronic headaches
- Changes of mood: lack of ability to concentrate; feelings of sadness, weariness, frustration, animation, euphoria, aggressiveness, anger, panic, violence, silliness, and/or "spaciness"
- Inappropriate laughter
- Crying spells
- Depression
- Constant anger
- Impairment of speaking and reading ability
- Lack of coordination
- Loss of balance
- Excessive hunger or thirst
- Sleepiness or insomnia
- Phobias, delusions, hallucinations
- Amnesia
- Convulsive seizures
- Blackouts
- Psychosis such as manic depression or schizophrenia
- Night terrors: scream in the middle of night, eyes open staring
- "Jekyll and Hyde" reaction
- Make clucking noise
- See a difference in handwriting just after eating a food or meal

---

22 Alan Scott Levin, M.D., and Merla Zellerbach. The Type 1/Type 2 Allergy Relief Program, 18–19.

23 Jerry Springer. Allergies—Making Kids Crazy. Interview with Doris Rapp, M.D. Air Date: December 17, 1992. 45 min., Multimedia Entertainment, Inc., 1944, videocassette.

A clinical ecologist, internist, or allergist who treats food allergies can perform some tests in an attempt to help you discover your food allergies. These tests could include skin testing and/or a blood test called RAST which measures food-specific immunoglobulins. None of these tests are perfect, but they may help you discover which foods may be causing problems. Also, there are some health-care professionals who closely supervise a special fasting, elimination, and rare food diet to help you determine your particular food allergies. Read The E.I. Syndrome by Sherry Rogers, M.D. if you desire to learn more about this diet.[24]

Eating on Rotation

By following a rotational diet, you gain control over your exposure to the foods that cause you cyclical food reactions. You may choose a 4-, 5-, 6-, 7-, or 8-day rotational diet. Whichever length you choose, each food eaten on a particular day is not eaten until that day repeats again in the rotation. For example, in the sample 4-day rotation in Table A, the broccoli and rice on Day 1 will not be eaten again until the following Day 1 (with three days in between). The same holds true for a 5-day or longer rotation. In the sample 5-day rotation in Table A, broccoli and rice are eaten on Day 2 and are not eaten again until the next Day 2 with four days in between their consumption. The same holds true for other foods in the two sample diets in Table A.

Table A

Four-Day Rotation

Day 1	Day 2	Day 3	Day 4	Day 1	Day 2	Day 3
broccoli	shrimp	carrot	orange	broccoli	shrimp	carrot
rice	potato	turkey	beans	rice	potato	turkey

Five-Day Rotation

Day 1	Day 2	Day 3	Day 4	Day 5	Day 1	Day 2
quinoa	rice	amaranth	buckwheat	beans	quinoa	rice
carrot	broccoli	tomato	spinach	asparagus	carrot	broccoli

Four days is generally a long enough rotation to assure maximum bowel transit time (the amount of time your body takes to move food through the complete digestive tract and eliminate the waste part of the food from your body). If you have chronic constipation, you may need more than a 4-day cycle. For example, you might choose a 5-, 6-, or 8-day rotation. I do not recommend a 7-day rotation because it becomes too monotonous eating the same foods every Monday, Tuesday, etc. If you need a longer cycle than four days, it might be easiest to choose an 8-day rotation. First, this allows maximum bowel transit time. Second, once you become healthier, you can easily switch to the most popular 4-day rotation.

When you first start, you may find, as I did, that the 4-day rotation will be long enough for some foods but not long enough for others. If this is the case, you can use the basic 4-day rotation but rotate some foods every eight days. In Table B, notice that rice, spelt, cod, shrimp, potato, amaranth, beans, and asparagus are only eaten on one day in eight, whereas broccoli, turkey, carrot, and orange are eaten every four days.

Table B

Day 1	Day 2	Day 3	Day 4	Day 1	Day 2	Day 3	Day 4
broccoli	cod	carrot	orange	broccoli	shrimp	carrot	orange
rice	potato	turkey	beans	spelt	amaranth	turkey	asparagus

[24] Sherry A. Rogers, M.D. The EI Syndrome (Syracuse, NY: Prestige Publishers, 1986).

The 4-Day Rotational Diet

This cookbook is designed for a 4-day rotation which, if needed, could be converted to an 8-day. Each day has a list of foods to be consumed on that day. Also, each of the four days has a wide variety of recipes to choose from—breads ("hamburger" buns, tortillas, muffins, pancakes, crackers, etc.); cereals; soups, stews, and meat or vegetarian casseroles; meats or poultry; fish and wild game; vegetable side dishes; salad side dishes and salad main courses with a salad dressing; and, of course, healthy, naturally sweet desserts and snacks. You can enjoy many all-American food favorites such as tacos, pizza, gravy, sandwiches, brownies, and cookies. The recipes may have many different ingredients than those to which you are accustomed, but there are only slight changes in flavor and texture. Before you know it your taste buds will not crave or need the original. Begin by simplifying your diet. Learn to enjoy the individual flavors of foods.

What Is a "Day"?

While an expected definition of a day would be the meals you eat between sunrise and sunset (breakfast, lunch, dinner), for the purposes of a rotational diet this 24-hour period can be adjusted to fit individual needs.

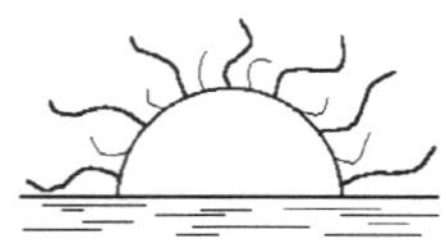

For example, persons who cannot handle preparing breakfast may prefer to use *plan*overs (planned leftovers) from dinner the previous evening and would define their rotational day as lunch, dinner, and breakfast the following morning.

If you work outside your home and carry your lunch, you may wish to define your day as dinner, breakfast, and lunch. This will allow you to prepare extra servings for your lunch on the following day while you are preparing your evening meal.

Basically, then, a "day" consists of any 24-hour period and the meals consumed during that time frame. This can be from midnight to midnight, 3 p.m. to 3 p.m., or any other cycle that works for your particular needs or situation. With careful planning, you can easily and successfully maintain your rotation and enjoy nutritious, delicious meals. (For ideas in planning and cooking meals, see Chapter 7—Menu Planning.)

Basic Rules to Follow on a 4-Day Rotational Diet

Rule 1. Simple is better. Eat whole foods, not highly processed foods that have lost much of their nutritional value and may contain hidden ingredients such as corn, soy, or egg. Eat a wide variety of foods. Diversify your diet by using many different types of fish and other protein sources, vegetables, whole grains, and grain substitutes.

Rule 2. Do not eat the same food item more often than every fourth day. For example, you can eat rice on Day 1. You will not eat rice again until the next Day 1, with three days in between. This means that rice will not be consumed on a schedule of every Sunday or Thursday, but that it will be eaten on whichever day of the week Day 1 of the rotational cycle falls. See Table C.

Table C

Sunday Day 1	**Monday Day 2**	**Tuesday Day 3**	**Wednesday Day 4**	**Thursday Day 1**	**Friday Day 2**	**Saturday Day 3**
rice	potato	millet	beans	rice	potato	millet

Sunday Day 1	**Monday Day 2**	**Tuesday Day 3**	**Wednesday Day 4**	**Thursday Day 1**	**Friday Day 2**	**Saturday Day 3**
beans	rice	potato	millet	beans	rice	potato

Rule 3. Within a rotation, food families are also rotated. Foods are grouped into botanical food families based on their biological origin. Each food family is assigned a name and a number for identification. You should rotate using the food families because foods in the same family tend to share common allergens and could react similarly in your body. If you eat rice on Day 1, spelt on Day 2, oat on Day 3, and millet on Day 4 you are not really rotating foods but are eating a member of the Grass Family every day. Table D shows how all foods from a particular family are eaten on an assigned day.

Table D

Day 1 Grass Family	Day 2 Lily Family	Day 3 Mustard Family	Day 4 Legume Family
rice	garlic	cauliflower	peas
spelt	onion	Brussels sprouts	pinto bean
oat	leeks	broccoli	garbanzo bean
millet	asparagus	cabbage	lima bean
etc.	etc.	etc.	etc.

For a complete listing of food families, see Appendix A: Food Families. This listing also includes nonedible plants because you may need to avoid foods in a family when you are allergic to a weed or plant included in the family group. For example: if you have an allergy to pigweed, be cautious of amaranth; if you have an allergy to poison ivy, be cautious of cashews, pistachios, and mangoes; and if you have an allergy to lamb's-quarters, be cautious of quinoa, spinach, chard, and beets.

Rule 4. Different foods within the same food family may be rotated every other day. As explained in Rule 3, within a 4-day rotation a particular food is eaten at least four days apart. However, Rule 4 gives more flexibility in that foods in the same food family may be eaten two days apart. Notice in Table E that each food is eaten every four days and foods in the same family are eaten two days apart. Examples include rice and spelt on Day 1 and oat and millet on Day 3 (from the Grass Family); garlic and onion on Day 2 and leeks and asparagus on Day 4 (from the Lily Family); etc. This allows for more flexibility and variety in planning meals.

Table E

Day 1	Day 2	Day 3	Day 4
Grass Family	**Lily Family**	**Grass Family**	**Lily Family**
rice	garlic	oat	leeks
spelt	onion	millet	asparagus
Mustard Family	**Legume Family**	**Mustard Family**	**Legume Family**
broccoli	garbanzo bean	cauliflower	peas
cabbage	lima bean	Brussels sprouts	pinto bean

One exception to Rule 4 which you should be aware of involves the Grass Family (number 6). Wheat, spelt, and Kamut® are very closely related and should always be eaten on the same day—not divided and used two days apart. In addition, if you have an allergy to wheat, you should be very careful when trying to add spelt or Kamut® to your rotation. Be sure to do a food challenge to learn if you react to either of these grains. (See the section What Is a Food Allergy? in this chapter for a description of a food challenge.)

If you have severe food allergies, you may need to add additional restrictions to your 4-day rotation. Two such restrictions may be:

1. Do not repeat foods or food families twice within one day unless at the same meal.
2. Do not incorporate Rule 4 in your rotation.

Because of mild allergies, I do not use Rule 4 for all of the food families. For example: Nightshade Family (number 14) and Bovine Family (number 137) are only eaten every four days rather than members of the family being split and eaten every other day.

Rule 5. Foods may be moved to another day providing that the complete food family is also moved.

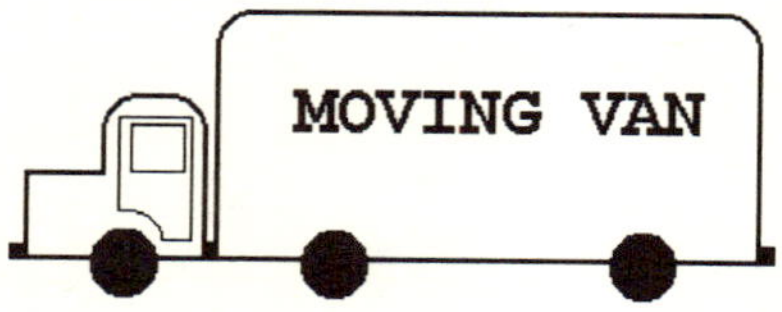

Example 1. Moving foods on a permanent basis. You may move cabbage (member of the Mustard Family) from Day 1 to Day 2 providing that you move the other members of the Mustard Family from Day 1 to Day 2. You will also need to move the Day 3 members of the Mustard Family to Day 4.

Example 2. Use "Floating Foods" to allow yourself to be creative and flexible within the regular 4-day rotation. A "floating food" is any food that you may sometimes desire to eat on a day which is two days later than its assigned day. It works best if the "floating food" is one that you consume less often because when you properly "float" a particular food you end up eating the food six days apart (five days in between). See Table F for an example using wild rice.

Table F

Day 1	Day 2	Day 3	Day 4
Wild & Brown Rice with Herbs & Pecans			

Day 1	Day 2	Day 3	Day 4
		Wild Rice Pasta Salad	

When I planned my rotation diet and began developing the recipes, I gradually added foods that I desired to "float" between Days 1 and 3 and between Days 2 and 4. If you look at the food lists for each day, such as Day 1 and Day 3 (pages 97 and 197), you will find parsley and cinnamon listed in the right hand column under "Foods That Float Between Days 1 & 3." Also, if you look at the food lists for Days 2 and 4 (pages 147 and 237), you will find garlic and the spices oregano and chili powder in the column labeled "Foods That Float Between Days 2 & 4." For the rotational diet outlined in this cookbook, these are the few foods that I have defined as "floating foods." Each of the recipes in which these foods occur does not have a warning asterisk to remind you to omit them for four days before eating them again.

There are other foods in this rotational diet that I occasionally "float" from Day 1 to 3 or from Day 2 to 4 or vice versa. As one example, you will find wild rice in recipes on Day 1 as well as on Day 3. Remember, when you use a "floating food" it is important for you to avoid eating it for four days before using it again. See Table F for an example of the ways I enjoy eating wild rice. However, I do not eat wild rice quite as often as this table lists. To assist you with your meal planning, every attempt has been made to asterisk (*) any foods in these recipes that are temporarily moved ("floated") from another day. You can assign any foods you wish to float between days as long as you follow Rules 2, 3, and 4.

“Fun Foods”

Example 3. Allow "Fun Foods" to brighten your day. There are some foods that I call "Fun Foods" because they are members of a food family with no other or only a few other foods in their family. These foods can be moved with ease as long as you remember to allow three days between the times you consume them. Below is my list of "Fun Foods" along with their food family number and the day on which I normally eat them. One example of how I use two different nuts as unassigned "Fun Foods" are Brazil and macadamia nuts. Since these nuts are each a member of a different food family and there are no other foods in their family, I can enjoy them on any day as long as I have not consumed them within the last four days. I usually use macadamia nuts in Day 4 recipes and Brazil nuts in Day 2 recipes. However, there are also a few recipes on Days 1 and 3 that include these nuts. Again, to assist you with your meal planning, every attempt has been made to asterisk (*) any unassigned "Fun Foods" in these recipes.

Also, since macadamia nuts are sometimes difficult to find as well as more expensive, I will use Brazil nuts in recipes on any day when I have not consumed them in the past four days and do not plan to consume them in the next four days.

List of Fun Foods

Food Family Number	Food	Day Assigned in Rotation
1	agar-agar and kombu	Day 4
10	pineapple	unassigned
16	banana and plantain	Day 2
17	ginger	unassigned
20	vanilla	unassigned
23	filberts (hazelnut)	Day 3
26	macadamia nut	unassigned
33	nutmeg	unassigned
35	poppyseed	unassigned
44	flaxseed and flaxseed oil	unassigned
50	maple granules	unassigned
54	okra	Day 2
59	papaya	unassigned
62	Brazil nut	unassigned
100	swordfish	Day 4

Example 4. Moving foods on a temporary basis. Occasionally I like to eat asparagus with chicken on Day 1. This can be accomplished if I plan ahead and make modifications within my rotational diet. Usually I eat the Lily Family on Days 2 and 4 as shown in Table E. To temporarily move asparagus from Day 4 to Day 1, omit eating the Lily Family on Day 4 before and Day 2 after you eat chicken and asparagus on Day 1. In addition, you must avoid eating asparagus on the Day 4 after you eat this food combination on Day 1. See Table G for a visual example to better understand this.

Table G

Day 1	Day 2	Day 3	Day 4
	Lily Family		Lily Family
	garlic		omit
	onion		

Day 1	Day 2	Day 3	Day 4
Lily Family	Lily Family		Lily Family
asparagus	omit		leeks
			omit asparagus

On the next repeat of the rotational cycle return to eating foods from the Lily Family as Table E on page 29 describes.

Example 5. Choose to substitute other foods rather than move foods. Sometimes moving foods is more difficult than creatively substituting. Carefully evaluate any move to be sure it does not cause too many problems and seriously consider adapting to the regularly used foods on a particular day before attempting a move. As an example, when I desired to develop a stuffed green pepper recipe, I needed to move rice from Day 1 to Day 2. This meant I would have to move or omit eating all other foods from the Grass Family such as Kamut®, rice, spelt, teff, etc. on Day 1. In addition, I would have to omit eating all food items from the Grass Family such as barley, oat, millet, rye, wild rice, etc. on the following Day 3. I decided that this particular move was too restrictive and instead chose to use garbanzo beans in my Stuffed Green Peppers. Happily, my family and I love them prepared this way.

Rule 6. Be your own best friend and helper. Relax, be understanding, and be kind to yourself. You may be feeling overwhelmed by your health situation and the many changes you know you will be making to help your system heal. But you can better deal with dietary and lifestyle changes if you develop a **positive sense of helping yourself.** Rest your mind; be flexible, optimistic, and calm; and give yourself time to retrain your taste buds and to learn

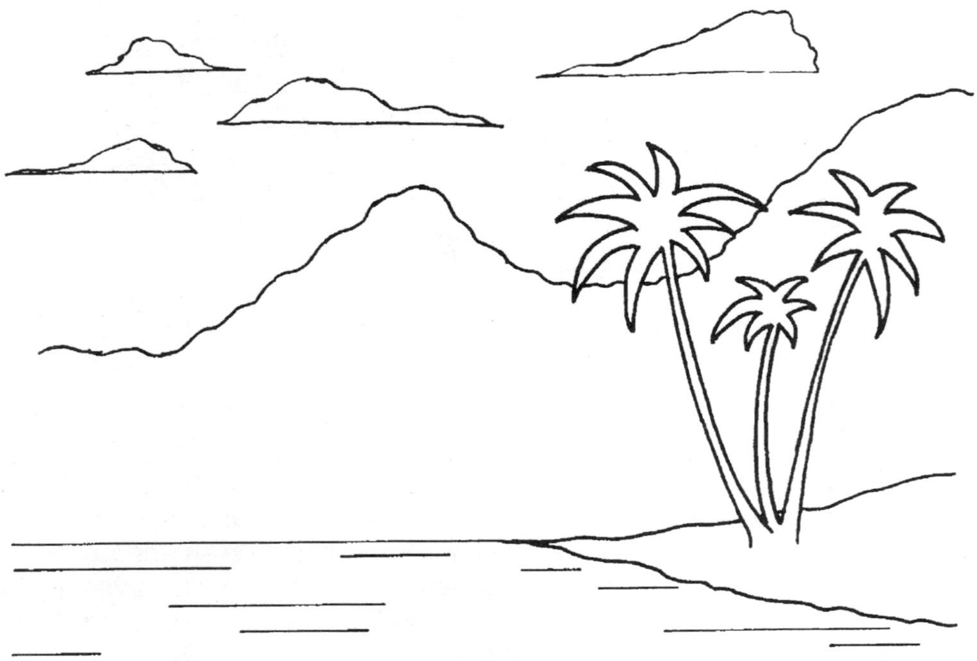

to use the many new foods and cooking techniques offered in this cookbook. Do not dwell on what you cannot eat. Instead, concentrate on how the foods you can eat are leading you to a well-nourished, healthy lifestyle. This will help you develop a positive outlook on how you are guiding yourself toward greater health. After eating on rotation for a while, you will realize it is an achievable and extremely healthy way to eat. I have now reached the point where many foods often do not taste or look as good when eaten on a day other than the regularly assigned day. Nor are they interesting or tempting to try.

To accomplish rotating foods successfully, you need to define your commitment level. You may need to start gradually and work up to a higher level of commitment. One way to do this would be to start with rotating your grains, then add meats to the rotation followed by vegetables and then fruits. Finally, add your spices to the rotation.

If you get off rotation, for whatever reason, don't become discouraged and drop all of it because you cannot do it all or do it as quickly as you might wish. Don't worry about the past. Just stop what you're doing, look forward, and start fresh. You may have added things too soon for your commitment level and may have to go back to just rotating your grains, then adding the other foods gradually. Do not try to be a "one hundred percenter." Allow yourself some freedom, especially when traveling or on special occasions.

This is a personal commitment that you are making and your individual time and energy levels need to be a factor in the decision. Make it realistic for you and your situation. But remember, you are changing your lifestyle **to benefit yourself**. Only you can truly define and set your personal commitment level and ultimately only you are responsible for following through on this commitment. You need to work with what you can handle and soon, with support, you can accomplish more than you ever dreamed.

Rule 7. Seek support. Seek nonprofessional help from understanding friends or family, a local HEAL support group (see section 4 of Appendix C: Resources for the HEAL address), or a food cooperative (see Appendix E: Cooperative Food Warehouses in the United States). Also, an overeaters support group may help. If necessary, seek professional help from a counselor. Other than the support of a friend, I have found the best solution for myself is in self-education. Read and reread information about *Candida* Related Complex (CRC), food allergies, rotational diet, etc. until you fully understand, visualize, and conquer it.

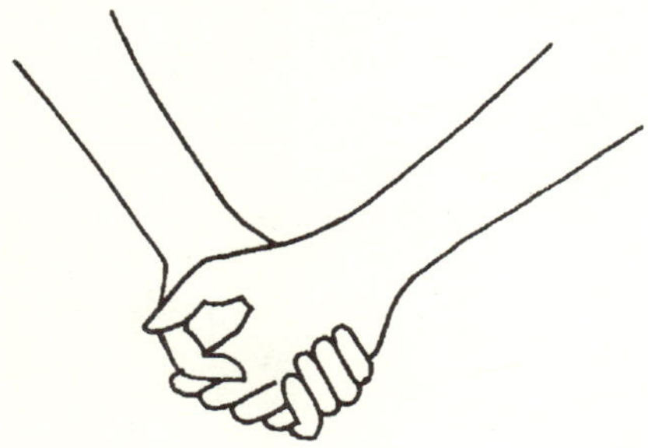

Success with a *Candida* control and/or rotational diet does not come overnight. Build your personal support system as you are able. It may take time to find the people and services that will benefit you, but the end result will be well worth it.

About This Cookbook

This cookbook offers you a food allergy, *Candida* control, and rotational diet that will enhance your health and well being with the use of a wide variety of foods. In addition, this cookbook introduces you to several "new" foods and teaches you how to prepare them as well as where to purchase them. Many quick and easy recipes are developed so you can prepare them with a minimum of time and energy.

As you work with the rotational diet offered in this cookbook and the food family charts in Appendix A, you will learn to recognize food families and be able to vary your diet according to your individual food allergies and/or to suit your taste. Soon after using a rotational diet, you may be able to safely tolerate foods that previously caused you a moderate to severe reaction. This is possible because you have allowed your body's immune system to have an appropriate rest period and to recover to the point where you have regained a tolerance to many previously offending foods. You may regain tolerance to some foods in as little as 3–4 weeks where for other foods it may take 2–6 months or longer. However, do realize that some food allergies may be permanent or fixed. Soon after following the rotational diet and recipes in this cookbook, you will realize good, tasty, nutritious meals are available and you will not miss the foods you cannot eat.

Happiness is not a state to arrive at, but a manner of traveling.
Margaret Lee Runbeck

Few of us do as much as we want to for others. But there is always one gift we can bestow—a smile.
Marjorie Holms

Things do not change—we do.
Henry David Thoreau

4. SPECIALTY FOODS

This chapter is devoted to the different specialty foods in various forms that you can purchase and learn to use in your cooking. They can be an important part of your diet if you are eating on rotation and/or are allergic to foods such as wheat and corn. The chapter includes an introduction to grains and nongrains and individual description sections on grains, nongrains, starches, sugar substitutes, and miscellaneous foods. The descriptions within each section are listed alphabetically. Each individual listing is divided into sections on Properties, History, Uses, and Sources. In some cases there is also a section entitled "Sondra's Thoughts" where I have included some of my personal thoughts and suggestions on the specific food item.

Introduction to Grains and Nongrains

Whole grains and whole-grain products have been staple foods for thousands of years in almost all cultures. Grains today are a common source of carbohydrates and an inexpensive source of protein.

The differentiation of nongrain is given to amaranth, buckwheat, and quinoa. This is because although they are prepared and act a lot like a grain in both whole-grain and flour form, they are not a part of the Grass Family (number 6). They are in distinctly different food families: amaranth in the Pigweed Family (number 30); quinoa in the Goosefoot Family (number 28); and buckwheat in the Buckwheat Family (number 27). (See Appendix A: Food Families.)

Whole grains are seeds that contain these three natural components:

- **the bran layer**: a tough outer coating, which protects the grain and is rich in fiber and minerals.
- **the germ**: contains vitamin E, essential fatty acids, and proteins. These nutrients provide food for the plant seed to develop a root system and to sprout.
- **the endosperm**: the starchy bulk layer of the grain, which is rich in complex carbohydrates and proteins. The nutrients in the endosperm nourish the seedling during the early growth period before the leaves begin to photosynthesize.

Refined grains have been degermed or polished, which removes the germ and bran layers and lowers the nutritional value. For example, "pearled" barley is a refined barley product that has undergone six scourings between Carborundam wheels. This process removes the bran and germ, and as a result the barley loses between 74–97% of its protein, fat, fiber, and minerals.[25] Another example of refined grain is the white (wheat) flour that is common in American diets. Wheat loses up to 80% of its nutrients in this refining process. Persons who use refined white flour commonly respond by saying it is "enriched." But why do we pay more money to have more than twenty nutrients removed and to have four added back—thiamin, niacin, riboflavin, and iron?[26] You should also be aware that the B vitamins used to "enrich" refined flour often have a yeast growth source which CRC patients should avoid. In addition, refined flours are subjected to a bleaching process, which destroys the essential amino acid or protein part of the flour.

---

[25] Sheila Phillips. "Natural Foods Primer: Grains." Information sheet from Blooming Prairie Warehouse, 2340 Heinz Road, Iowa City, IA 52240.
[26] Ibid.

Another property of flour is gluten, a type of protein that controls a bread's ability to raise. When flour containing gluten is mixed with water, kneaded, and beaten, it forms an elastic framework that stretches as either yeast or another leavening agent causes it to grow. When you bake the dough this gluten framework sets up to form the structure of the baked good.

Grains that contain gluten are wheat and other wheat relatives (spelt and Kamut®), rye, oats, and barley. This list is in descending order of more-to-less gluten. Grains and nongrains that are essentially gluten-free are amaranth, buckwheat, corn, millet, quinoa, rice, sorghum, and teff.

According to the Rodale Research Center in eastern Pennsylvania, all grains and grain-like foods do contain some traces of gluten.[27] However, these foods that are essentially gluten-free should be all right for celiacs who cannot digest gluten. This is because the gluten in these essentially gluten-free grains and nongrains is chemically bound and unavailable to enter into any reactions in the body.

A Special Note: Celiacs are unable to digest gluten. According to Marjorie Hurt Jones,[28] celiacs who continue to eat gluten-containing foods develop abdominal symptoms such as gas pain, bloating, cramping, etc. because the gluten is not digested and erodes their intestinal villi. The intestinal villi are very important for absorption of soluble nutrients in our body. Celiacs who continue to ingest gluten-containing foods show signs of malnourishment no matter what they eat.

Washing Whole Grains and Nongrains

Before cooking grains, they should be rinsed to remove dirt and hulls. My method of rinsing grains is to place in the cooking pan 2–3 times more water than the amount of grain to be cooked. Add the measurement of grain and gently stir with a spoon or your hand. If immature grains, hulls, or other debris float to the water surface, skim or gently pour off and discard. To drain smaller or medium-size grains, pour water and grain into a fine-mesh strainer. For larger grains such as spelt and Kamut®, a small-holed colander can be used. One important thing to keep in mind when rinsing grains and nongrains is the porous or nonporous nature of the grain. Quick-cooking grains such as quinoa, buckwheat groats, and millet are very porous and should be rinsed very quickly to keep them from absorbing too much of the rinsing water. If too much water is absorbed during rinsing, it can change the texture of the cooked product. With whole quinoa the rinsing process should be repeated 2–3 times to remove the saponin layer that causes a bitter taste.

Cooking Whole Grains and Nongrains

A rule of thumb in cooking is to use one cup of grain or nongrain to two cups of water or broth (vegetable or meat). Combine rinsed grain and liquid with salt or other added seasonings in a stainless steel, 2 1/2 quart saucepan. Bring to boil on high, cover, reduce heat to between low and medium, and allow to simmer for designated cooking time. (See chart on the next page for liquid amount and simmering time.) For the best results, do not uncover or stir during the cooking process. If it is necessary to check progress during the cooking time, do so quickly to minimize the steam loss. DO NOT STIR because it will disrupt the even cooking of the grain. If tasting for doneness, use a fork to gently remove a small amount from the surface of the cooking grain or nongrain. Different stoves and different pans may require adjustments in time, temperature, and amount of liquid used. The cooking chart on the next page was developed using stainless steel waterless cookware.

---

[27] Marjorie Hurt Jones, R.N. "New Foods and How to Use Them," The Human Ecologist, no. 52 (Winter 1991), 1. Referenced as a "telephone conversation with Rodale Research Center, Kutztown, Pennsylvania."
[28] Marjorie Hurt Jones, R.N. Super Foods (Coeur d'Alene, ID: Mast Enterprises, Inc., 1990), 27.

Grain and Nongrain Cooking Chart

	Amount of Grain or Nongrain	Amount of Liquid	Simmering Time	Yield
Amaranth	1 cup	2 cups	30 minutes	2 1/4 cups
Barley, hulled	1/2 cup	2 cups	45 minutes	2 1/4 cups
Buckwheat Groats, unroasted	1 cup	2 cups	15 minutes	3 cups
Kamut®	1 cup	3 cups	2 1/2 hours	3 cups
Millet, hulled	1 cup	2 cups	15 minutes	4 cups
Quinoa	1 cup	2 cups	15 minutes	4 cups
Rice—Brown Basmati	1 cup	2 1/4 cups	30 minutes	3 cups
Rice—Long or Short Grain Brown	1 cup	2 1/4 cups	35 minutes	3 cups
Rice—White Basmati	1 cup	2 cups	15 minutes	2 1/2 cups
Spelt	1 cup	3 cups	2 1/2 hours	3 cups
Wild Rice	1 cup	2 1/2 cups	40 minutes	3 cups

Another excellent method for cooking grains and nongrains is in a slow cooker. (See cereal recipes in the Table of Contents for each day under Cereals, Grains, and Nongrains.)

Purchasing and Storing Whole Grains and Whole-grain Flours

The key to purchasing fresh whole grains is to look for products that are unbroken. Unbroken grains can last for a long time if properly stored. Store grains in glass jars with tight-fitting lids and keep them in a cool, dry, dark place. For grains that I use often and do not store for a long period of time, I store the glass jars in the basement or in a cupboard. I place grains that I may store for a longer period of time in glass jars in the freezer. Once you store a grain in the freezer remove only the amount you want to cook. Do not allow it to stand out and warm up and then refreeze. This can create a mold problem.

A pleasant aroma is the best clue to freshness in whole-grain flours. If you smell any "off odors" this could indicate mold or rancidity in the flour. This rancid odor comes from the flour being stored too long at an improper temperature. The germ part of the whole grain and its oil become rancid if exposed to air and heat for any length of time. Rancid flour has a distinct bitter taste. I recommend that you store whole-grain flours in glass jars with tight-fitting lids in the freezer.

Grains

Kamut®

Properties A member of the Grass Family (number 6), Kamut® (pronounced Kah-moot) is a trade name associated with a variety of an ancient Egyptian gluten-containing grain related to durum wheat. Each golden-colored kernel is two to three times the size of a wheat kernel and has a distinctive hump in the middle. Kamut® has a wonderful, rich, and almost-buttery taste. It is commonly found in the form of whole grain (berries), flakes, puffed, cold breakfast cereal, flour, and pastas.

Though it is related to durum wheat, studies have indicated that many wheat-sensitive persons can tolerate Kamut®, especially on a rotational basis. However, since Kamut® and wheat are closely related, persons who react allergically to wheat should do a food challenge to assess the advisability of adding Kamut® to a personalized rotational diet since Kamut® could cause a similar allergic response. (See the section What Is a Food Allergy? in Chapter 3—Rotational Diet for a description of a food challenge.)

Kamut® is higher in nutritional value than any other strain of wheat. It has 30% more protein than common wheat varieties as well as having more of eight out of nine minerals, especially magnesium and zinc. Of the 18 amino acids found in wheat, Kamut® contains higher levels of 16 of them. Also, Kamut® has significantly higher levels of all of the major fatty acids.

History

It's believed that Kamut® originated in the Tigris and Euphrates area of the Middle East, possibly in Egypt. It first came to the United States in 1949 when a U.S. airman stationed in Portugal was given 36 kernels of Kamut®. He was told that the kernels were gathered from some sort of stone box found in an excavated tomb from an Egyptian pyramid. (This account of where the grains were found is questionable since there is no documentation that ancient and mummified seeds found in the pyramids were able to grow.) Intrigued, the airman mailed the seeds to his father, a Montana wheat farmer. When they were planted, 32 of the 36 seeds germinated and within 6 years 1,500 bushels of Egyptian wheat filled a Montana granary. It received some local attention at the county fair as "King Tut's Wheat," but eventually the novelty diminished, the large wheat went for cattle feed, and the grain was all but forgotten.

In 1977, a Montana agricultural scientist and wheat farmer (Bob Quinn, Ph.D.) and his father (Mack) launched a search to find some of the ancient grain they remembered as "King Tut's Wheat." The Quinns saw a future for the ancient strain of wheat and, by scouring the barns and cellars in the Montana wheat belt, they located a one-pint jar of seeds. For the next ten years they worked to increase the grain, carefully selecting and propagating it on their ranch near Big Sandy, Montana. Quinn named the grain Kamut® which is an ancient Egyptian word for wheat.

Unlike modern-day wheat, Kamut® has not been hybridized and "scientifically improved." Since it is self-pollinating, the Kamut® plants grown today are replications of the ancient ones. They can grow in a field right next to common wheat and not interbreed or "cross" with it.

Uses

Kamut® flour resembles finely ground cornmeal, and you can use it for almost any purpose where you would use whole-grain wheat flour. Most baked goods made with Kamut® flour turn a pretty golden brown. As a good rule of thumb, when replacing whole-wheat flour in a recipe with Kamut® flour, use one tablespoon less Kamut® per cup of flour. Since Kamut® is a whole grain, it is more like whole-wheat flour than white flour and would probably not be an accurate replacement in recipes using white flour.

Kamut® pasta has a delicious firm texture and does not get waterlogged like normal wheat pasta. Kamut® flakes are similar in appearance to oatmeal and can be cooked for a hot cereal or used to make delicious granola bars and "stove-top" stuffing. See Day 1 recipes for more uses for this versatile grain.

Sources

Kamut® in its many different forms can usually be purchased in health-food stores, through mail-order companies, and through other outlets that carry specialty foods (see Appendix C: Resources). If you do not find it in your local health-food store, ask the manager to stock this wonderful grain so that others can also learn to use and appreciate it.

Millet

Properties Millet is a tiny, gluten-free, bright yellow seed that is covered with a hull that has a dull shine. The hulls are removed before the grain is used in cooking. Even though it is from the Grass Family (number 6), many who do not tolerate other grains can eat millet without experiencing grain-like allergic reactions. This may possibly be because they have not eaten this grain as much as other grains or have never eaten it.

The gentle, lightly sweet flavor of millet is enhanced by herbs and spices, vegetable and meat stocks, and fruits. Since it is rich in iron, potassium, calcium, B vitamins, and protein, millet has many nutritional benefits.

History Millet is a hardy plant that survives most any growing conditions from drought-dry to water-logged soil and it appears in as many as 6,000 variations around the world. Millet was considered a "holy plant" in China around 2800 B.C. and was a popular ancient staple of India, Egypt, and North Africa. In Java, millet was grown as a border around rice fields to activate growth and encourage abundance in the rice crop. Today, millet is still a major food source in Asia and North Africa. However, in Great Britain and the United States it is mostly recognized as bird seed and cattle feed.

The key element in millet, silica, is a crystalline compound also found in quartz crystals. The silica is responsible for opening the millet plant to light and warmth. This factor may also have contributed to the legend that millet has the ability to transmit spiritual energy.

Uses Millet is available in several forms such as hulled grain, flour, flakes, and puffed millet. Cooked hulled millet has a soft, dry texture, but it can also be cooked to a creamy texture such as in Creamy Millet Cereal, Millet Pudding, and Salmon Millet Dinner. Dry roasting millet before cooking brings out more flavor and helps to blend in the flavor of other combined foods such as in Basic Millet with caraway. Some of my favorite Day 3 combinations are to flavor millet with apples and cinnamon in Millet Pudding or to add it to turkey and vegetables in Millet Turkey Vegetable Stew. Puffed millet is a dry cereal similar to puffed rice. Millet flour can be used in baking, but I have found that it must be used with egg as a binding agent for the end product to hold together.

Since millet turns rancid quickly after hulling, it should be stored in glass jars in the refrigerator or freezer.

Sources Hulled millet and other millet products may be purchased in health-food stores as well as through food-buying cooperatives and mail-order sources (see Appendix C: Resources).

* *

Rice

Properties Rice, a gluten-free grain in the Grass Family (number 6), is the second most produced food in the world. There are many varieties available in a range of colors from off-white to black. Generally rice has a rather plain flavor that provides an excellent canvas waiting to be colored with other foods and spices. The only limiting factor is the imagination of the cook. Natural rice is a great source of B vitamins.

History Rice originated in India, Southeast Asia, and China around 4000 B.C. Today it is grown in many parts of the world, including Italy, Spain, Asia, China, India, South America, Africa, Australia, and the United States. It likes warm, moist growing conditions and has the most water content of all grains.

Some of the various rice varieties you may encounter are short-, medium-, and long-grain brown rice; sweet brown rice; Basmati; Texmati; Calmati; and specialty rice varieties such as mahogany, black japonica, field run japonica, royal, and wehani.

Uses

Brown rice is available in many forms including whole grain, flour, puffed, rice cakes, flakes, pastas, and creamy hot cereal. Brown rice flour generally has a drier consistency than wheat flour, but it is very popular with people who cannot tolerate wheat. An especially tasty form of puffed rice is produced by Lundberg Family Farms of Richvale, California. The only ingredients in Lundberg Organic Brown Rice Crunchies are puffed organic brown rice, organic brown rice syrup, and sea salt. I enjoy Crunchies plain as a snack or with chilled Almond Milk (page 104) as a cold breakfast cereal.

Some of my favorite Day 1 recipes for rice found in this cookbook are Wild & Brown Rice with Herbs; Raspberry Rice Granola; rice pastas in Pasta Primavera, Chicken Spaghetti, and Chicken Vegetable Salad; and the many casserole dishes that use rice as a main ingredient.

Sondra's Thoughts

You should avoid using such products as polished rice, Minute Rice, and other highly processed rice products. This is because they are usually not organically grown and most of the natural vitamins and fiber are removed during processing. In addition, there is no way of knowing if the re-added nutrients in these products include yeast-based vitamins.

Sources

Organic rice products may be purchased in health-food stores as well as through food-buying cooperatives and mail-order sources (see Appendix C: Resources).

* *

Spelt

Properties

A member of the Grass Family (number 6), spelt is a gluten-containing grain related to wheat. The nutrients in spelt dissolve rapidly in liquid and become more readily available to the body with only a minimum of digestive work.

Possibly due to its high level of solubility, this delicious, easily digestible grain may be tolerated by many wheat-sensitive persons. However, recent research has indicated that wheat-sensitive persons should be very cautious when attempting to add spelt products to their diet.[29, 30] Since spelt and wheat are closely related, spelt products can cause similar responses for persons who react allergically to wheat. A food challenge should be used to assess the advisability of adding spelt to a personalized rotational diet. (See the section What Is a Food Allergy? in Chapter 3—Rotational Diet for a description of a food challenge.)

Spelt grain is a light golden brown in color and closely resembles wheat grain in appearance and size. It may be found in several forms such as whole grain, flour, flakes, and pastas. Spelt has a nutty flavor which is similar to whole wheat, and the flour is an excellent substitute, with minor adjustments, for whole wheat flour in recipes.

One of spelt's most outstanding features is its high nutritional value. It contains all of the basic materials for a healthy body, including protein (it contains up to 40% more than commercial wheat), fats, carbohydrates, vitamins, trace

---

[29] Harold M. Friedman, M.D., Robert E. Tortolani, M.D., John Glick, M.D., and Richard T. Burtis, M.D. "Spelt is Wheat," Allergy Proceedings, Vol. 15, no. 4 (July-August 1994), 217-218.

[30] John W. Yunginger, M.D. "Food Ingredient Labeling: How Many Ways Can Wheat Be Spelt?" Allergy Proceedings, Vol. 15, no. 4 (July-August 1994), 219-220.

elements, and minerals. Spelt is particularly rich in B vitamins and in polyunsaturated fats (essential fatty acids). It has a higher content than wheat in several amino acids (up to 65% more).

History Spelt is not a hybrid like commercial wheat. It is among the first original, natural grains known to man. Spelt originated in central Asia (the Tigris-Euphrates River valley) and was later brought to Europe where it gained great popularity. It can be grown without fertilizer and pesticides and requires a minimum of care. It grows in varying terrains and in any climate, even those with difficult winters. Due to its resistance, spelt is not sensitive to typical grain diseases. The spelt kernel is tightly surrounded by a strong husk or hull, which must be removed before the grain can be used for cooking. This protective covering guards the spelt grain against all types of pollutants in the air, even radioactive fallout. It also protects the grain during storage, ensuring the freshest possible product after dehulling and milling.

Modern research has proven that spelt was grown in Europe more than 9,000 years ago. It is also mentioned by name in some translations of the Bible (Exodus 9:31–32 and Ezekiel 4:9).

According to lore, in the Middle Ages St. Hildegard of Bingen, a Benedictine nun, received a vision that she should feed spelt to the patients under her care. Soon "terminal" patients were recovering and, as word spread of her work, people began to flock to her clinic. Writings on her life state that many were helped by her special nutritional regimen, which is a testimony to the valuable nutritional characteristics of spelt.

Today, spelt is very popular in European countries, specifically Germany, Italy, France, Switzerland, and Austria, where it is considered a "gourmet" food. It was introduced into the United States food market by Purity Foods of Okemos, Michigan in 1990 and is steadily gaining popularity as people learn of its incredible benefits. Before it gained more recognition, spelt was used mostly in cattle feed in the United States.

Uses To substitute spelt flour for whole-wheat flour in a recipe, a good rule of thumb is to either increase the amount of flour used by 20–25% or to start with only 3/4 of the liquid called for in the recipe. (You can add small additional amounts of liquid if needed.) Spelt products are excellent when used to make Almond-Sesame Granola Bars, Spelt Crackers, and Tuna or Chicken Noodle Casserole (see Day 1 recipes).

Sources Spelt products can be purchased in the natural foods section of better grocery stores and in health-food stores as well as through food-buying cooperatives and mail-order sources (see Appendix C: Resources).

* *

Teff

Properties Teff is an ancient, gluten-free grain. Even though teff is from the Grass Family (number 6), it is not related to any of the other foods we eat. For this reason many who do not tolerate other grains can eat teff without experiencing grain-like allergic reactions.

There are many varieties of teff, but only brown, ivory, and red are grown in the United States. The word teff means "lost" and is appropriate since the seeds are very tiny, even smaller than amaranth or quinoa. Being the smallest grain, it takes 150 grains to equal one wheat kernel. Harvesting is very labor intensive since teff is so small and is easily lost in the fields. Also, the crop can be lost should water fall prematurely on the seed panicles, causing the water-soluble bran to decompose.

In appearance, brown teff flour seems to have both brown and white particles. However, finished food products have a very dark, rich, brown color like the cooked brown teff grain.

Teff's mild, pleasing, slightly molasses-like flavor is so delicate that it allows the flavor of other ingredients to come through. This effect is seen in recipes from this cookbook where the sesame flavor of the seeds and/or oil in crackers and pancakes or the pear flavor in Teff Pear Cake can be distinguished. The cooked grain has a gelatinous texture. Ivory teff has an even milder flavor but turns a faint green color when cooked.

In addition to its versatile flavor and basically nonallergic properties, teff helps to promote good nutrition. Rich in iron, calcium, and potassium, teff has as much as five times the amount of these elements as may be found in other grains. Teff is high in copper and zinc as well as in protein and soluble and insoluble fiber.

History

Teff comes from Ethiopia and has been loved by Ethiopians for thousands of years. Ethiopia and teff survived invasions by the Egyptians, Romans, Arabs, and Europeans. Even though the teff fields were burnt, the Ethiopians could easily carry the tiny seed into hiding because only about two pounds of seed were needed to plant the next year's crop.

When Wayne Carlson was a Public Health worker in Ethiopia, he learned about and enjoyed eating teff. When he returned to the United States, he missed having teff in his diet and decided to try to grow teff in the United States. In southwestern Idaho, near the Oregon border, Mr. Carlson found a valley with a terrain and climate similar to Ethiopia and began raising teff there. For the first five years he raised teff for a limited market. Now, since 1988, he grows enough to sell to the health-food markets. Arrowhead Mills distributes his brown teff to health-food stores. Brown and ivory teff are marketed by direct mail from Mr. Carlson's company (see address in Appendix C: Resources).

Uses

The tiny grain seed is dried for cooking into cereal or for grinding into flour. You can prepare crackers, tortillas, muffins, pancakes, and desserts with teff flour. Most recipes using teff that I have read in published cookbooks, newsletters, and booklets contain ingredients such as a gluten-containing grain, eggs, starch, some type of sweetener, and/or milk. However, I have successfully developed recipes without many added ingredients. This is especially helpful when rotating and/or eliminating foods due to allergies. Some say that teff acts as a mild laxative, so do add it to your diet slowly as with any other new food.

Sondra's Thoughts

When I first tried teff, I did not enjoy the flavor of either the brown or ivory forms. But because I did not have an allergic reaction to it, I continued to eat teff cereal every four days, and before I finished eating my first pound I was in love with it. In clarification, I first tried teff very early on in my change in dietary habits and my taste buds were still clouded with *Candida* and a desire for heavy sweets. This probably influenced my initial reaction to the teff flavor. Now, I enjoy teff's slight molasses taste especially for breakfast—either as pancakes, muffins, or cereal and often without adding any sweetener.

Sources

Include teff in your diet today by trying my delicious Day 1 recipes. Ask your health-food store to stock brown teff seed and/or flour (distributed by Arrowhead Mills) or order directly from the grower or Arrowhead Mills.

To order from the grower, contact Mr. Carlson for current prices and ordering instructions at The Teff Company (see Appendix C: Resources).

Wild Rice

Properties While wild rice is a member of the Grass Family (number 6), it is in a different subgroup than rice and is technically an aquatic grass seed. Brown-black in color, it is a very thin grain that can be as long as one inch in length. It has a very strong flavor so a little goes a long way when it is included in recipes. Wild rice has a greater concentration of B vitamins, magnesium, and zinc than rice and has one of the highest protein contents among grains. It is low in fat and rich in carbohydrates, which are easily converted to energy in the body.

History Wild rice is indigenous to the lakes and rivers of Minnesota and Canada where it is still harvested today. It has been a staple food of the Chippewa Indians and an important part of their heritage for centuries. Because wild rice is harvested by hand, its price reflects its scarcity and labor-intensive processing. Considered a gourmet food by many, wild rice aficionados maintain that it is well worth the cost.

Uses Wild rice is available in the whole grain and in 100% wild-rice pasta. As wild rice cooks, the grains open to show a soft white-gray inside against a curling brown-black cover. Some of my favorite wild-rice recipes on Day 3 are Salmon or Turkey Vegetable Salad with 100% Wild-Rice Pasta and Pasta Salad for Day 3. Occasionally I move wild rice temporarily to Day 1 to make Wild & Brown Rice with Herbs. Also, I enjoy Northwest Natural brand Halibut Medallions, which are made with wild rice and are delicious served on a Kamut® bun.

Sources Wild rice may be purchased in health-food stores as well as through food-buying cooperatives and mail-order sources (see Appendix C: Resources).

Nongrains

Amaranth

Properties Amaranth is a gluten-free nongrain from the Pigweed Family (number 30), which is tolerated by many who are allergic to grains. However, if you are allergic to the pollen of pigweed, be aware that you may have a sensitivity to amaranth. Amaranth can be purchased in four forms—whole grain (referred to as seeds so it does not get confused with true grains from the Grass Family), flour, roasted bran flour, and puffed.

Amaranth grows best at low altitudes with Kansas and Nebraska offering the best growing conditions in North America. While amaranth has many advantageous growth characteristics, its nearly wild nature offers many challenges for farmers. The seeds need a lot of moisture for approximately three weeks to germinate and to support early growth. But the mature plants require very little moisture and thrive on neglect and drought. It grows in straight lines, and wild pigweed is commonly found among the plants. The seeds will mold on the stalk with too much moisture in late summer and early fall or will fly away in the wind if the air is too dry. The six-foot seed stalks survive best when picked by hand. As an added advantage, amaranth roots are shallow (just below the surface) and they crowd out most of the weeds making chemical herbicides unnecessary.

The small amaranth seeds are slightly smaller than alfalfa seeds. They range in color from tan to black. The cooked whole seeds have a gelatinous texture and are coated with a thick, shiny film that makes them shimmer like caviar.

Amaranth has a wonderful, nutty, slightly sweet flavor that is intensified if the seed is dry-roasted before cooking. The black seeds can add a bitter taste, so attempt to purchase amaranth with as little black seed in it as possible.

Including amaranth in your diet contributes to good nutrition because it has a high level of vegetable protein with a good balance of amino acids. It is especially high in lysine which is low in most grass grains. Also, when compared to grains from the Grass Family, amaranth is low in carbohydrates. It is rich in vitamins and minerals, including vitamin B complex, iron, calcium, and phosphorus. Puffed amaranth is very high in dietary fiber, much higher than grains from the Grass Family.

History Amaranth originated with the Aztecs in Mexico and in South America centuries ago. In 1521, Cortez banned amaranth and it nearly vanished, but four and a half centuries later in 1972 a botanical team found it growing wild in Mexico. They collected some of the seeds and were successful in growing it in the United States. Also, amaranth was known in ancient China, and today China is the major producer of amaranth, followed by Mexico and Central America. Amaranth means "immortality," an appropriate name considering its history.

Uses Amaranth seeds are harvested and dried to be cooked as cereal or used as a thickening agent. The seeds can also be sprouted and used as you would alfalfa sprouts or ground into flour for baked goods (see Day 2 recipes). For those who are not allergic to grains and do not need to follow the rotational diet in this cookbook, you may substitute amaranth flour for a portion of the flour called for in your favorite recipes. In this way you can gain the nutritional value, sweetness, and moisture of amaranth. Replace the amount of flour called for with 1 part amaranth flour to 3–4 parts wheat flour.

However, when using only amaranth in your recipes, this gluten-free flour needs the addition of a starch or a natural gum to compensate for wheat's gluten properties. As a general rule of thumb, use 75% amaranth flour and 25% potato starch, arrowroot starch, tapioca starch, soy flour, pea flour, or ground nuts. Amaranth flour feels very fine and delicate. The soft, smooth texture and high moisture content of the dough require a lot of tender loving care. Amaranth tortillas seem to be the hardest to make. Amaranth works best in thin and/or crispy products such as my delicious tortillas, crackers, and pizza crust. However, I have been successful in making cookies by using lots of additional tender loving care so the centers are not doughy. Puffed amaranth can be used as breading, as a snack, or as a texturizer in recipes such as cookies or granola.

Home gardeners can grow amaranth and harvest the leaves to eat. For the home gardener it is not beneficial to grow amaranth for the seeds because it is too labor intensive to harvest and dry. But when you harvest the leaves, they grow back and the plant produces fewer seeds. Just strip the leaves from the heavy center stalk and cook 10–15 minutes—steam, stir fry, or toss into soup or stew approximately 10–15 minutes before serving. Also, you may freeze the leaves to eat year round; simply blanch as you would spinach.

Sondra's Thoughts During the summers of 1993 and 1994 I succeeded in growing amaranth in my garden. I enjoyed experimenting with the dark green leaves and have included several Day 2 recipes that use them—Vegetarian Lasagna, Vegetarian Pizza, Low Carbohydrate Lasagna, and Steamed Amaranth Greens. I would encourage you to add this interesting crop to your garden. You can obtain seeds from Nu-World Amaranth, Inc. and Seeds of Change (see Appendix C: Resources).

Sources Purchase whole seed, puffed amaranth, and flour from your local health-food store. Also, various mail-order sources carry all four forms (see Appendix C: Resources). Some mail-order sources also freshly grind the flour to order. However, the freshly ground flour that I have purchased does not seem to be as fine as the organic flour distributed by Arrowhead Mills. The more coarsely ground flour seems to be okay for preparing crackers, but I do not like it as well for preparing other food products, especially tortillas. The flour seems to be the hardest form to find, probably because if it stands for many weeks the oils can go rancid, become bitter, and develop a strong odor. When you purchase the flour, store it in glass jars either in the refrigerator or freezer. Also, ask when new shipments are expected. For the freshest source, you may choose to order all four forms plus the garden seeds directly from the grower, Nu-World Amaranth, Inc. (see Appendix C: Resources).

* *

Buckwheat

Properties

Despite its name, buckwheat is not related to wheat but is instead a gluten-free nongrain from the Polygonaceae Family, sometimes known as the Buckwheat Family (number 27). Other members of this family are rhubarb, garden sorrel, and dock (a weed).

Grown in northern climates, buckwheat does well in adverse conditions. In fact, it thrives in locations where other crops fail. The bush-like plant grows quickly, adapts well to poor soils and moist cool climates, and can even be planted in July and harvested in 70 days.

Buckwheat has a shallow root system and smoothers out the weeds around it. In addition, no known insects harm the fruit of the plant (seeds). Because of these two factors, little or no chemical application is needed to grow buckwheat.

The plants have many glorious white and pink blooms. Each flower produces one interesting triangular-shaped seed (fruit of the plant) covered with a protective hard outer black hull. This fruit, called groats, is white with hints of green, gray, and tan. If you roast the buckwheat groats, then called kasha, they become a deep brown color with a strong aroma. Besides producing groats, a field of fragrant buckwheat blossoms attracts many bees to produce buckwheat honey, which is darker and more flavorful than clover honey.

Buckwheat has a strong earthy flavor. Some say that you either love it or hate it, but I feel you can learn to love the flavor if you do not enjoy it at first. When you are first getting used to the flavor of buckwheat, be sure and try the raw groats because roasting intensifies the flavor as well as the color and aroma.

Adding buckwheat to your diet also contributes to good nutrition. Buckwheat groats are rich in the B vitamins, especially thiamin and riboflavin. It also has large amounts of vitamin E, is rich in phosphorus and potassium, and is high in iron and calcium. Buckwheat is the best food source of rutin, a bioflavonoid which functions in the body to strengthen the walls of the blood vessels and to help prevent arteriosclerosis. A good source of protein, buckwheat has seven usable amino acids, is especially high in lysine, and is best complemented by combining it with peas, beans, or dairy products. You will notice that buckwheat is assigned to Day 4, which also includes several varieties of beans and peas.

There are three grades of buckwheat flour: whole grain, dark, and light. Whole-grain flour is made by grinding groats still covered with the protective outer black hull. Dark buckwheat flour is made by again using hull-covered groats. However, additional hulls are added before grinding into flour. Commercial light buckwheat flour is made from groats with most of the hulls removed.

History

Originally buckwheat came from the plains of China and Siberia. The Chinese cultivated this ancient nongrain for hundreds of years. Traders took it from Asia to Europe and then the early-American settlers transported it to the United States. By the 1800s it was an important crop in the United States, but then wheat and corn became more widely used and buckwheat faded in popularity. Buckwheat is the basis of many delicious whole-food dishes in Asia and Europe (piroshki, kasha varnishkas, kasha knishes) and in Japanese cuisine, mostly in the form of a pasta called soba.

Uses

There are various ways to prepare buckwheat to create delicious recipes, e.g., pancakes, brownies, and stir fries. The groats are very porous and cook quickly (about 15 minutes). Because of this porous nature, when you rinse the groats before cooking them you should do so quickly (see Washing Whole Grains and Nongrains on page 36). Raw or roasted whole groats may be cooked by simmering or baking and served as a potato substitute or used in other Day 4 recipes. You may coarsely grind the groats into grits to cook for breakfast as Creamy Buckwheat Cereal. Or finely grind them into White Buckwheat Flour (page 249) to prepare Day 4 recipes such as Blueberry Buckwheat Muffins, Orange Buckwheat Cake, Carob Cake Brownies, and Buckwheat Pancakes. Raw buckwheat groats may be stored in an air-tight container in a cool, dry place for eight months or longer.

Sondra's Thoughts

I have been told by some wheat-sensitive people that they are also sensitive to buckwheat. If you are reacting to whole-grain or dark buckwheat flour, it may be because the hard outer hull has not been removed from the seed and it is adding too much fiber to your diet. At one time I felt that I was sensitive to buckwheat when I was only eating foods cooked with whole-grain buckwheat flour. When I made the switch to using mostly buckwheat groats with the outer hull removed and/or grinding the groats into White Buckwheat Flour using my blender, I noticed that my problems with buckwheat disappeared. An added advantage was that I had much better success in cooking with the White Buckwheat Flour than with the whole-grain buckwheat flour.

Another reason why you may feel you are allergic to buckwheat is that you may be eating buckwheat pancakes made from a prepared mix. Be sure to read the label because many buckwheat pancake mixes include other ingredients such as wheat flour instead of using buckwheat flour only. Be aware also that allergic reactions to buckwheat may be due to a sensitivity to the weed "dock."

Sources

Purchase buckwheat groats and whole-grain buckwheat flour from your local health-food store or food-buying cooperative. If you cannot find buckwheat locally, purchase buckwheat groats (either raw or roasted) from various mail-order sources or order directly from the main producer of buckwheat products, Birkett Mills (see Appendix C: Resources).

If you do not desire to prepare your own White Buckwheat Flour (see Day 4 recipe), check with your mail-order sources to locate one which grinds freshly ground flours to order or purchase directly from Birkett Mills (see Appendix C: Resources).

For more general or nutritional information on buckwheat and the various buckwheat products available, contact: Buckwheat Institute, P.O. Box 440, Penn Yan, NY 14527.

* *

Quinoa

Properties

Quinoa (pronounced keen-wa) is a gluten-free nongrain from the Chenopodium or Goosefoot Family (number 28) and is tolerated by many who are allergic to grains. There are 2,000 known varieties of quinoa. Other members of this family are spinach, beets, chard, and a weed called lamb's-quarters.

The highest quality quinoa only grows at high altitudes—6,000–15,000 feet. It can thrive in thin, dry air and poor, sandy soil. In addition, it is able to withstand the strain of intense radiation from the sun at high altitudes as well as the below-freezing temperatures.

All of the 2,000 varieties have very elliptical seeds, approximately the size of millet. The color ranges from off-white to black. Imported quinoa is an off-white plump kernel whereas domestic quinoa is gray and slightly smaller. Black quinoa is truly black with a hint of purple, very small, not readily available, and considered a delicacy like wild rice.

Quinoa has a slightly bland character that can easily be enhanced with vegetables, apple, meats, etc. to create a delicious, light, fluffy dish. The subtle, nutty taste makes it a great side dish with almost any meal, or add it to soups, salads, and casseroles (see Day 3 recipes).

Quinoa is a complete protein source, containing all eight essential amino acids. In fact, this protein source is so good that The National Academy of Sciences has called it "one of the best sources of vegetable protein in the vegetable kingdom." Also, this essential amino acid balance is close to the ideal set by the United Nations Food and Agriculture Organization. Quinoa protein is equal in quality to that of dried milk and close to that of mother's milk. Quinoa is also high in Vitamin E, B vitamins, calcium, phosphorous, and iron.

History

Quinoa has been cultivated in South America in the Andes Mountains since 3000 B.C. The Inca Indians named it quinoa, meaning "the mother grain," for its life-giving properties. Quinoa was as important to the Incas as the buffalo was to the American Indian. The Incas used the whole plant in their daily life. The young plants supplied deep, green, leafy vegetables. The seeds were their staple nourishment. The stalks were used for fuel in high altitude areas where wood was unavailable. Finally, the ash from a quinoa fire was used with coca leaves in a manner similar to chewing tobacco, producing a mild narcotic effect.

The Incas realized quinoa's life-giving properties to such an extent that they encouraged pregnant and lactating mothers to eat quinoa every day for healthy babies and an adequate milk supply. Also, if needed, mothers made a thin gruel for their babies from cooked quinoa flour to supplement their milk.

Quinoa was so important to the Incas that it was considered sacred, and as part of their ceremonial rights the Inca ruler planted the first row each year with a gold planting stick. Also, the grain was mixed with blood to form dolls for religious rituals.

In 1982, Steve Gorad, founding president of the Quinoa Corporation, traded an Andean farmer the shirt off his back for quinoa seeds. This launched the Colorado quinoa growing program under the supervision of Colorado State University. Some quinoa is grown in the Rocky Mountains, but most of our supply comes from the plant's original home—Peru and Bolivia. These low-income-South American farmers do not use chemicals because they either do not have access to them or cannot afford them.

Quinoa seeds have a bitter coating called saponin. This coating functions as a natural repellent to insects and birds plus it protects the seeds from the high intensity of the altiplano sun. Before cooking the seeds you need to wash this coating off (see Washing Whole Grains and Nongrains on page 36). The tiny wet seeds will not slip through a mesh strainer because the seeds rest on top of each other when you pour slowly. The saponin coating is not harmful, just very bitter. Interestingly, the Incas saved the foam from washing quinoa to use as shampoo.

To remove the bitter saponin coating so the seed can be ground into flour, the Quinoa Corporation prewashes their quinoa in South America prior to importation. In addition, they have developed a system of belts along which they jostle the whole seeds. This method, called pearling, uses friction rather than chemicals to buff off the saponin (outer-most edge of the kernel).

Uses

Quinoa can be considered a fast food within whole-grain cookery since the seeds cook very quickly. Whole seeds are delicious cooked and served several different ways. My favorites are Quinoa Salad and Quinoa Pudding (see Day 3 recipes). As the whole quinoa cooks, the germ (outside of the grain) unfolds, resembling a partial spiral. This glistening translucent spiral resembles caviar. Also, pancakes and muffins made from quinoa flour with the addition of a starch are delicious.

Sources

Whole quinoa seeds can be purchased at most health-food stores, food-buying cooperatives, and mail-order sources. However, if your local health-food store or cooperative does not carry the flour, ask them to stock only the flour from Quinoa Corporation or order directly from them yourself (see Appendix C: Resources).

Starches

Arrowroot

Properties

Arrowroot is an edible starch made from the rootstocks of the *Maranta arundinacea* (West Indies or "true" arrowroot) plant. It is a fine, silky white powder with a faint licorice aroma. Its fine texture allows it to thicken quickly when cooked at lower temperatures and for a shorter time period than other starches. When boiled in water, it yields a transparent, odorless, pleasant-tasting jelly. Being almost pure starch, arrowroot supplies no vitamins and contains only 0.2% protein. However, it is easily digested and is an excellent thickening and binding agent for use by persons requiring a bland, low-salt, and/or low-protein diet. *Maranta arundinacea* is the only food in the Arrowroot Family (number 19) and has been assigned to Day 2 in this rotational diet.

History

"True" arrowroot is probably a native of Guyana and western Brazil and is cultivated throughout the West Indies, Southeast Asia, Australia, and South Africa. The plants reach a height of 5–6 feet and have large, arrow-shaped leaves and a few short-stalked white flowers. The plants are harvested when the root tubers are gorged with starch just before the plant's dormant season. The peeled roots are grated in water, the resulting mixture is dried to a powder, and the powder is then purified by several washings.

Uses

Arrowroot can be used as a thickening and binding agent in foods where you may have previously used cornstarch or tapioca starch. In this rotational diet, it is used as a thickener in Day 2 stews and casseroles and as a binding agent in amaranth baked goods. Arrowroot thickens to produce a clear, nongummy texture. An appropriate ratio would be to use 1 tablespoon of arrowroot to thicken 1 cup of liquid. Use 2 tablespoons to achieve a firmer texture for your final product. To reduce crumbliness in nongluten baking, substitute 3/4 cup of arrowroot for 1 cup flour as a binder.

Sondra's Thoughts

Arrowroot is also produced from plants other than *Maranta arundinacea*, which can involve seven other families. Since it can be difficult to determine the exact source for arrowroot, I have assigned most of the possible source families to Day 2. The Cyad Family (number 4), Tacca Family (number 13), and Canna Family (number 18) have arrowroot as their only member and are easily assigned to Day 2. The Ginger Family (number 14) includes the spice ginger that is an unassigned "Fun Food." I normally use ginger in Day 2 and Day 4 recipes, making it easy to use a possible arrowroot from this family on the correct day. The two families that have the most-used foods to be aware of are the Banana Family (number 16) and Spurge Family (number 47). Bananas are assigned to Day 2 so an arrowroot source from this family would not be a problem. However, there is a possibility that tapioca starch flour from the Spurge Family (number 47) could be marketed as arrowroot. The Spurge Family is assigned to Day 3 and tapioca is a thickener used in recipes on that day. Tapioca starch flour is very similar in texture and appearance to arrowroot, but does not have as strong an aroma and may have a slightly finer texture.

It is also possible that an arrowroot product could be diluted with potato starch. Since the Potato Family (number 74) is also assigned to Day 2, this should not cause a problem unless you are allergic to potatoes.

The best advice I can give you regarding arrowroot and its sources would be to be aware of any possible reactions you may have when you consume it. If you do have a reaction, you may wish to research the plant source used to make the arrowroot product you purchased. Try changing to a different brand, particularly one that uses a different source. As with most food products, be sure to read labels and make the best possible choice you can given the information you have.

Sources

Arrowroot is available in health-food stores, through food-buying cooperatives, and from mail-order sources (see Appendix C: Resources).

* *

Kudzu (Kuzu)

Properties

Kudzu (also spelled kuzu) is an oriental culinary thickener that is popular in macrobiotic cooking. Usually sold in a white chunk form, kudzu is a starch powder extracted from the roots of the wild kudzu vine. It may be used for the same thickening purposes as arrowroot or tapioca starch. As a member of the Legume Family (number 41), kudzu is assigned to Day 4 with most of the rest of this family. In addition, since it is more expensive than other thickening agents, using kudzu on this day actually is more economical since there are fewer recipes requiring a thickener.

History

Kudzu is a tenacious, perennial vine which thrives naturally in the rugged, volcanic, mountainous terrain and rural regions of Japan and other areas of eastern Asia as well as in the southeastern United States.

Japanese folklore attributes this deep-rooted plant's strong thickening characteristic to its ability to grow through hard mountain soil, splitting bedrock in its path. For centuries skilled craftsmen have followed a time-honored process, which takes over 100 days, to extract the kudzu starch. The roots are hand harvested at full maturity during the cold winter months. To extract the starch, the roots are crushed and the resulting mash is washed and filtered several times, using pure mountain water. The resulting kudzu cakes are set in wooden boxes to dry naturally and are then crumbled into a chunky powder.

In addition to its culinary uses, kudzu is also used in traditional folk medicine in Japan. However, in the United States its primary use is for thickening puddings, gravies, clear soups, sauces, and jellied fruit desserts.

Uses

Since the chunks are difficult to measure accurately, I have found that grinding them into a powder in my blender greatly simplifies measuring kudzu for a recipe. Store the white powder in a glass jar and measure as the package or recipe directions say for the chunks. A good ratio is 1 tablespoon of kudzu powder for 1 cup of liquid. The kudzu must be cooked for its thickening power to work. The powder may be added directly to cold foods before cooking or may be dissolved in a small amount of cold liquid before being added to hot food and simmered for 10–15 minutes. Kudzu produces a slightly thinner gel, but it is clear, not cloudy like cornstarch.

Sources Kudzu (kuzu) may be purchased in health-food stores as well as through food-buying cooperatives and mail-order sources (see Appendix C: Resources).

* *

Tapioca

Properties Tapioca is a starch prepared from the root of the cassava plant (*Manihot esculenta* [bitter cassava] or *Manihot aipi* [sweet cassava]). As a member of the Spurge Family (number 47), it is assigned to Day 3 for use as a thickener or binder. The familiar granular "pearl" form of tapioca is commonly used in puddings. Also, a fine white tapioca starch flour similar in behavior and consistency to cornstarch or arrowroot is available. Tapioca is quite nutritious and digestible.

History The cassava plant is native to the West Indies and to South America. After the cassava was introduced into Asia during the 19th century, it became a common food in that part of the world as well.

Uses When cooked, granular tapioca swells, thickens, and becomes translucent. Tapioca granules and starch flour are used as a thickener in soups, sauces, and puddings. The starch flour is also used as a binder in baked goods, especially in my Day 3 recipes using quinoa flour (Quinoa Applesauce Muffins, Quinoa Pancakes). A general rule of thumb is to use 1–2 tablespoons of flour or 4 teaspoons of pearls per 1 cup of liquid to be thickened.

Sources Tapioca granules may be purchased in regular grocery stores and health-food stores as well as through food-buying cooperatives and mail-order sources. Tapioca starch flour may be labeled as tapioca starch or tapioca flour and is not as easy to locate as the granules. Good options for locating this product are health-food stores, food-buying cooperatives, and, especially, mail-order sources (see Appendix C: Resources).

Sugar Substitutes

FOS (Fructo-oligo-saccharides)

Properties FOS (Fructo-oligo-saccharides) is a relatively fine white powder that has a clean taste about half as sweet as regular sugar with no aftertaste or bitterness. Also known as NutraFlora™ or neosugar, it consists of natural sugar (sucrose, common table sugar) to which an additional molecule has been attached. Because of the extra added molecule, the resulting FOS molecule is too big for humans to digest.[31] This means that it is essentially noncaloric because it is not broken down in the digestive process. Because of this, the blood sugar level remains stable (no sugar spike).

Because FOS is not broken down in the digestive process, it reaches the intestines intact where it is broken down and used by the beneficial bacteria. Because it "feeds" the beneficial bacteria, FOS is categorized as a probiotic enhancer. At the same time, FOS cannot be used by *Candida* and other yeast, or

[31] Peter J. Perna, Ph.D. "Fructooligosaccharides (FOS)—An All Natural Food Which Promotes *Bifidobacteria* and *Lactobacillus*" (Broomfield, CO: Center for Applied Nutrition, ZeaGen, Inc., 350 Interlocken Blvd), 1.

by salmonella, *E. Coli.*, and certain other harmful bacteria.[32, 33, 34, 35] Due to this characteristic, FOS is often beneficial in the treatment of "leaky gut" syndrome as well as *Candida* Related Complex (CRC).

FOS is a naturally occurring substance found in small amounts in a variety of fruits, vegetables, and grains.[36] It is produced commercially by using a special enzyme to add an extra molecule to sucrose. It does cost more than other sweeteners, but the benefit of having an easy-to-use sweetener that is also good for you far outweighs the price consideration. In this rotational diet, FOS has been assigned as a Day 3 sweetener. However, many people use it more often than every four days for its therapeutic properties.

History FOS has been used in Japan as a low-calorie, "non-nutritive" sweetening, bulking, and health-promoting agent for nearly a decade with no adverse reactions or effects to date.[37] However, as with many supplementary substances, overingestion of FOS (5 teaspoons/day for men, 6 teaspoons/day for women) may result in the development of diarrhea.[38]

Uses FOS is a pleasure to eat. For maximum health benefit, a good time to take it is on an empty stomach before meals, but it can be added to almost any food. Perhaps the simplest way to enjoy FOS is to place 1/4 teaspoon (or more, if desired) directly in your mouth. With the addition of moisture, the FOS will tend to form a small ball and dissolve like a piece of candy. In fact, except for the lower sweetness level, FOS tastes and dissolves a little like cotton candy and is helpful in satisfying a "sweet tooth" craving.

FOS does not dissolve as readily as sugar so it takes a little more stirring to dissolve when added to cold liquids. You will find it included in such Day 3 recipes as Quinoa Biscuits, Quinoa Cereal, and Basic Quinoa. In addition, you can move it to Day 2 to use as a sweetener in plain yogurt.

Sondra's Thoughts As a probiotic enhancer, FOS is an ideal addition to your health-care regimen, especially when you are taking an *acidophilus* supplement. There are some *acidophilus* supplements on the market that have FOS included in them. I would recommend that you not use these combined products since you have no control over the ratio of FOS to *acidophilus* supplement. Also, FOS has an indefinite shelf life while the *acidophilus* product has a limited one.

To learn more about the health benefits that can be achieved through including FOS as a regular part of your health-care regimen, you can contact me at Canary Connect (see Appendix G). Request the FOS information packet that includes information on dealing with CRC and food allergies through using FOS on a regular basis. Appendix G also contains a list of available research articles/abstracts on the use and benefits of FOS. To keep abreast of the most up-to-date information on FOS, subscribe to the Canary Connect News newsletter (see Appendix G).

---

[32] H. Hidaka, T. Eida, T. Takizawa, T. Tokunaga, and Y. Tahiro. "Effects of Fructooligosaccharides on Intestinal Flora and Human Health," *Bifidobacteria* Microflora Abstract (Vol. 5, issue 1, 1986), 37-50.
[33] R.C. McKellar and H.W. Modler. "Metabolism of Fructooligosaccharides by *Bifidobacterium sp.*," Applied Microbiology Abstract (Vol. 31, 1989), 537-541.
[34] T. Mitsuoka, H. Hidaka, and T. Eida. "Effect of Fructooligosaccharides on Intestinal Microflora," Die Nahrung Abstract (Vol. 31, issue 5-6, 1987), 436.
[35] H.W. Modler, R.C. McKellar, and M. Yaguchi. "*Bifidobacteria* and *Bifidogenic* Factors," Journal of Canadian Institute of Food Science and Technology (Vol. 21, issue 1, 1990), 29-41.
[36] Peter J. Perna, Ph.D. "Fructooligosaccharides (FOS)—An All Natural Food Which Promotes *Bifidobacteria* and *Lactobacillus*." 1.
[37] J.E. Spiegel, R. Rose, P. Karabell, V.H. Frankos, and D.F. Schmitt. "Safety and Benefits of Fructooligosaccharides as Food Ingredients," Food Technology (January 1994), 85-89.
[38] Ibid.

Sources FOS is available by mail order (see Appendix G: Canary Connect). However, it may be available in your local health-food store.

Honey

Properties Honey, probably the most commonly used natural sweetener, is 99% naturally predigested and therefore requires little additional processing by the digestive tract. The resulting absorption and energy boost occurs quickly and there is little or no strain on the digestive system. Honey is a thick, sticky syrup in texture. The darkness or lightness of its golden color indicates how strongly it is flavored and how rich it is in mineral content. In addition, a honey's base source plant affects its individual flavor and color (buckwheat honey is probably the "darkest" honey available). Darker honeys have a much stronger, distinctive flavor and contain higher levels of minerals such as iron, copper, sodium, potassium, magnesium, manganese, calcium, and phosphorous. In addition, honey contains small amounts of C and B vitamins.

Honey generally is the least chemically contaminated sweetener available because bees exposed to pesticides usually don't make it back to the hive. Labeling such as "U.S. Grade A" or "Fancy" refers to the level of filtration used in processing and does not give any indication of quality or freedom from chemical contamination.

Honey can come from many different floral sources. For rotational purposes it is important to know the source of any honey you wish to use and to purchase only honey that is labeled with this information. Be sure to read the label carefully because it is also a common practice to mix different source honeys to create a marketed brand.

The source for Berry Honey can be from raspberries, blackberries, or a combination of both. Orange Blossom Honey can be from a variety of citrus fruits such as orange, grapefruit, tangerine, and tangelo. Clover Honey and Alfalfa Honey also may contain pollen from other source plants. Baker's Honey may include titi, oil seed, goldenrod, Brazilian pepper, Chinese tallow, purple loosestrife, salt cedar, horsemint, and buckwheat and is not a good choice for persons on rotation.

Tupelo Honey is light amber in color, has a mild pleasant flavor, and, if it is pure, never granulates. It has a low glucose-to-water ratio and is likely to remain liquid with no special treatment. The tupelo tree is mostly found along the Apalachicola River in northwestern Florida and southern Georgia.

As a general rule, for honey the best processing is the least processing. You should avoid honey that has been subjected to heat or chemicals or that comes from beehives that are sprayed with antibiotics or other chemicals. Be sure to choose honey that is labeled "undiluted" because some marketed honey is diluted with corn syrup.

Uses Because honey is 20–50% sweeter than sugar, substitute 2/3 to 3/4 cup of honey for 1 cup of sugar. However, recipes in this cookbook have been developed using much less honey and they are still enjoyed by those who normally eat sweets. To facilitate the measuring process, moisten the measuring cup or spoon with water or oil. This will help the honey slide out without sticking. In addition, you should decrease the amount of liquid in the recipe by 1/4 cup for each 3/4 cup of honey used. An addition of a pinch of baking soda to baked goods will help neutralize the natural acidity of honey. Honey browns more easily than sugar so the oven temperature should be decreased by 25–30°F, and the pan should be placed on the middle or top oven rack.

Due to its ability to absorb and retain moisture, honey has a "keeping" quality which retards the drying out that occurs in baked goods. The flavor of baked goods made with honey is actually better the day after baking. Because using honey as a sweetener will add an additional flavor factor to your end product, it is better to use a lighter, more mildly flavored honey.

Honey should be stored at room temperature in a dry place. Be sure to keep the lid and rim of the jar clean so that the lid will close tightly. Almost all honey naturally crystallizes over time. It is easy to reliquify honey by placing the container in a pan of warm water (not hot) until the crystals disappear. This process does not affect the taste or purity of the honey.

Honey has been assigned as a Day 4 sweetener. To use honey in this rotational diet, you must remember that it contains bee protein and can be used only once in four days regardless of its base source plant. Because of the bee protein, you cannot use a rotation of Berry Honey on Day 1, Sage Honey on Day 2, Avocado Honey on Day 3, and Orange Blossom (citrus) or Buckwheat Honey on Day 4 even though these base source plants come from different families. In addition, you may wish to avoid honeys with a base source plant to which you are allergic.

Sources Honey is readily available for purchase from many different sources. The main concern regarding which type and brand to purchase revolves around the processing system used and the primary plant source involved.

* *

Maple Granules

Properties and Uses Maple granules are a dehydrated form of 100% pure maple syrup. Maple syrup, a concentrate of maple-tree sap, has been used as a mainstay natural-food sweetener for years. Pure maple syrup is a member of the Maple Family (number 50). Because it is in a family by itself, it is listed as an unassigned "Fun Food" in this rotational diet (see explanation on pages 30–31).

I prefer to use maple granules to sweeten Day 3 oat cereals and apple crisps.

Sources Maple granules are available through health-food stores, food-buying cooperatives, and mail-order sources (see Appendix C: Resources).

* *

Brown Rice Syrup

Properties Brown rice syrup is a rather opaque golden liquid with a consistency similar to honey. It has a pleasant, lightly sweet taste, but is only about 20% as sweet as sugar. A member of the Grass Family (number 6), brown rice syrup is an excellent sweetener when only a touch of sweetness is needed.

Lundberg Family Farms is one source for this product. Their Sweet Dreams Organic Brown Rice Syrup is made by grinding organic brown rice into a meal, cooking it to a slurry, and mixing it with a small amount of natural cereal enzymes (less than 1%). This process converts the starches to complex natural sugars (maltoses). The liquid is then squeezed from the slurry and cooked until thickened. No artificial additives, stabilizers, or chemicals are used in the Lundberg process.

Uses Brown rice syrup may be used to top your favorite Day 1 pancake recipes, toasted Kamut® or Spelt Yeast-Free Bread, or rice cakes. One of my favorite Day 1 desserts is Amazing Sugarless Cookies sweetened with brown rice syrup.

Sources Brown rice syrup may be purchased in health-food stores as well as through food-buying cooperatives and mail-order sources (see Appendix C: Resources).

* *

Stevia

Properties Stevia is a natural herbal sweetener that is approximately 100 times sweeter than sugar. Having a faintly licorice-like flavor, the white powder extract form of stevia is most commonly used in cooking and baking. This white powder extract is its purest available form. It is also available as a brown liquid extract and as crumbled *Stevia rebaudiana* leaves. A member of the Composite Family (number 80), *Stevia rebaudiana* is a small shrub which grows wild in the province of São Paulo near the southern border of Brazil, on the frontier with Paraguay. While a teaspoon of white stevia extract powder has the same sweetening power of 2–4 cups of sugar, it contains only 8 calories. Since it is not absorbed by the body and has such a low caloric content, stevia does not trigger a rise in blood sugar levels. It has been researched extensively since l899 and found to be completely nontoxic, in contrast to many artificial sweeteners available today. Because of these properties, stevia has been used effectively in the treatment of diabetes, high blood pressure, and infections, as well as in weight-loss programs.

History The *Stevia rebaudiana* plant was first scientifically studied in 1899 by Moises S. Bertoni, a Paraguayan botanist who recognized its highly concentrated sweetening power. Stevia has long been used by the Guarani Indian tribes to sweeten teas and foods. In the city of Birigui, in São Paulo province, Brazil, stevia is so popular that it is used to sweeten milkshakes, juices, and coffee in almost all bars and restaurants. During World War II there was some speculation among scientists that stevia might be useful as a sweetener in the United States because sugar was at a premium. Unfortunately, the plant was not cultivated for industry outside of South America and the idea never materialized. More recently the Japanese have been using stevia to sweeten their diet foods since all artificial sweeteners are banned in Japan.

Uses Unlike some artificial sweeteners, stevia is stable at any temperature and is very useful in foods from the sweetening of beverages and cereals to baking. Because of its concentrated sweetness, typically no more than 1/4 teaspoon of the powder extract is needed to sweeten a whole recipe. In fact, adding too much stevia to a recipe can make it bitter. For a cup of tea a few grains (less than a "pinch") are usually sufficient. Because of its high potency as a sweetener, it is best to move cautiously when you first begin using stevia. Start with slightly less than is called for until you learn how much to use to satisfy your personal taste. All of the recipes in this cookbook that call for stevia use the white powder extract, referred to as “white powder concentrate.”

Sources At the publication date of this cookbook stevia is very difficult to acquire in the United States. I have included recipes using stevia for those persons who may have it on hand and with the hope that it will be more readily available in the future. The only mail-order source for stevia that I am aware of at this time is Body Ecology Diet (see Appendix C: Resources).

Miscellaneous Foods

Carob

Properties

A member of the Legume Family (number 41), carob is a naturally sweet, high-protein, low-fat, low-calorie, caffeine-free tropical bean that is an excellent substitute for chocolate or cocoa. Unlike cocoa, which has a naturally bitter taste, carob's natural sweetness allows you to use much less sweetener while having cocoa's rich brown color and consistency. Carob powder is slightly lighter in color than cocoa, but its aroma and flavor are very similar. An additional advantage of using carob is that it usually costs about one-fifth as much as chocolate.

History

The carob tree is an evergreen which can reach a height of fifty feet. They are found in hot climates with an abundance of rain, primarily near the shores of the Mediterranean Sea. Also, carob trees can be found in the semiarid regions of the United States. The trees require very little pruning, need no spraying because they are remarkably free from fungus diseases and insect pests, and in most soils need no fertilization until the tree begins bearing fruit. The fruit is a fat leathery pod which averages from three to twelve inches in length and contains five to fifteen brown seeds in a sweet pulp. Most trees start bearing fruit five years from budding with an average yield of 250 pounds per acre. At eight years the yield increases to 2,500 pounds per acre, and at twelve years the yield may be as much as 5,000 pounds per acre.

The name carob seems to have no single, accepted origin. The plant is also variously known as the honey locust, the algarroba, the caroubler, and the Egyptian fig. Many believe that the "locust" mentioned in the Bible as the food John the Baptist ate were carob pods, and that is why the carob is still known as St. John's bread and sometimes as locust pod.

Carob powder in raw or toasted form contains the entire seed pod except for the seeds. The pod is processed into pulp, dried, toasted, and pulverized into the final product. Carob powder has been available in the United States since the 1920s as a roasted cocoa replacement.

The ovate carob seeds are extensively used in the manufacture of gum tragacanth, a widely used food additive. In addition, they are used for animal feed, and an oil is extracted, called algarroba oil, which is used for medicinal purposes. Carob seeds, uniform in weight, are thought to have been the original carat weight used by jewelers.

Uses

Carob, an excellent chocolate substitute, can be used to make such treats as Carob Cake Brownies, Carob Shake, and Carob Pudding (see Day 4 recipes). Carob chunks can be used as a naturally sweet snack treat. It is important to remember that carob should only be used in the powder or the chunk form. Commercial "carob chips" usually include ingredients such as sweeteners, whey, nonfat milk solids, hydrogenated palm oil, cottonseed oil, and lecithin (soy) most of which should be avoided on a *Candida* control diet.

Sources

Carob powder and chunks can be purchased in health-food stores and through mail-order companies and other outlets that carry specialty foods (see Appendix C: Resources).

* *

Clarified Butter (Ghee)

Properties

Clarified butter (also known as ghee) is the pure oil derived from butter when the milk solids are separated and removed and the water is cooked out (butter is over 16% water). Since it eliminates the milk sugar that may affect persons with *Candida* Related Complex or lactose intolerance, clarified butter is a versatile oil that is beneficial even for persons on a dairy-free regimen.

History In India and the Middle East, ghee has been a staple oil and a practical way to preserve butter for many centuries. Often called "royal oil," ghee was used as a medicinal supplement for healthy skin, mental alertness, good digestion, and improved memory and was renowned for its rejuvenating properties. For a deep restful sleep, a teaspoon of ghee stirred into warm milk was prescribed. Traditional herbal remedies were usually mixed into a small amount of ghee and then eaten, which allowed the herbs to be assimilated into the cells more quickly. Placed into tiny vessels with cotton wicks, ghee was also used for candles in special ceremonies and on festive occasions.

Uses Since clarified butter is a pure oil it may be used as you would other oils assigned to Day 2. Use it for sautéing and frying since it does not burn or smoke like other oils. For a rich buttery flavor in baked dishes, replace the butter listed in the recipe with half the amount of clarified butter. It adds a special touch to Fried Potatoes. You can also use it plain or with Day 2 herbs and spices mixed in to top baked potatoes, spaghetti squash, purchased amaranth pasta, shrimp, crab, or lobster. Take it along with you when dining out to use on your baked potato or as a dipping sauce for shellfish. Experiment with topping various Day 2 foods with clarified butter with or without herb combinations. Let your imagination be your guide.

Sources While Clarified Butter is relatively simple to make (page 195), it is also available commercially at health-food stores and through mail-order sources under the product name Ghee (see Appendix C: Resources).

* *

Flaxseed and Flaxseed Oil

Properties A member of the Flax Family (number 44), flaxseeds are flat, oval, and pointed at one end. Seeds range in color from light to dark reddish brown or yellow. Ground flaxseed, which is made by grinding the seeds in a blender, is brown in color and is a good source of dietary fiber. Flaxseed oil has a fairly bright yellow color, relative little odor, and has a light buttery taste.

Flaxseed oil is an important food substance because of its high levels of essential fatty acids, Omega 3 and 6. These are essential to proper body function and are not produced by the human body. These essential fatty acids (EFAs) are key factors in the regulation of cholesterol metabolism; the maintenance and regulation of the functions and integrity of cell membranes; and the production of prostaglandins, which are the very active biological substances that regulate nearly every body function. Prostaglandins have an active role in the inflammatory process, the healing and repair process, the immune system, the neural circuits in the brain, the cardiovascular system, the digestive and reproductive systems, and the body thermostat and calorie-loss mechanism. It is easy to understand why a deficiency in Omega 3 EFAs can contribute to such ailments as water retention; dry, scaly, or oily skin; goose flesh (bumps on back of arms and buttocks); high cholesterol; high blood pressure; arthritis; dry eyes; breast tenderness; premenstrual symptoms; and severe menstrual cramps. To adequately process the Omega 3 EFAs found in flaxseed oil so that they can be used in the production of prostaglandins, the body must also have adequate amounts of magnesium, B vitamins (B_3, B_6, B_{12}), selenium, zinc, iron, and vitamin C.[39, 40]

As stated in the book Chronic Fatigue Syndrome and the Yeast Connection by Dr. William G. Crook, "During the past decade, almost without exception, physicians treating patients with yeast-connected health problems have used EFA (essential fatty acid) supplements as an essential part of their treatment program."[41] The usual recommended amount of flaxseed oil to be taken daily is one or two tablespoons.[42, 43] It may be taken by tablespoon, but because most oils are not palatable in their individual forms, it is easier to consume the flaxseed oil by including it in or on the food you eat. When used primarily for its nutritive qualities, flaxseed oil should never be cooked because the heating process destroys the essential fatty acids.

History Flaxseed and flaxseed oil have been used for 5,000 years. However, it is only recently that the extent of the beneficial effects of these substances has been uncovered. Flaxseed oil is common in Europe and was common in the United States until the beginning of World War II. Flax is an annual plant that is grown mostly in the colder regions of the world. Because of the cool, long days common to its northern latitudes, Canada is the world leader in high-quality flax production. The majority of the world's flax production (about 85%) is centered in Canada, the United States, Argentina, India, and the Soviet Union.

The name "linseed oil" used to be interchangeable with "flaxseed oil." But in recent years there has been an international effort to separate the use of "flaxseed" and "linseed." "Flaxseed" refers to products from the flax plant that are produced for human consumption. "Linseed" is used when referring to products that have been denatured, made unfit for human consumption, and used commercially in paints, varnishes, and other like substances.

Uses Ground flaxseed can be cooked in water to create a flour binder for use as an egg substitute in baking. Flaxseed oil is excellent for use in uncooked salad dressings and for a topping on pancakes, biscuits, cooked vegetables, or any other food on which you would like to have a buttery taste. It can be blended half-and-half with butter or clarified butter to form a "soft" spread. Since the heating process destroys the EFAs, add flaxseed oil to any dish after it is cooked when using it for its nutritive qualities.

Heat, light, and air (oxygen) must be eliminated during processing and storage for flaxseed oil to maintain its freshness. Purchased flaxseed oil should have an expiration date stamped on the container indicating its effective shelf life. In addition, both ground flaxseed and flaxseed oil go rancid very quickly so they should be refrigerated or frozen.

Sondra's Thoughts Since I use flaxseed oil for its nutritive qualities and I have no problems with consuming it on a continued basis, I include it on all four days of my personal rotation. However, if you need to rotate flaxseed oil in your personal plan, it can be placed on any day you choose because it is in a family by itself (number 44).

Sources Purchase flaxseed products through health-food stores, mail-order sources, and food-buying cooperatives (see Appendix C: Resources).

---

[39] Ingeborg M. Johnston, C.N., and James R. Johnston, Ph.D. Flaxseed (Linseed) Oil and the Power of Omega-3: How to Make Nature's Cholesterol Fighters Work for You (New Canaan, CT: A Good Health Guide, Keats Publishing, Inc., 1990), 26.

[40] "Fresh Flax Oil" (Monument, CO: A pamphlet published by Allergy Resources, Inc.).

[41] William G. Crook, M.D. Chronic Fatigue Syndrome and the Yeast Connection (Jackson, Tennessee: Professional Books, 1992), 256.

[42] Ibid.

[43] "Fresh Flax Oil."

Guar Gum

Properties Guar gum is a fine white powder derived from the seed pod of the guar plant, *Cyamopsis tetragonolobus*. As a member of the Legume Family (number 41), guar gum has been assigned to Day 4. Guar gum adds fiber to foods and is used commercially as a binder in low-gluten or no-gluten flour baked goods to help them rise and hold moisture. It is also used in the production of ice cream to promote a smooth, soft texture and to keep ice crystals from forming. Because of its highly absorbent character, guar gum thickens instantly when mixed with cold liquid.

History The guar plant is native to India and is cultivated in the United States today for use as forage as well as for the production of guar gum.

Uses I use guar gum as a binder for buckwheat baked goods and tortillas. Since guar gum thickens so quickly, the following tip will help you use it effectively in your baking. If you are making a recipe which will require a good amount of mixing, you can add the guar gum to the dry ingredients before combining them with the liquid ingredients. However, since the guar gum will have a tendency to clump when combined with liquids, in recipes where only minimal mixing is required add the guar gum to the liquid ingredients, quickly whisk it in, and immediately add the liquids to the dry ingredients. The recommended ratio is to use 1 teaspoon of guar gum to thicken 1 cup of liquid.

Sources Guar gum may be purchased at health-food stores, through food-buying cooperatives, and by mail-order (see Appendix C: Resources).

* *

Tahini

Properties and Uses Tahini is a light colored butter made by grinding raw whole or skinned sesame seeds. It has its own interesting flavor, different from the flavor of plain sesame, and can range in consistency from very oily to somewhat dry. Tahini is a member of the Pedalium Family (number 75), and it can be used to replace peanut butter as a spread on rice cakes or on Kamut® or Spelt Yeast-Free Bread or Dinner Rolls. It also makes an excellent topping to replace jelly on your favorite Day 1 muffin or pancake recipe. In addition, it can be used as an egg substitute in recipes by using a mixture of 1 tablespoon tahini and 3 tablespoons of water.

Sources Tahini may be purchased in health-food stores as well as through food-buying cooperatives and mail-order sources (see Appendix C: Resources).

5. BASIC EQUIPMENT

Recommended Basic Equipment

Having and properly using the correct equipment is by far one of the best ways to save time in the kitchen and therefore to save energy and money. Here is a list of equipment that I would recommend you have to facilitate meal planning and preparation. If you do not have this equipment, you may desire to gradually add it to your kitchen.

<u>Digital timer</u>:

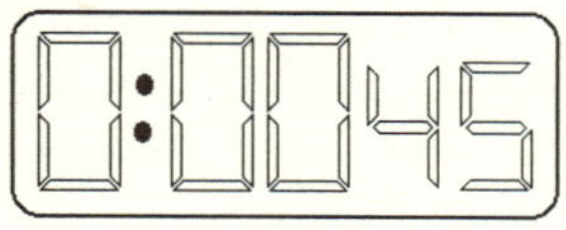

I recommend that you purchase a digital timer with the following two features:

1. Digital timer that measures in hours, minutes, and seconds. You need the seconds for tortillas.
2. Memory feature: This is an interesting feature in that after your time is up and you turn off the timer, it can automatically reset back to the amount of time that you just finished. This feature is great for making tortillas.

<u>Measuring Equipment</u>:

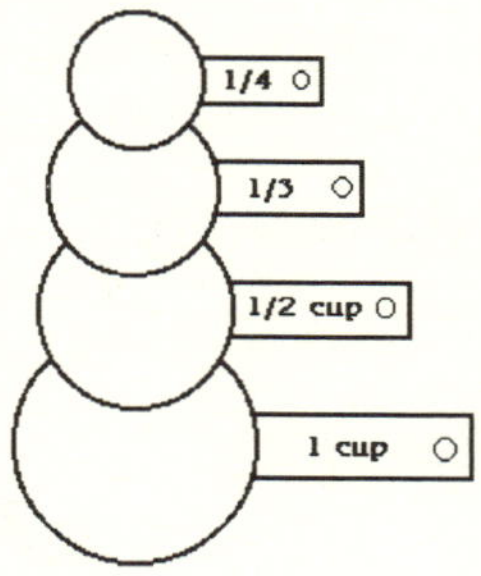

⇒ At least two sets of metal dry-measuring cups (1/4, 1/3, 1/2, and 1 cup).

⇒ At least one 1/8 cup metal dry-measuring cup. This may be a coffee measure that is sold separately and usually measures approximately 1/8 cup.

⇒ Clear glass measuring cups of various sizes to measure liquids and foods such as cooked meats and vegetables, especially if measuring over 1/2 cup. I recommend Pyrex brand since they have handles that allow you to nest them inside of each other for storage. Another advantage of this brand is the easy-to-read red painted increment markings. They make measuring accurately easier than using the indentation markings found on other brands. I would recommend that you have at least the following:

- two 1-cup measures
- two 2-cup measures
- one 4-cup measure
- and possibly one 8-cup measure

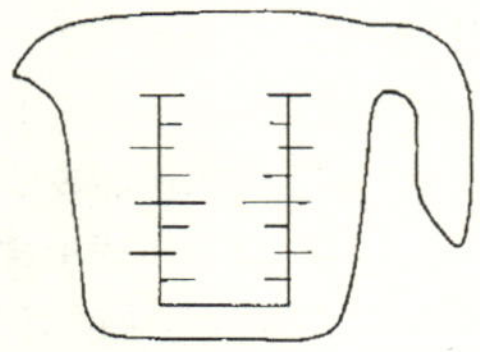

⇒ At least two sets of metal, long-handled measuring spoons. The long handles (approximately 5 inches in length) work well for measuring and are helpful in getting small amounts of spices, etc. out of narrow-neck bottles. These spoons are also much handier to use and clean if you take them apart and store them on four separate small hooks conveniently located in the mixing area of your kitchen.

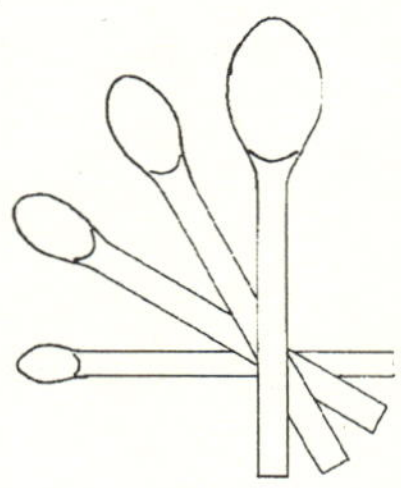

⇒ At least one 1/8 teaspoon measure. I have only seen a 1/8 teaspoon measure in a set of short-handled plastic measuring spoons. The 1/8 teaspoon measure is the only spoon from my plastic set that I use because of the petroleum factor of the plastic. In addition, I have noticed a lot of static cling between many cooking products and plastic so it is difficult to get an accurate measurement of food, especially when measuring in such small amounts.

Curved-Sided Bowl:

Mixing bowls can be found in two basic styles: A straight-sided bowl has a larger flat surface in the bottom before the side comes up at a right angle. A curved-sided bowl has a smaller flat surface at the center of the bottom before beginning a gradual curve that continues to the lip of the bowl. I feel that the curved-sided bowl works best for stiffer doughs and/or batters that you need to work with your hands or a spatula to knead in additional amounts of flour (e.g., tortillas, noodles, crackers, biscuits, etc.). I also prefer the curved-sided bowl for thinner batters such as pancakes because a whisk used for blending ingredients moves smoothly along the curved sides. Previously, Pyrex sold a set of four increasing-size bowls with nice curved sides that nested inside each other. These bowls also have two lips, one for use as a handle and a smaller lip for pouring. If you can acquire these at a garage sale, I recommend that you do so. If not, I recommend that you acquire one each of the Anchor Hocking 4-cup and 8-cup mixing-measures. These measures have an adequate curved side, a nice-sized handle for comfort, and a pour spout. These two mixing-measures can also double for the two large measuring cups on the recommended measuring equipment list on the previous page.

Strainers:

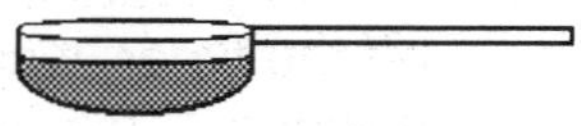

You should have a set of various sizes of fine-mesh strainers to wash small-size to medium-size grains such as quinoa, amaranth, teff, millet, rice, and buckwheat. These strainers can also be used to strain meat broth or to sift carob powder.

Colanders:

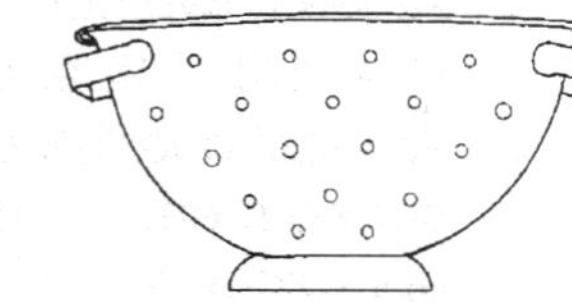

You should have at least one or more colanders for washing dried beans and larger grains such as Kamut® and spelt.

Two Splatter Screens:

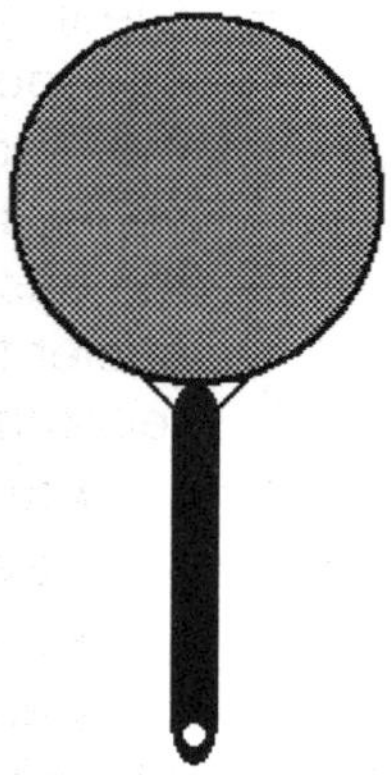

A splatter screen is a fine-mesh screen approximately 11–12 inches in diameter with a circular frame and a handle. Cost in a discount department store is usually under $3. A splatter screen is listed in those recipes in this cookbook where its use would be beneficial.

Most often I use a splatter screen to prevent oil or liquids from splattering out onto the stove, which makes cleanup easier. I could use a lid for this purpose, but I also want to prevent moisture from building up in the food that I am cooking (basically dry heat cooking). Also, I may desire to cook off some of the liquid, such as in thickening tomato sauce as well as blending the flavors of the spices in Picante Sauce.

Another use for a splatter screen is to reheat muffins and thaw or heat tortillas (see Reheating, page 91). You may find other uses for this inexpensive, versatile kitchen tool.

Knives:

A set of good quality cooking knives is an important asset for your kitchen. I recommend having at least a good paring knife and a French knife. They will help make your food preparation easier and faster.

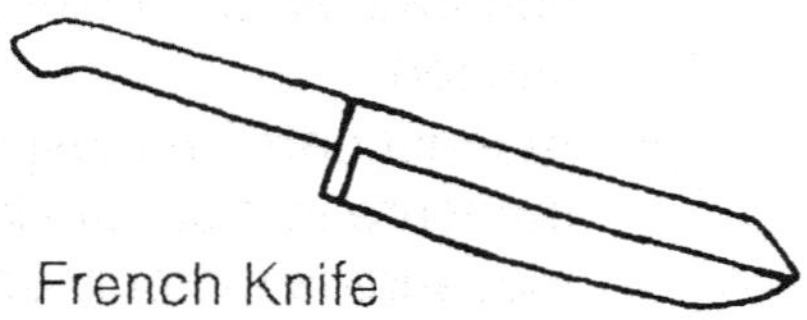

French Knife

Although I am chemically sensitive, I purchased a full set of white-handled Cutco cutlery and was able to tolerate the materials immediately. Explore your available options and choose a brand that will work well for you. You may wish to build your knife set over a period of time instead of investing in a complete set immediately.

Cutting Board:

Cutting boards can be used for several food preparation purposes. The most obvious use is in preparing and cutting up vegetables, but they can also be used to roll out noodles, tortillas, pie crust, biscuit dough, etc. A pebble-like-surfaced acrylic cutting board, at least 12 x 13 inches in size, is recommended for preparing large amounts of vegetables. An over-the-sink style of cutting board is handy if you have limited kitchen space. If you plan to use a cutting board to roll out doughs, I recommend a smooth-surfaced, tempered-glass cutting board at least 16 x 20 inches in size.

I do not recommend using a wooden cutting board. It is the worst sanitation problem you probably have in your family kitchen. Since wood is porous, any liquids or juices from the food products being prepared on it can seep down into the board's surface. This is especially unsanitary when using the board for preparing raw meats.

One 10-inch Cast-Iron Skillet approximately two inches in depth:

See "How to Season Cast Iron" starting on page 63.

One or Two 10–12 Inch Cast-Iron Griddles:

See "How to Season Cast Iron" starting on page 63.

One Blender with Glass Jar:

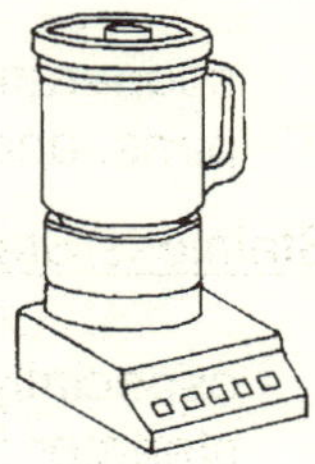

I recommend KitchenAid brand because it comes with a glass jar and the motor is very heavy duty and will work for nut chopping and grinding. Another advantage is that the base of the jar is wider than most other brands. If you cannot purchase a KitchenAid, the next brand I would recommend is the Oster because of its durability over some of the less expensive brands. In addition, you may wish to have a second glass blender jar.

One Stand Mixer with Beaters and Dough Hooks:

I recommend KitchenAid or Oster brand. A stand mixer uses less of your energy than a hand-held mixer and gives you more control of the batter. The dough hooks are especially helpful for preparing Kamut® or Spelt Yeast-Free Bread, "Hamburger" Buns, and Dinner Rolls.

Food Processor:

You may desire a large food processor if you will be doing an extensive amount of canning or freezing. However, for just the basic recipe needs in this cookbook, I recommend the Black and Decker® Handy Shortcut™ because it is easier to clean than a larger model. Since the container holds two cups you often can use it as your measuring guide in many recipes such as Scalloped Potatoes.

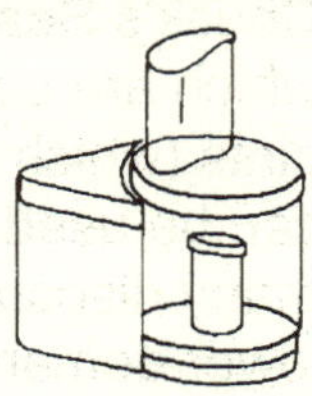

Another benefit is that it doesn't take the Handy Shortcut™ very long to accomplish the task you are using it for and you can set it under an exhaust fan to quickly clear any new-motor smells that may bother a chemically sensitive person. The base of this food processor is plastic and when you first acquire it the motor may need to outgas. I outgassed mine by putting it in another room near an air purifier and letting it run for a little while then turning it off to let it cool. I repeated this procedure 4–6 times until I could no longer smell an odor when it was operating. By following this procedure, a chemically sensitive person should be able to use it with little difficulty relatively soon.

Slow Cookers:

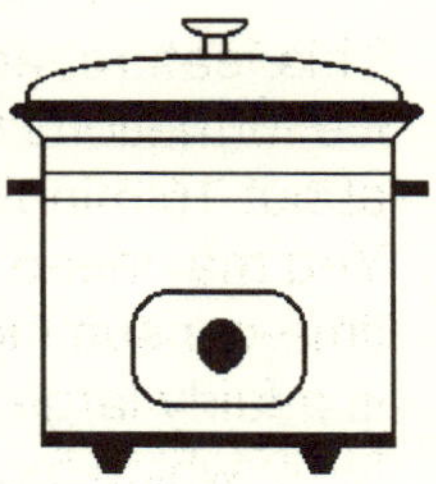

⇒ One 1-quart size slow cooker: I recommend Rival brand Crockette mainly because the crock insert lifts out of the heating base, which makes it easier to clean. This size is especially useful for the various cereal recipes in this cookbook.

⇒ One regular-size slow cooker: Again I would recommend the Rival brand or any other brand where the crock insert lifts out of the heating base to make cleanup easier.

Toaster Oven:

Having a toaster oven allows you to heat only the cooking space you need since you do not need the entire stove oven for one small casserole dish or to reheat a few pieces of pizza. If you are chemically sensitive, I would recommend that you not acquire a toaster oven that has a continuous cleaning feature. The odors from this process may be a problem for you. When you shop for a toaster oven, take along the dishes you are likely to use in it to be sure they will fit.

Counter-top Grill:

An electric thermostat-controlled counter-top grill is a handy addition to your kitchen. It can be used to grill steaks, burgers, fish filets, pork chops, and other foods to give them that special grilled flavor without using charcoal or gas grills that can cause problems for chemically sensitive persons. Be sure to look for a model that disassembles and reassembles easily for cleaning.

Stainless Steel Cookware and Bakeware:

There are many brands on the market. Check also with food-buying cooperatives for purchasing some good quality bakeware—such as baking sheets, muffin pans, and square baking dishes—at a lower cost.

Stainless Steel Steamer Pan:

Used for steaming vegetables and heating some leftovers, this pan is especially useful for persons who cannot tolerate using a microwave oven. Be sure the steamer insert has an inside diameter of at least 7 3/4 inches and a height of at least 3 1/4 inches. This will allow you to use Grab-It bowls for thawing and reheating leftovers. I recommend a steamer pan over a collapsible steamer basket since it is easier to clean.

Covered Casserole Dishes:

You will want several in your kitchen. I highly recommend having at least four to six Corning Grab-It bowls with glass lids as well as the plastic lids and one Corning 10-inch square casserole with glass lid (about 2–3 inches deep).

An Assortment of Glass Jars:

An assortment of glass jars with tight-fitting lids is useful for storing and/or freezing leftovers such as meat and/or vegetable broths, cooked beans, soups, salad dressings, "Mayos," etc. You can begin by saving jars that you purchase food in, such as Chuck's Seafood brand tuna or salmon, or you can purchase wide-mouth canning jars which are easier to use and to clean. They come in various sizes such as half-pints and pints (which are handy for freezing leftovers), to quarts, tall half-gallons, and gallons (that can be used to store grains and flours). These jars are available in the canning sections of many discount, hardware, and grocery stores. The half-pint and half-gallon sizes are in lower demand and may need to be special ordered.

A Wide-Mouth Funnel:

A wide-mouth funnel to use when filling jars makes the process easier and helps prevent spills.

One or Two Food Freezers:

I recommend a chest freezer that has a push button manual defrost feature. This feature facilitates defrosting by heating the sides of the chest freezer and melting the ice formations very quickly. When defrosting my freezer, I am ready to replace the food in about 15 minutes time. With a chest freezer you only need to defrost it about once a year. You may need to straighten or rearrange the food a few times in between, but the more time-consuming emptying and defrosting process is kept to a minimum. My chest freezer is a fairly large Sears and Roebuck model. I also purchased a few extra hanging baskets for it, which facilitates storing more food in better order.

If you can afford or need more than one food freezer, I also recommend an upright manual defrost model so you can store grains in gallon glass jars. This will allow you to buy in larger quantities at a lower price and to have more on hand to cut down on trips to the store. You can also store leftovers in glass jars in this freezer to give you a "quick and easy meal" supply for the days when you do not have as much time to cook.

How to Season Cast Iron

Items needed:

- ◊ griddle, skillet, or other cast-iron cookware to be seasoned
- ◊ electric burner that is close to the size of the heating surface of the cookware
- ◊ oven
- ◊ roll of paper towels
- ◊ stiff brush—a fingernail brush will work
- ◊ liquid lecithin

1. Place cookware on cold range burner. Turn range on low and warm the cookware just enough to peel off the label and the glue. Remove cookware from heat and turn off range burner.
2. Wash cookware thoroughly with mild soap and stiff brush. Rinse and dry thoroughly with paper towels.
3. Return cookware to cold range burner. Turn burner on medium-low.
4. Pour a thin stream of liquid lecithin onto cookware in a circular motion similar to pouring syrup on pancakes. Pour the most liquid around the outer edge.
5. Using a paper towel, spread the lecithin evenly over the top surface of the cookware. Be sure to include corners and crevices. You only want a thin layer of lecithin left on the cookware. The cast-iron surface may be a little rough and damage the paper towel. If so, use another towel to finish spreading the lecithin. Be sure to remove any pieces of paper towel from the cookware. Also, spread lecithin on the entire handle if it is cast iron. (Special Note: If your handle is wooden, remove it during this seasoning process.)
6. Place coated cookware in **cold** oven. Turn oven on and set at 300°F. Heat cookware for 30 minutes.
7. Remove cookware from the oven and, while it is still warm, wipe off the excess lecithin with paper towels. Do not turn off the oven.
8. Repeat steps 4 through 7 ten times making sure your cookware remains warm enough to spread the lecithin. Also, since your cookware is warm, you can return it to the warm oven rather than taking time to cool the oven for each repeat. If you do not have time to immediately repeat the steps while your cookware is warm, you will need to restart the process beginning with step 3—with cold cookware and oven.

Special Notes: You only need to season the handle a couple of times. Often the directions with your cookware will tell you to season the outside edge and bottom. I do not recommend this because of the oily mess it makes on the range burner and in the oven. Also, to help eliminate oven spills, I suggest placing an old large baking sheet on the lower rack and the cookware to be seasoned on the upper rack of your oven. I also clean my oven immediately after I have completed the seasoning to remove the burnt odor and any spills that occur.

Using Cast-Iron Cookware

When you first begin using your seasoned cast-iron cookware, you may need to use slightly more oil than called for in my recipes. But as you use and reuse your cookware, it becomes more seasoned and will require less oil.

Foods that I enjoy cooking and that work best on a cast-iron griddle are my recipes for pancakes, tortillas, griddle breads, and fried eggplant. In this cookbook testing of the recipes that use a griddle was done on a seasoned cast-iron griddle with the electric range control set on low to medium. Other griddles and ranges may vary. Making a large quantity of tortillas, which uses very little oil, removes some of the seasoned finish from the griddle. But after preparing other foods which use oil, the seasoned finish will be restored.

I use my cast-iron skillet to dry roast small amounts of grains and nongrains. Also, I use the skillet to prepare stir-fry vegetables and simple fried meats that do not require the addition of liquid for steaming. Cast iron is especially good for stir-fry vegetables because you need less oil. This allows the natural flavor of the vegetables to emerge. Avoid cooking acidic foods such as tomatoes in cast iron because the acid can remove the seasoned finish.

Daily Care of Cast-Iron Cookware

To protect your cast-iron cookware it is important to heat it slowly beginning with a cold burner or oven. Never place cold cookware on a preheated burner or in a preheated oven.

Most people will tell you not to wash cast-iron cookware after each use. However, I prefer to wash the cooled cookware quickly (do not leave it to soak) with mild soapy water and a sponge similar to the type recommended for nonstick-coated cookware. Rinse and dry immediately with paper towel. To save on paper towel usage, I dry my cookware with a small old cloth that I use only for this purpose. I wash this cloth about every three months. Cast-iron cookware should not be washed in an automatic dishwasher.

When storing cast-iron cookware, always put it in a warm dry place with the lids off to prevent collection of moisture. The drawer under the oven on your electric range is excellent for storage of cast-iron cookware.

The control center of your life
is your attitude.

6. HELPFUL HINTS

General Helpful Hints

1. When making dietary changes in your life, do so gradually whenever possible to allow yourself time to adjust. As you are able, make changes in the following areas:
    - Eat organic foods. See Chapter 12—Organics—The Only Way to Go!
    - Drink some type of "purified" water or consider purchasing a home water-purification unit. See page 11 and Appendix C: Resources.
    - Can and freeze organic produce for use during seasons when it is not available. See section on Canning and Freezing in Chapter 12 starting on page 290.
    - Experiment with new foods and recipes. See Chapter 4—Specialty Foods.
    - Rotate foods. When beginning to rotate foods, start with an achievable level of commitment. Begin by rotating grains, then add meats, vegetables, fruits, and spices to your rotation as you are able. See Rule 6 (pages 32–33).

2. It is essential to make the dietary changes that are most important **immediately**. These changes include:
    - Avoid sugar, yeast, etc. in your diet. See listing of "Foods You Must Avoid" beginning on page 14.
    - Omit foods to which you are allergic.

3. Remember that it takes time to change your taste buds and food cravings. As you kill off the *Candida* yeast, your food cravings will decrease. Be patient with yourself.

4. Plan your meals ahead of time. Make a shopping list for the needed items and shop only from that list. Diverting from your shopping list without careful consideration (e.g., impulse buying) may cause you to divert from either the *Candida* control or the rotational diet. See Chapter 7—Meal Planning.

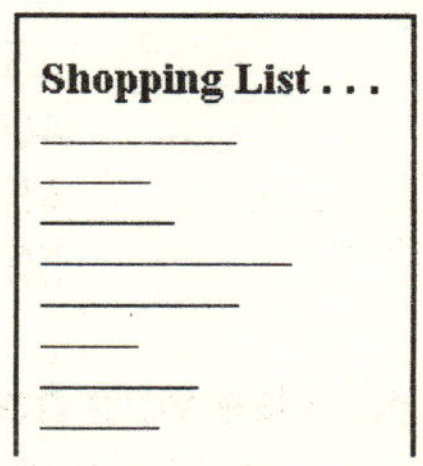

5. When incorporating organic fruits, vegetables, meats, grains, etc. into your diet, order these products by mail if they are not available in your area. See Appendix C: Resources.

6. Organize the food in your cabinets, shelves, refrigerator, and freezer according to days. You may wish to use different-colored tags or labels to color code foods for each day.

7. Organize your kitchen to make meal preparation easier and more efficient. Use as many of the following steps as you can in your kitchen.
    - Keep measuring and mixing equipment in the same cupboard.
    - Set up your food staples cupboard as close to your measuring and mixing cupboard as possible.
    - Arrange counter top space for food preparation steps. Have your measuring and mixing counter space near your measuring and mixing equipment cupboard. Set up a food cleaning and chopping area near the sink.
    - For storage of kitchen items that you use less frequently, use the higher cupboard shelves or hard-to-reach corners. Save the more accessible storage areas for the items you use most often.
    - Assign storage areas or counter top space for specific food and equipment items and always return the items to their assigned area.

- Store long-handled measuring spoons on hooks under the overhead cupboards near the mixing area. Use a separate hook for each spoon size.
- Keep hot pads or mitts and trivets for hot pans or dishes near the stove area.
- Store your serving and eating utensils near the table.

8. During meal preparation, clean up your kitchen and dishes throughout the preparation and cooking stages.

9. Read through each recipe before starting to prepare it. Make it a habit to check for the availability of necessary ingredients. Place them in your mixing area and, after you use each item, set it aside or put it away. Use a table knife or other straight edge to mark your place in the recipe. Following these tips will help you keep your place if you are interrupted.

10. In several recipes you are instructed to make a "well" in the center of the combined dry ingredients. To accomplish this, distribute the dry ingredients in the mixing bowl so there is an indentation (hole) in the center where the liquid ingredients will be poured.

11. When preparing a fraction of (1/2, 1/4) or multiplying (doubling, tripling) a recipe, I suggest you first calculate the measurements of ingredients needed. Write the amounts down in the margin of the cookbook or on a separate piece of paper.

12. The oven temperatures found in the recipes are given in degrees Fahrenheit (F.). At times you may find a recipe from another source which does not list a specific oven temperature but which instructs you to use a "slow" or other level of oven. The following chart gives the temperature ranges associated with these descriptions to aid you in adapting recipes.

Temperature	Descriptive Term
250° and 275° F.	very slow
300° and 325° F.	slow
350° and 375° F.	moderate
400° and 425° F.	hot
450° and 475° F.	very hot
500° and 525° F.	extremely hot

13. Use your freezer to your advantage. Fix double recipes and freeze the extra portions to use for "instant" meals later. Try to always keep one or two meals for each day in the freezer for those lazy-feeling days.

14. There are several ways to test the doneness of baked goods.
    - Insert a toothpick into the center of a baked good such as cake or muffins. The toothpick will come out clean when the baked good is done.
    - For a recipe such as Orange Buckwheat Cake, the cake is done when the center bounces back when lightly tapped.
    - For a recipe such as Soy Bread, the bread is done when it sounds hollow when lightly tapped on the surface.

15. Scrub the skins of all vegetables and fruits before peeling or cutting to avoid spreading the mold which may have accumulated on the surface during the growth or storage process.

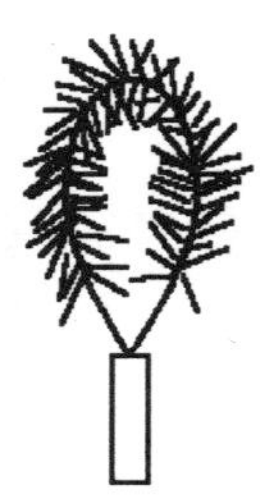

16. When a recipe calls for leeks or onions, chop or slice the complete vegetable and freeze the unused portion for later use when your time is limited. (No blanching required.)

17. Snip and measure parsley and other fresh herbs all in one step by clipping them with kitchen scissors over a clear liquid measure. This will allow you to cut up only the amount you need.

18. Save the cooking water from vegetables and meats to use as broth in future soups and casseroles. Freeze in amounts that you would most likely use in recipes.

19. Oils may be stored in the freezer in their original containers to extend their shelf life. This is especially helpful if you purchase a quantity of oils at one time. To use the oils, thaw and store in the refrigerator.

20. Oils that become thick at refrigerator temperatures, such as olive and sesame oil, are easier to measure if you store them in a wide-mouth jar. This enables you to measure the thicker consistence of these oils by spooning them out rather than warming to reliquify them and then pouring them out.

21. Store syrups (e.g., brown rice syrup and honey) at room temperature in a container with a tight-fitting lid. Wash the rim of the container after each use before replacing the lid.

22. When measuring syrups (e.g., brown rice syrup and honey), lightly coat the measuring utensil with oil first. This makes the removal of the syrup from the utensil much easier. If the recipe calls for oil, simply measure the oil before the syrup. If the recipe does not call for oil, use water on the measuring utensil. However, water does not work as well as oil.

23. For easier cleanup, use a dry cloth to wipe dough particles and flour off the rolling surface and rolling pin before wiping with a wet cloth.

24. If your hand temperature is normally warm, you may have difficulty with dough batters that require handling and/or rolling, e.g., tortillas, homemade noodles, biscuits, crackers. To solve this problem, you can cool your hand temperature by rinsing with cool water before handling batters that require hand manipulation and rolling. Also, you may find success using a rolling pin designed to be filled with cold water. The difficulty in handling batters with hands that are too warm is that the batter remains too sticky to work successfully no matter how much additional flour is added. Also, after adding too much flour, the dough and end product become tough.

25. Sometimes persons with *Candida* Related Complex will react to flours but have no problem eating the whole grain. There are two reasons for this reaction.
    - The oil in flour stored at room temperature starts to deteriorate and mold multiplies.
    - The surface dirt, mold, and pollens that are removed when washing the grain before cooking are not removed before the grain is ground into flour.

    Before you give up on flours and baked goods, try purchasing freshly ground flour and freeze it immediately. If this does not help, try grinding your own flour. Before grinding, sort through the grain to remove any debris and immature grains which otherwise would float to the top when washing the grain. Also, do what you can to remove dirt from the grain surface by shaking the grain in a mesh strainer or wiping it with a dry cloth.

26. Most *Candida* Related Complex sufferers are mold-sensitive and may not be able to tolerate supermarket nuts and seeds. I recommend organic nuts and seeds purchased directly from the grower, such as Jaffe Brothers (see Appendix C: Resources). After picking and shelling, the organic growers immediately freeze or refrigerate their nuts and seeds. By purchasing direct from organic growers, you omit various handling steps and time when the product is stored at room temperature. Therefore, you eliminate the steps where the original low mold count on the nuts and seeds begins to multiply.

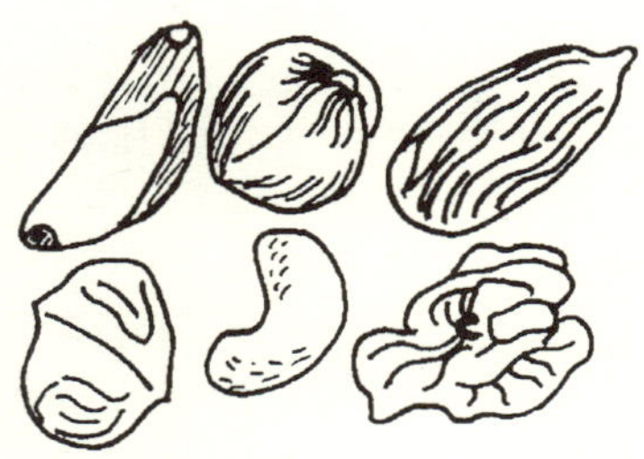

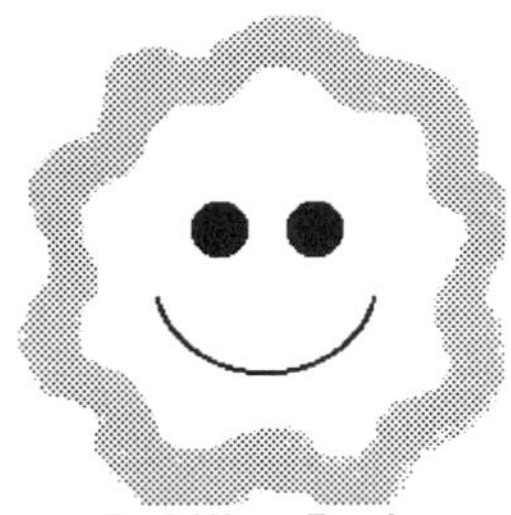

27. If you feel "stuck" on your limited diet, begin to change your attitude by focusing on what you **can** eat and enjoy. This will help you stay on your food allergy, *Candida* control, and/or rotational diet.
28. Remember, it is the *Candida* yeast that is controlling you and the feelings that you are experiencing. You need to change your attitude to "**I can beat this**!" Then **you** will be in control.
29. For additional helpful hints, read the section entitled "General Tips to Follow in the *Candida* Control Diet" found in Chapter 2 starting on page 15.

Helpful Hints on Accurate Measuring

I have found that the accurate measurement of ingredients is the best guarantee of success in baking, especially when using wheat-free, gluten-free flours and thickeners. In contrast, for some recipes amounts are given as a guide (e.g., casseroles, stir fries, salads, Millet Pudding). After preparing these recipes a couple of times, you can exercise your own creative cooking skills and use the "dump" or "sprinkle" method of measuring.

A. To measure dry ingredients such as flour, starch, etc. use a set of dry measuring cups (1 cup, 1/2 cup, 1/3 cup, 1/4 cup).
   1. Choose measuring cup appropriate to the amount you desire to measure.
   2. Fill cup a little over full with the dry ingredient, especially on the back side (side nearest the handle).
   3. Using a table knife held vertically, move the back side (straight edge) across the top of the measuring cup to level off the dry ingredient. Be sure to have some type of container underneath to catch the excess ingredient.

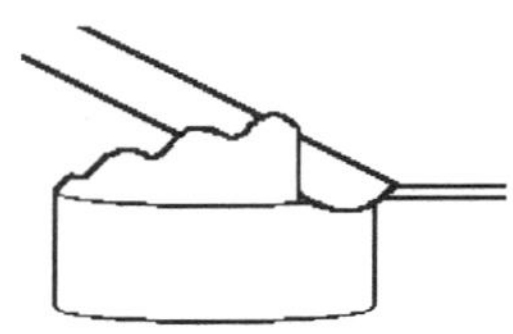

B. To measure small amounts of dry ingredients such as starch, leavening agents (e.g., vitamin C crystals, baking soda, baking powder), salt, seasonings, etc., use a set of measuring spoons (1 tablespoon, 1 teaspoon, 1/2 teaspoon, 1/4 teaspoon).
   1. Choose measuring spoon appropriate to the amount you desire to measure.
   2. Dip measuring spoon into dry ingredient until it is a little over full, especially on the back side (side nearest the handle).
   3. Using a table knife held vertically, move the back side (straight edge) across the top of the spoon to level off the dry ingredient. Be sure to have some type of container underneath to catch the excess ingredient.
   4. Special Note: Usually salt and seasonings do not need to be measured as accurately. You may just shake the spoon gently to level the ingredient.

C. To measure very small amounts (1/8, 1/16, 1/32 teaspoon) of a dry ingredient such as white powder stevia:
   1. Fill a 1/8 teaspoon measure with the stevia and level it off as described above.
   2. Using the tip of a very thin-bladed knife, divide the stevia in half. The stevia will hold its form well enough to then take the tip of the knife and push half of the 1/8 teaspoon (1/16 teaspoon) of the stevia out of the measuring spoon and into the bowl, etc.
   3. If you need to measure 1/32 teaspoon, divide the 1/16 amount in half and then only push off one fourth of the amount in the 1/8 teaspoon measure.
   4. Special Note: When you are first learning to measure in these very small amounts, you may wish to measure into a small separate container before adding the ingredient to your mixing bowl.

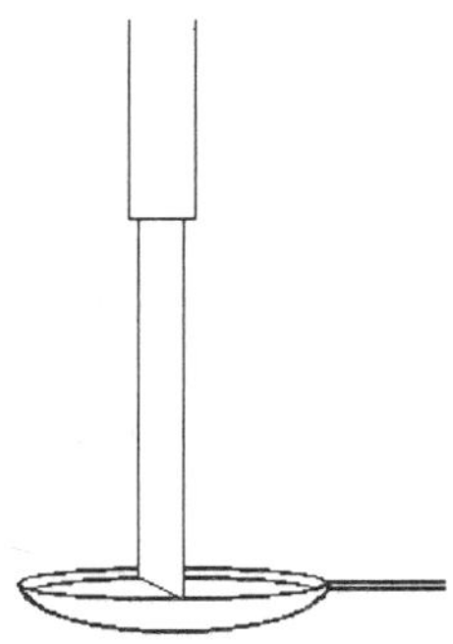

D. To measure very small amounts of a dry ingredient such as salt or seasonings, use the pinch method. A pinch is the amount that you can pinch between your index finger and thumb. My recipes are based on an approximate equivalent of 10 pinches of sea salt per 1/4 teaspoon.

E. To measure liquid ingredients such as water, juice, syrup, oil, etc., use a clear liquid measuring cup which has red painted lines to mark the fractional divisions of the measure.
   1. Place liquid measure on a level table or counter.
   2. Bend down so your eyes are level with the red lines on the measure.
   3. Liquids are measured at the bottom of the meniscus (ma-NIS-cus). The meniscus is the saucer-like depression which you see along the top edge of the liquid. Add the liquid gradually until the meniscus is lined up with the desired red mark on your liquid measuring cup.

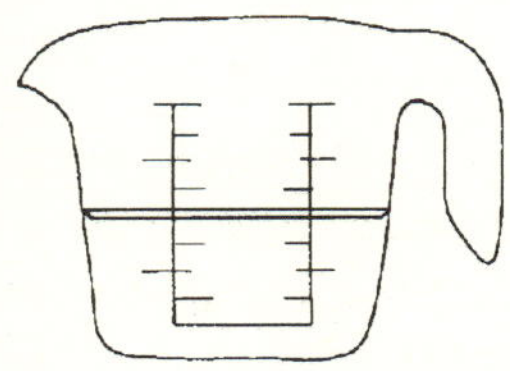

   4. Special Note: The difference in the amount of liquid measured at the top versus the bottom of the meniscus is only a small additional amount and does not make a significant difference in some recipes. However, in many wheat-free baked products the difference in the amount of liquid can cause doughy centers as well as other problems. This very simple measuring tip is easy to learn and can make all the difference in your success with these recipes.

F. To measure small amounts of liquid ingredients you may use measuring spoons, but be careful that your measured liquid does not "round up" on the spoon and add additional liquid.

<u>Measuring Equivalents</u>

Here are some simple fractional equivalents to assist you when you are measuring odd amounts (such as 3/8 teaspoon, 5/8 teaspoon, 7/8 cup, etc.) and preparing one-half or double a recipe:

1 gallon	=	4 quarts or 8 pints or 16 cups
1 quart	=	2 pints or 4 cups
1 pint	=	2 cups
1 cup	=	16 tablespoons
7/8 cup	=	14 tablespoons or 1 cup less 2 tablespoons
1/2 cup	=	8 tablespoons
1/3 cup	=	5 1/3 tablespoons or 5 tablespoons + 1 teaspoon
1/4 cup	=	4 tablespoons
1/8 cup	=	2 tablespoons
1 tablespoon	=	3 teaspoons
1/2 tablespoon	=	1 1/2 teaspoons
7/8 teaspoon	=	1/2 teaspoon + 1/4 teaspoon + 1/8 teaspoon
3/4 teaspoon	=	1/2 teaspoon + 1/4 teaspoon
5/8 teaspoon	=	1/2 teaspoon + 1/8 teaspoon
3/8 teaspoon	=	1/4 teaspoon + 1/8 teaspoon
1/8 teaspoon	=	one half of a 1/4 teaspoon
1/16 teaspoon	=	one half of a 1/8 teaspoon or one-fourth of a 1/4 teaspoon
1/32 teaspoon	=	one fourth of a 1/8 teaspoon

Measuring Abbreviations

To assure accurate interpretation of measurements, there are very few abbreviations used in this cookbook. For your reference, the following is a list of common abbreviations.

T. or Tbs. or Tbsp.	=	tablespoon
t. or tsp. or teas.	=	teaspoon
c. or C.	=	cup
pt.	=	pint
qt.	=	quart
gal.	=	gallon

Bean Cookery

Many people shy away from cooking beans, but they are one of the easiest foods to cook, especially when preparing them in the slow cooker. Yes, beans do take a long time to cook, either over low heat on the stove or cooking in a slow cooker. However, the actual preparation time that you spend with the beans is very, very low in comparison with many other foods you prepare.

Often I hear people mention that they experience intestinal gas after eating beans. For some time I experienced intestinal gas so severe that I believed I was allergic to beans, but no tests confirmed this. After experimentation and reading, I realized that I was not allergic to beans, but that I did need to cook them in a special way to help diminish the intestinal gas I was experiencing. Following are general rules of thumb for cooking beans, especially to diminish intestinal gas. Learning this simple method will help you add delicious variety to your diet.

- **Step 1**: Purchase beans that are not shriveled. Organic beans are handled less, so they may not be as clean as other beans. Beans are generally sorted by machine and occasionally you will find some shriveled ones as well as stones and dirt clods in your purchased beans. You can save time later if you sort through the beans and discard any shriveled beans, large stones, dirt clods, or other debris before storing them. Beans store well in a tightly covered glass jar in a cool dry place.
- **Step 2**: Measure beans according to recipe or amount you wish to cook.
- **Step 3**: Wash beans thoroughly. This removes surface mold, dirt, and other debris. Add enough water to cover beans and use a spoon or your hand to stir them around. If beans and debris float to the top, skim off and discard. Drain and discard water. Add fresh water and repeat procedure. Repeat two or three times until the rinse water is clear.
- **Step 4**: Place rinsed beans in a very large bowl or a very large measuring cup. For 2 cups of dried beans, I use an 8-cup measuring cup and fill it with water. Place container in refrigerator and allow beans to soak for 8–12 hours. Washing the beans and starting the soaking process can easily be accomplished in very little time while you are preparing your evening meal the night before you plan to cook the beans.
- **Step 5**: When you are ready to cook the beans, drain off the water. Again thoroughly rinse beans using a spoon or your hand to stir them around in the water to remove the filmy (starchy) substance that formed when the beans were soaked. Repeat two or three times until the rinsing water is clear.
- **Step 6**: Follow individual recipe directions regarding the required size of slow cooker, cooking temperature, amount of water, and seasonings. **NOTE: It is IMPORTANT that you do not add salt at this time.** If you wish, you may choose to wait until the beans are cooked to add the spices that are indicated in the recipe.

- **Step 7**: Cook beans until tender but not mushy. Three methods of testing for doneness are described by Marjorie Hurt Jones in the Mastering Food Allergies newsletter.[44] In all three methods the test beans should be discarded once the test is completed.
    1. Remove three or four beans on a spoon and blow on them. If the skins burst, the beans are done.
    2. Put a sample bean in your mouth and press it against the roof of your mouth. If you are able to break it up with your tongue without using your teeth, the beans are done.
    3. Bite into a bean. If it is tender without firm resistance, the beans are done.

    If the beans finish cooking ahead of the time you plan to serve them (e.g., an hour or so early), turn the slow cooker setting to low or off for a while and allow the beans to set. Turn the heat on near serving time to heat the beans back to serving temperature.

- **Step 8**: IMPORTANT! Add the salt listed in the recipe within the last ten or fifteen minutes of cooking. This is usually when I am doing the last minute meal preparations. Stir the salt into the amount of beans you feel you and/or your family will eat for this meal and allow them to simmer either in the slow cooker or on the stove until ready to serve.

    Since I usually cook double or triple batches of beans to freeze for quick and easy meals later, I don't add the salt to the leftover beans until I thaw and warm them for a later meal. If there are leftover salted beans, I freeze them and warm them up later for my family only. I have found that adding the salt during the last ten to fifteen minutes before serving and not eating leftover salted beans helps me avoid intestinal gas problems. This may help you also. Experiment with this procedure to see if it will aid you in incorporating beans into your diet.

Three other methods that can be used to help make beans tender and to aid in alleviating intestinal gas problems are:

1. Begin soaking the beans earlier in the day. After two hours, drain and rinse the beans and add new soaking water. Repeat the procedure every two hours or so throughout the day.
2. Add kombu to the beans while they are cooking.
3. Start cooking the beans by simmering on the stove top for 30 minutes with no seasonings added. Drain water from beans, rinse thoroughly, and transfer to slow cooker with appropriate water and seasonings for remaining cooking time.

You may wish to try these additional methods as you learn to cook beans. Experiment with the different cooking procedures to learn which works best for you.

If you soak too many beans, you may drain and freeze them in a cellophane or plastic bag. To cook, simply pull them from the freezer and cook as directed.

If you forget to presoak your beans, you may use the following procedure:

- Place beans in a large saucepan, Dutch oven, or large kettle. Cover with water.
- Bring to a boil on the stove top and boil for approximately two minutes.
- Remove pan from heat, cover, and let stand for one hour.
- Drain water and thoroughly rinse beans.

The beans are now ready to continue with the normal cooking steps.

You will notice that my recipes for lentils and split peas call for presoaking them. While these two legumes do not need to be presoaked before cooking as beans do, I follow this procedure to aid in eliminating intestinal gas problems.

---

[44] Marjorie Hurt Jones. "Bean Cookery," Mastering Food Allergies (Vol. IV, No. 3, issue 33 [March 1989]), 1.

For those who do not wish to use a slow cooker to prepare beans but prefer the stove top, use the following method.

1. Place soaked, rinsed, and drained beans in a large kettle or Dutch oven.
2. Cover with approximately three to four inches of water.
3. Bring to a boil, reduce heat, and simmer for appropriate time according to the following chart.

Bean Cookery Chart

Type of Legume	Simmering Time
Anasazi Beans	1 1/2 – 2 1/2 hours
Adzuki Beans	1 1/2 – 2 1/2 hours
Black Turtle Beans	1 1/2 – 3 hours
Black-eyed Peas	1 – 1 1/2 hours
Garbanzo Beans (Chickpeas)	2 – 3 hours
Kidney Beans	2 – 3 hours
Lentils, Green	1 – 2 hours
Lentils, Red (do not soak)	25 minutes
Lima Beans	45 minutes – 1 1/2 hours
Mung Beans	2 – 3 hours
Navy Beans	2 – 3 hours
Northern Beans	2 – 3 hours
Pinto Beans	1 1/2 – 2 hours
Soybeans	2 1/2 – 3 hours
Split Peas	1 – 2 hours

Many factors affect the cooking time of beans. These factors include the variety, maturity, age, and moisture content of the beans as well as altitude. Even the kind of water you use can affect the cooking time (e.g., beans take longer to cook when hard water is used).

Leavening Agents

A leavening agent consists of an acid and an alkaline substance. It is the reaction between these two substances which causes the food to "raise."

Most people are familiar with baking powder. Often the ingredients of a nonalum baking powder are calcium acid phosphate, baking soda, and corn starch. Another type of baking powder is Featherweight brand whose ingredients are potato starch, calcium phosphate, and potassium bicarbonate. When using Featherweight brand baking powder, substitute 1 1/2 teaspoons for 1 teaspoon of regular baking powder.

You can also make your own baking powder by using:

1 teaspoon of baking soda
2 teaspoons of some type of starch or flour
2 teaspoons of cream of tartar

Mix the three ingredients together and store in an air-tight container. It can be used like regular baking powder at an approximate ratio of 1 1/2 to 1 3/4 teaspoons of the homemade to replace 1 teaspoon of regular baking powder.

Baking powder contains both parts of the leavening agent—the acid and the alkaline. However, for many people with allergies using regular baking powder (especially on a daily basis) is a problem because of an allergy to corn. The Featherweight brand of baking powder, which has a potato starch base, may cause a problem for persons who are allergic to the Nightshade Family (number 74). Homemade baking powder may be a problem for persons with CRC because cream of tartar is made from the fermented residue in wine barrels.

Another available leavening agent is unbuffered, corn-free vitamin C crystals combined with baking soda. You will find that almost all of the bakery product recipes in this cookbook that need a leavening agent use this combination. If you would like to convert some of your recipes from baking powder to use the vitamin C crystals and baking soda, the formula to start with is:

1/4 teaspoon of vitamin C crystals	+	1 teaspoon of baking soda	=	1 1/2 to 2 teaspoons of regular baking powder

Since most of my baked goods recipes call for vitamin C crystals and baking soda, this is one combination of ingredients that I do not rotate. If you have reaction problems when using vitamin C crystals, you may need to research the source used to make the brand you are using. You may wish to locate different brands that use different sources and rotate them or use other leavening agents instead. At publication date, very little testing has been done toward using other leavening agents in these recipes. If you need to use something other than vitamin C crystals, I highly recommend that you purchase the back issue of Mastering Food Allergies newsletter where Marjorie Hurt Jones discusses leavening agents and the different acid and alkaline substitutes (Volume VII, No. 2, Issue 62, February 1992). See the Newsletters section of Appendix D: Recommended Reading for her address to order this back issue.

Preparation of Muffin Pans, Baking Dishes/Sheets, and Loaf Pans for Baking

Use the same kind of oil that is used in the recipe. Use the amount of oil that the recipe directs for oiling the pan. If the recipe does not give a specific amount, begin with 1/4 teaspoon of oil and add more only if needed. Follow recipe instructions for oiling the pan. (Some recipes, such as crackers and pizza crust, emphasize spreading the oil with your fingertips so that your fingers become lightly coated with oil, which aids in spreading the dough.) If the recipe does not give specific instructions, follow the procedure below.

- Use 1/4 teaspoon of oil for 12 muffin cups.
- Drop a very small amount of oil into each muffin cup. If you run out of oil before adding it to all 12 cups, do not add more oil until after completing the next step.
- Take a 2-inch square of cellophane (cut several at a time to have handy to use) and spread the oil around in each cup, making sure to completely coat the bottom and sides with oil. Extra oil may remain on your cellophane square and it may be used to coat any muffin cups that did not have oil placed in them.
- Add more oil if needed to coat each cup.
- If the recipe calls for the muffin pan to be floured, immediately sprinkle each cup with a small amount of the flour. Again use the same flour as used in the recipe.
- Immediately, shake the muffin pan quickly from side to side and front to back to spread the flour at least around the bottom. The amount of flour needed varies depending on the kind of flour used, but I usually use 1 teaspoon per 6 muffin cups.
- Add more flour if needed.
- Remove excess flour, if any, by turning the oiled and floured muffin pan upside down over the sink and gently tapping on the bottom.

Use this same principle with baking dishes except that you dribble the 1/4 teaspoon of oil around in the pan before spreading with a cellophane square.

Food Storage Wraps

It is best to avoid using wax paper because it may be dusted with a corn product. This may be a problem for the corn-sensitive person. Likewise, you should avoid using plastic wrap or bags since they are made from petroleum and may be a problem for the chemically sensitive person. In addition, a chemically sensitive person should not use aluminum. Use cellophane instead. Cellophane can be purchased on a roll similar to wax paper or in bag form. Use scissors to cut the cellophane roll. The plant fiber bags come in various sizes as well as in pleated and flat styles. They may be purchased at your health-food store, through a food-buying cooperative or mail-order source, or directly from a supplier such as Pak Sel (see Appendix C: Resources).

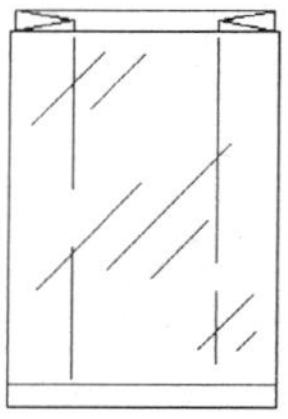

Cellophane rips very easily, so handle it with care. The bags also deteriorate over time so do not purchase too large a supply at one time. When I use a cellophane bag to freeze fruits or vegetables for use during winter months, I place a self-adhesive label on it and then place another slightly larger bag over it. During the off season when I use the frozen product, I do not throw away the outside bag if it is in good condition. I keep it in the freezer for use in freezing something else before I dispose of it. Once you have kept a cellophane bag in the refrigerator or freezer, you must keep it at that temperature if you wish to save it for possible future reuse.

Substitutes

Substitutes for Wheat Flour in Baking and Thickening

Various cookbooks that I have read have different lists of flour and thickener substitutes. The following is a compilation of the options listed in several of them. This list helped me convert some recipes. However, you should be aware that often I was also substituting many other ingredients (e.g., sugar, egg, baking powder, yeast, etc.). When converting recipes there is often a need for lots of testing and retesting to get a quality product. I have included this listing so if you desire you can substitute different flours and thickeners in your favorite recipes.

Substitute for 1 Cup Wheat Flour in Baking

Amount	Substitute
1 cup	amaranth flour with the addition of a starch
1/2 cup	barley flour
3/4 cup	brown rice flour plus 1/4 cup sweet rice flour
1 cup	buckwheat flour
3/4 cup	garbanzo bean (chickpea) or other bean flours
1 cup	millet flour
1 1/3 cups	oat flour
1 cup	quinoa flour with the addition of a starch
7/8 cup	rice flour
1 1/4 cups	rye flour

Substitute for 1 Cup of Whole-wheat Flour in Baking

1 cup	Kamut® flour
1 cup	Spelt flour—however, reduce the amount of liquid by 25%.

Substitute for 2 Tablespoons of Wheat Flour for Thickening:

Amount	Substitute
1 tablespoon	arrowroot starch
1 tablespoon	bean flour
1 tablespoon	cornstarch
1 teaspoon	guar gum
1 tablespoon	kudzu
1 tablespoon	nut flour
1 tablespoon	potato starch
1 tablespoon	rice flour
1 tablespoon	tapioca starch flour

For thickening, use a whisk to dissolve the substitute starch or flour in cool or room temperature liquid (not hot) before adding to hot food. The above measurements are the amounts required to thicken 1 cup of liquid for sauces. Double the listed amount when using these substitutes to thicken puddings.

Cook as little as possible to thicken food. Prolonged cooking of starches tends to break them down and the mixture looses the thickening effect and sometimes becomes watery. When this happens you may need to add more thickener.

Egg Substitutes

You will notice that most of my recipes do not call for eggs. They are designed without eggs or have an egg substitute alternative for you to use.

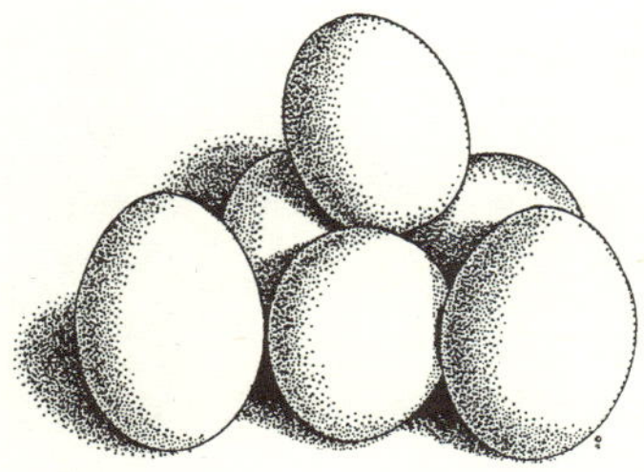

Eggs are needed in recipes for three main reasons:

- flavor
- binding quality
- raising quality

It seems like each cookbook I read has a different list of egg substitutes. This section includes a compilation of the options listed in several cookbooks. You will find some of these substitutes used in this cookbook. However, I have used the flaxseed substitute most often.

Some of these substitutes are more useful for their binding property, others for their raising property, and some work well in both areas. I have included this listing so you can experiment with other egg substitutes if needed.

Due to different likes, dislikes, or food allergies, you may find these substitutes helpful in adjusting your current favorite recipes or modifying some of the recipes in this cookbook.

To Replace 1 egg in a recipe use:

- 1 tablespoon ground flaxseed or flax meal mixed with 3 tablespoons of water. Dissolve and mix with recipe. Good for leavening.
- 1 tablespoon ground flaxseed combined with 1/4 cup water in a saucepan. While stirring constantly, bring to boil on high, then cook on medium-high for 1–2 minutes until thickened to the consistency of egg white. Good as a binder and for leavening.
- 1 tablespoon psyllium seed husk mixed with 3 tablespoons of water. Let it stand briefly before adding to recipe. Good as a binder.
- 1 tablespoon tahini with 3 tablespoons of water.
- 2 tablespoons arrowroot starch with 2 tablespoons water. Good for dipping food product in before breading. Should be able to replace the arrowroot with other starches and flours (e.g., tapioca starch, potato starch, soy flour, and other bean flours).

- 1 tablespoon lecithin granules with 3 tablespoons water.
- 1/4 cup tofu. Good as a binder.
- 1 tablespoon garbanzo bean flour with 1 tablespoon oil.
- 3 tablespoons thick pureed fruit.
- Ener-G Egg Replacer by Ener-G Foods (see Appendix C: Resources). For best results, mix the powder with the recommended amount of liquid and let it stand 10 minutes before adding it to the recipe. Ener-G Egg Replacer contains potato starch, tapioca flour, leavening (calcium lactate, calcium carbonate, citric acid), and carbohydrate gum.
- 2 teaspoons baking powder* mixed with 2 tablespoons water. For a second egg in the recipe add only an additional 1 teaspoon baking powder* and 2 tablespoons water.
- 1/2 teaspoon baking powder*, 2 tablespoons flour, and 1 1/2 teaspoons oil.
- 2 tablespoons water, 1 tablespoon oil, and 2 tablespoons baking powder*.
- 2 tablespoons apricot mixture (see recipe below). I do not recommend this for persons with *Candida* Related Complex (CRC). However, the idea and recipe are from Sally Rockwell's book Coping with *Candida* Cookbook.
- 1 teaspoon plain unflavored gelatin dissolved with 3 tablespoons water. Place in freezer. Take out when thickened and beat until frothy. Good as a binder.

To Replace 1 egg white in a recipe:

- 1 tablespoon plain unflavored gelatin dissolved in 1 tablespoon water. Whip. Chill and whip again.

Apricot Mixture for Egg Replacer

Measure 1 cup of dried apricots into a bowl. Cover with boiling water and let stand until fruit is soft. Puree in blender or food processor. Cover and store in refrigerator.

Milk Substitutes

Often persons with *Candida* Related Complex (CRC) need to omit dairy milk from their diet. This not only presents a problem in having a beverage, but creates a dilemma when preparing milk-based soups and casseroles and in making some baked products.

- For a beverage use:
  - ◊ some type of "purified" water
  - ◊ mineral water
  - ◊ carbonated water
  - ◊ Pau D'Arco tea
  - ◊ Dacopa (beverage from dahlia tubers)

- For a milk substitute in baking use:
  - ◊ an equal amount of water for the required amount of milk or buttermilk. If you are substituting water in a pancake recipe, start by using a direct substitution amount. Cook one pancake to test for raising properties and make any adjustments needed in the remaining batter—add more water to thin the batter or add more flour to thicken the batter to increase the raising properties of the pancakes.
  - ◊ an equal amount of fruit juice for the required amount of milk. This works especially well if you need a sweeter flavor for the recipe you are preparing—such as in Kamut® or Spelt Muffins, Oat Bran Muffins, and Orange Buckwheat Cake.

---

* Remember that regular baking powder contains corn so avoid these substitutes if sensitive to corn or following a rotation.

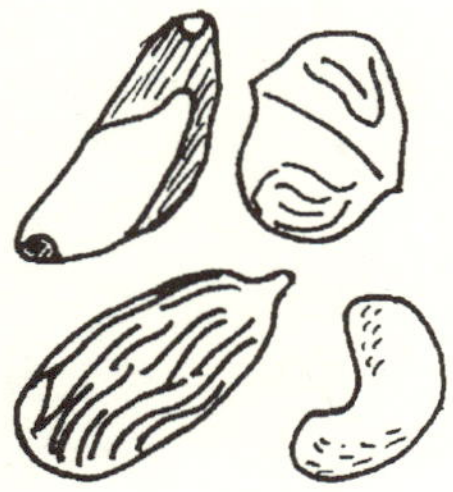

- For hot or cold breakfast cereals, you can use a variety of nut milks, such as:
    - ◊ Almond Milk in Day 1 cereals
    - ◊ Brazil Nut Milk in Day 2 Amaranth Cereals
    - ◊ Macadamia Nut or Cashew Milk in Day 4 Cream of Buckwheat Cereal

  These nut milks can be prepared ahead of time, frozen in ice cube trays, stored frozen in cellophane bags, and thawed in the amounts needed. This process will make using them for your breakfast cereals much easier.

- For soups, you can use the following nut milks as substitutes.
    - ◊ Brazil Nut Milk
    - ◊ Cashew Milk
    - ◊ Macadamia Nut Milk

  I do not recommend using Almond Milk. My experience with using Almond Milk to make soups has resulted in soups that are not very tasty.

- For creamy-based casseroles such as Chicken or Tuna Rice Casserole or Chicken or Tuna Noodle Casserole, use sesame milk.

- For custards and puddings, use almond, Brazil nut, or macadamia nut milk.

Most of the recipes in this cookbook have the milk substitute proportions incorporated into the ingredients and preparation steps so you do not need to make the nut milk separately ahead of time.

If you are experimenting with your own favorite recipes and need a milk substitute, use:

1/4 cup of chopped almonds, Brazil nuts, cashews, or macadamia nuts
1 cup of water

These amounts will yield slightly more than one cup of nut milk. For a description of an easy blender method to make nut milk, see the recipes for Almond Milk on Day 1, Brazil or Macadamia Nut Milk on Day 2, or Cashew Milk on Day 4.

To make sesame milk, use the following ingredient amounts and use the same blender preparation method as for the nut milks.

2 tablespoons hulled sesame seeds
1 cup water

Prepared soy milks in dry powder and liquid form are commercially available, but may not be a good choice for persons with food allergies or CRC. Soy is a common food allergen and may need to be avoided by persons with food allergies. Also, the dry powder form of soy milk is often not organic and the prepared liquid soy milks have other ingredients in them—such as whey and barley malt—which should be avoided by persons with CRC.

For more information on milk substitutes, I highly recommend that you acquire a copy of issue #53 of Mastering Food Allergies newsletter by Marjorie Hurt Jones (Vol. VI, No. 3, March 1991) which contains an article entitled "Alternatives to Milk." The address for ordering this back issue can be found in the Newsletters section of Appendix D: Recommended Reading.

Sugar Substitutes

Below is a list of sugar substitutes gathered from natural cooking sources.

- Substitute 3/4 cup of honey or rice syrup for 1 cup sugar, then reduce the liquid by 1/8 to 1/4 cup.
- Substitute 1 cup fruit juice for 1 cup of sugar and 1 cup of liquid.

- Omit sugar and substitute 1/4 teaspoon of stevia (white powder concentrate) per 1 1/2 cups of flour listed in the recipe.
- Omit the listed measurement of sugar and substitute with double the amount of FOS. Liquid may need to be adjusted (lowered) since FOS causes baking doughs to become sticky.

Since my taste buds are reeducated and my sweet tooth is now much lower, I reduce the amount of sweetener called for in regular recipes. If you have omitted sweeteners from your diet for a period of time, you may be able to do the same.

When working with recipes that call for honey, you can reduce the amount of honey and sweetness by using the following substitute.

- Replace 1/4 cup honey with a scant 3 tablespoons of water.

More Helpful Hints

Use the remainder of this page and the last page of this chapter to add more helpful hints as you learn them. If you discover any that are especially useful, and would like to share them with others, see Appendix G: Canary Connect for information on how to submit them to the Canary Connect News newsletter.

Helpful Hints on Tortilla Preparation

A. Assemble Needed Equipment: Before you begin tortilla preparation, assemble needed equipment in each work area. Here is a list of the four preparation areas and the equipment needed for each:

1. Equipment needed in the mixing area:
   - ◊ medium-size, curved-sided bowl
   - ◊ another small bowl
   - ◊ set of dry measuring cups & spoons
   - ◊ clear 1-cup liquid measure
   - ◊ whisk
   - ◊ table fork & knife
   - ◊ rubber spatula
   - ◊ recipe
   - ◊ ingredients

2. It is preferable that the rolling area be located within inches of the cooking area (see number 3 under Tips on Cooking Tortillas if this is not possible in your kitchen). Equipment needed in the kneading and rolling area:
   - ◊ clean rolling surface*
   - ◊ rolling pin
   - ◊ table knife
   - ◊ additional flour
   - ◊ pastry brush
   - ◊ solid metal spatula (a slotted spatula can tear the dough)

3. Equipment needed in the cooking area:
   - ◊ preheated, nonstick, unoiled griddle or skillet. I prefer a well-seasoned cast-iron griddle.
   - ◊ an electric range with a heat setting between low and medium
   - ◊ another metal spatula (slotted or solid)
   - ◊ timer that can measure time in seconds. A touch pad timer on a microwave oven will work, but a digital timer that has a memory feature is best when making tortillas.

4. Equipment needed in the cooling area located near the cooking area:
   - ◊ cooling rack
   - ◊ clean cotton muslin towel (at least 16 by 22 inches, folded in half so you can place tortillas between the layers to finish cooling) placed on a second cooling rack
   - ◊ large flat cellophane bags for storage

*Suggested rolling surfaces are:
   - ◊ clean, smooth kitchen counter (my preference)
   - ◊ smooth-surfaced, tempered-glass cutting board. The pebble-like acrylic cutting boards are not smooth enough to use to roll out tortillas.
   - ◊ clean, smooth, wooden bread board. If you choose the wooden bread board, be sure this board does not have any knife cuts on it and you have not used it to cut meat. A wooden bread board is the worst sanitation problem you may have in your family kitchen.
   - ◊ cotton muslin rolling cloth may be acceptable

B. Tips on Tortilla Preparation During Mixing:

1. Measure ingredients accurately. Until you become familiar with the proper feel of the dough, accurate measuring is your best guarantee of success.
2. I start with less flour than needed for some flavors of tortillas because the initial mixing of dry and wet ingredients is easier if you start with less and then add extra flour. Also, fewer crumbs of dough particles form.
3. After you have some experience with tortilla preparation, you may desire to double the basic recipe. When I do this, I divide the dough in half before I begin kneading.

C. Tips on Tortilla Preparation During Kneading:

1. Have rolling surface floured before you begin kneading and keep surface well floured during the entire process. See each recipe for amount of flour to start.
2. If you have warm hands you may want to run them under cold water before you begin the kneading. Hands that are too warm can cause the dough to become sticky and difficult to handle.
3. The purpose of kneading is to work additional flour into the dough to make it easier to roll. You may use any kneading method you wish.
4. Keep your hands well floured. You may sometimes need to clean off your hands. Use the back of a table knife to remove most of the dough residue.
5. Before you begin the rolling process, cut dough into equal portions amounting to the number of tortillas the recipe has been developed to yield.
6. Scrape rolling area with metal spatula to remove remaining dough particles (these particles tend to "mess things up" during rolling). Also, wash your hands. Again, if you have warm hands, you may want to run them under cold water before you begin to roll out the tortillas.

D. Tips on Rolling Out Tortillas:

1. Roll each tortilla separately.
2. Start each tortilla with a floured rolling surface. Each recipe tells you how much flour to use.
3. My preference is to pat out each dough portion as much as possible, but you only need to pat it evenly flat. If dough is still sticking a lot to the rolling surface as you pat it out, you may need to knead more flour into each dough portion. Then continue with the process.
4. Be sure both sides of dough are well floured before you begin rolling.
5. With a floured rolling pin, roll from the center out in all directions until dough is evenly thin and has the diameter suggested by the recipe. However, you may have more success with only a 6-inch tortilla when you are first learning. Try to keep the tortilla circular, but do not concern yourself if it is not perfect.

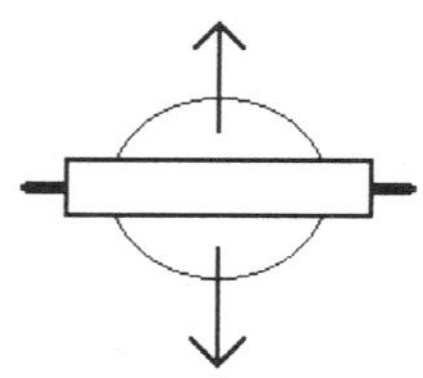

6. Keep dough well floured on both sides. When the underneath side is sticking, flip the dough to flour. Before you flip, use the metal spatula to loosen the edges and center of the tortilla from the rolling surface. To flip, place spatula under the center of the tortilla and your hand on top to support it. During this process, mend any cracked dough edges as they appear. Tiny cracks will become large ones if left unrepaired.

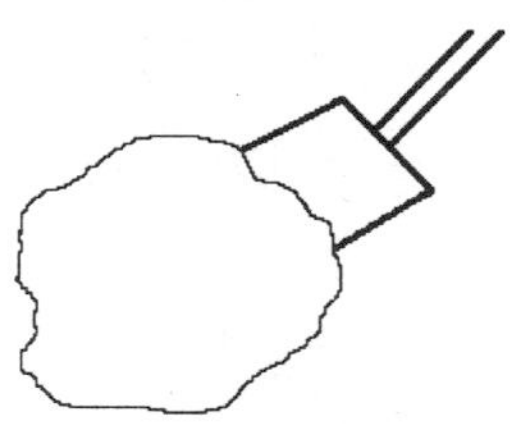

7. Before cooking the tortilla, gently brush excess flour from the top of the dough using a pastry brush or your hand. Flip tortilla. If there are moist areas on the dough surface, sprinkle some flour on the surface (if areas are too moist, they will burn when cooking) and then brush excess flour away. I prefer to use a pastry brush rather than my hand because the brush is gentler and does a better job. If you do damage any edges, mend them before cooking.

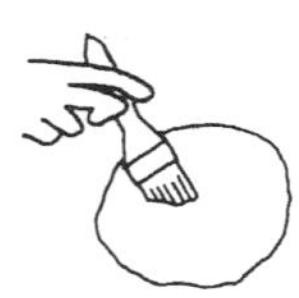

8. I always brush away the excess flour from the tortilla surface because I do not like the taste of the dry toasted flour on the surface of the cooked tortilla. Also, the excess flour will build up on the griddle, burn, and cause an unpleasant taste and smell.
9. Since spelt and Kamut® flour contain gluten, these tortillas are more durable than other tortillas. You may remove the excess flour by gently flipping the tortilla from hand to hand as stated in these recipes.
10. Before you begin to roll out your next tortilla, clean the flour off the rolling surface with the metal spatula. This excess flour usually does not work well to start another tortilla but can be used to flour moist areas on the tortilla surface during the rolling process. This means it is best to start each tortilla with a clean surface and a small amount of fresh flour (refer to each recipe for this amount).
11. There are slight differences in rolling out tortillas for the different flours (see individual recipes for details).
12. After you make a few tortillas you will need to clean off the build-up of raw dough on the spatula.

E. Tips on Cooking Tortillas:

1. Be sure your griddle or skillet is unoiled and preheated hot enough that water dances when sprinkled on the surface.
2. Transfer tortilla carefully to the griddle by first lifting the left side of the tortilla with metal spatula (see Diagram A). Then replace the spatula with your left hand (see Diagram B). Next place the spatula under the right side of the tortilla (see Diagram C). This will give adequate support as you use your hand and the spatula to lift the tortilla over and gently drop it onto the griddle (see Diagram D). These directions are for a right-handed person. A left-handed person would do just the opposite.

Diagram A *Diagram B*

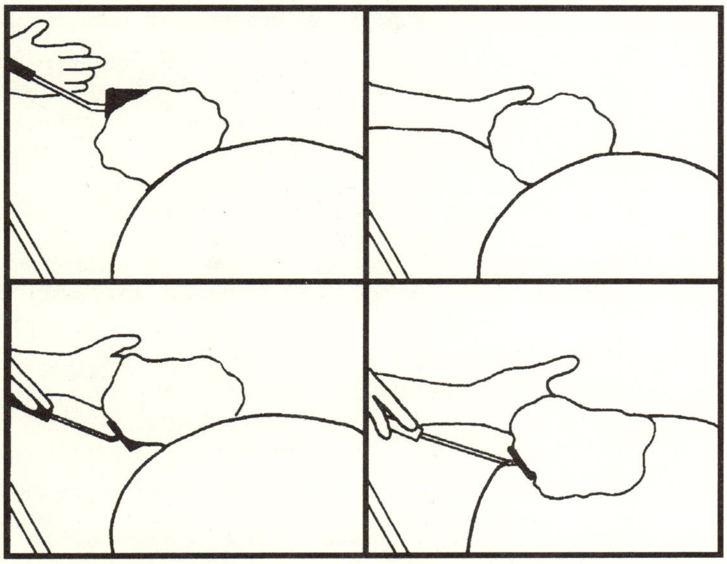

Diagram C *Diagram D*

3. Follow these directions if your kitchen does not allow your rolling area to be only inches away from the range. First, place a protective pad that is able to withstand the heat of the griddle on the counter surface near where you are rolling out your tortillas. I prefer a small metal cooling rack. When each tortilla is ready to cook, place the hot griddle on the protective pad, gently transfer the tortilla as described above, and immediately return the griddle to the range.

4. For timing during cooking, use a digital timer which measures in seconds and has a memory feature. This memory feature is great for making tortillas because you set the timer for 45 seconds, start it timing immediately after placing the tortilla on the griddle, then continue to roll out your next tortilla. When the timer tells you the time is up, you flip your tortilla over, stop the timer, and then restart it for another 45 seconds that the timer has automatically reset for you. When you are cooking something as delicate as tortillas for only 40–45 seconds per side and you have to take time to reprogram the timer, your tortilla is cooking an additional 5–10 seconds while you are fumbling to quickly reset it. Being hurried like this can cause mistakes and can lead to problems with the food you are preparing.

5. Cook first side of tortilla for 45 seconds, flip tortilla with cooking spatula, and cook the second side for 45 seconds. Occasionally the first side will feel a little moist and you may want to flip it back to the first side for 5 seconds or less. (Also, I personally feel that buckwheat tortillas are best when cooked for only 40 seconds on each side.)

6. There are slight differences in the way tortillas cook for the different flours (see individual recipes for details).

7 After you cook 2–4 tortillas you will need to clean off the build-up of browned flour from the spatula.

F. Tips on Cooling Tortillas:

1. With spatula, transfer the cooked tortilla to a cooling rack for 1–2 minutes. After this cooling time, the tortilla will not be completely cool, but it is easily cool enough to use your hand and transfer it to between the layers of cloth on the second cooling rack. I like this method of cooling the best because the tortillas can finish cooling without becoming dry. Also, notice how durable yet pliable the tortilla is after cooling.

2. Occasionally, if you cook the tortilla too long on the griddle, it may help to cool it completely between layers of the cotton cloth.

3. If you allow a tortilla to cool too long and become dry, follow these directions. First, transfer the dry tortilla between the layers of cloth. Then, place the next cooked tortilla directly on the top of the dry tortilla without allowing it to cool on cooling rack. This will help the dry tortilla to regain a little moisture.

G. Additional Tips on Tortilla Preparation:

1. After becoming experienced with tortilla preparation, you can dovetail your work. First, begin the rolling process of your next tortilla while one tortilla is cooking and another one is cooling.

2. When you get to this stage of success, set your timer for only 40 seconds. This will allow you 5 seconds to stop what you are doing, brush the flour off your hands, and get to the range to attend to the cooking tortilla.

3. For the dovetail process, while the first side of a tortilla is cooking, scrape and add flour to the rolling surface. Then pat out the next tortilla and start the rolling. After turning the tortilla that is cooking, put the tortilla that has been cooling between the layers of cotton cloth and return to the rolling process of the next tortilla. After the second side has cooked, transfer the cooked tortilla to the cooling rack. The griddle is now empty, but leave it on the range to stay hot because it will only take about one minute or so to finish the rolling process. Continue this process to prepare all the tortillas.

4. As you become more experienced you can learn a faster way to roll out the tortilla while keeping it well floured. Using the principle of rolling from the center out, keep your rolling pin moving by rolling back and forth. However, put the most pressure on the dough when you are rolling from the center to the outside. Also, you may lift the rolling pin off the dough frequently to use your other hand to twist the dough on the rolling surface. This way you know immediately if the underneath surface of the tortilla needs more flour.

5. For best results, do not make tortillas on days when you have a high humidity level in your kitchen. The dough will tend to be sticky and you may have to add too much flour to make it workable, which can result in tough tortillas.

H. Tips on Preparing Multiple Batches of Tortillas:

1. When you have some experience with tortilla preparation you may desire to prepare a double batch at one time. When doubling each recipe, you will have more success if you divide the dough in half in the mixing bowl just before you knead it.

2. Tortilla preparation takes time just to set and clean up the kitchen. So you may desire to prepare 4–8 tortillas of each desired flavor at one time. If you do this, I suggest that you remove the accumulated flour from the griddle surface after preparing 4 tortillas. Just hold the hot griddle over the sink and quickly brush off with a dry cloth.

3. Thoroughly clean the rolling surface between each flavor of tortillas. First, clean off flour with a dry cloth, then use a wet cloth to clean.

I. Tips on Storing, Freezing, Reheating, and Serving Tortillas:

1. Prepare tortillas when you have time and energy so you will have them available for a quick meal. A meal away from home is very easy to pack when you have tortillas available in the freezer.

2. **To store**, place the tortillas in a flat cellophane bag—one flavor per bag and usually no more than eight per bag. Use a self-adhesive label to mark the flavor. Then seal the bags in a square Tupperware container with a cover and place in freezer. If you desire, you may seal each cellophane bag in a sealable plastic bag instead of a Tupperware container. Also, you may place the tortillas directly in a plastic bag, but this is not my preference. Whatever you choose, store them flat in the freezer and in a safe place where other foods will not damage them.

3. **To thaw and/or reheat** tortillas as needed, begin by transferring the desired amount from the bag of frozen tortillas to another cellophane bag. Next, allow them to thaw:
   - at room temperature for approximately 30 minutes.
   - in microwave for 5–10 seconds.
   - on a splatter screen over top of a pan of steaming water for approximately 10–20 seconds.
   - in refrigerator for a few hours.

   Whatever way you choose, they will dry out if allowed to thaw outside a cellophane or plastic bag.

4. **To serve tortillas** as a deli sandwich, you may serve them whole folded over the ingredients or cut them in half easily with a pair of scissors. Buckwheat and Teff Tortillas sometimes crack when folded so I usually cut them in half and layer the goodies between the tortilla halves. Be creative with your sandwiches by using various fillings and combinations.
   - Meats: grilled chicken breast or leftover roast chicken, beef, turkey, venison, or pork.
   - Spreads: Almond, Sunflower, Filbert, Macadamia Nut, or Cashew "Mayo."
   - Greens: Swiss chard, lettuce, spinach, or garden sorrel.
   - Vegetables: shredded carrots and/or sliced celery, zucchini, or cucumber.
   - BLTs: bacon (fresh side meat), lettuce, tomato, and "Mayo."
   - PBJs: nut butter (almond, cashew, etc.) and 100% fruit sweetened jelly.
   - Sandwich Salads: tuna, salmon, egg, or shrimp salad.
   - Tortillas make great sandwiches for meals eaten away from home. When you do this, pack your tortillas separate from your fillings so the tortillas do not get moisture from the fillings and fall apart when you pick them up to eat.
   - Serve tortillas as hot dishes such as tacos, enchiladas, burritos, and various fajitas.

   Whatever filling you choose and however you serve them, tortillas are a special addition to any meal, especially for those who cannot tolerate yeasted breads. Simply fill, fold, and enjoy.

Special Note: If you are taking tortillas with you for a traveling meal and you are in a dry climate (e.g., Colorado, Arizona, etc.), you can help prevent them from drying out by placing your cellophane-wrapped tortillas in a resealable plastic bag.

Hopefully, between reading the individual tortilla recipes and these "Helpful Hints on Tortilla Preparation," you will have success in no time. If you need extra help, you may wish to purchase my forthcoming cooking video "Tortillas and More." (See Appendix G for more information.)

7. MEAL PLANNING

If you have read How to Use This Book and chapters 1–6 prior to beginning this chapter, you will have a good knowledge base for understanding the information included in this chapter on Meal Planning. If you have not read all of the preceding chapters, I do suggest that you at least read How to Use This Book, Chapter 5—Basic Equipment, and Chapter 6—Helpful Hints.

Basic Equipment outlines the equipment that I feel an efficient kitchen needs to make food and meal preparation easier and faster. If you do not have the advantage of being able to use commercially prepared food products, at least having the right equipment will assist you in preparing food in your own kitchen.

Helpful Hints outlines tips and suggestions that may be especially important for the "I Don't Cook" cook. The general methods and tips found in this chapter will help you with actual food and meal preparation.

Chapters 1–3 are also important to read—particularly for the information they contain on *Candida* Related Complex (CRC) and rotational diet. Chapter 4—Specialty Foods is an important source of information on the specialty foods used in this cookbook. It will give you a good background on the properties, history, and uses of the new foods that you will be adding to your diet, as well as enhance your enjoyment of them.

When planning a meal, be creative and use a wide variety of foods. The phrase "rotational diet" originally comes from the term "the rotary diversified diet" so remember to incorporate diversity into your meal planning. Your attitude and planning will make all the difference in the world. For instance, I do not feel deprived because I am allergic to foods. Instead I feel lucky because in many ways I have more choices and variety in my meals than many nonallergic people. If you are like many people, you are accustomed to using prepared foods and mixes or fast-food restaurants and carry out in your meal planning. You will find that starting a rotational and *Candida* control diet, as well as "cooking from scratch," is a challenge. However, if you are committed to improving your health, planning and preparing foods and meals within you dietary restrictions that complement your lifestyle is accomplishable.

The Basics

Meal planning is the core of following a rotational diet. Advanced planning can simplify your meal preparation and therefore help to simplify your life. By using advanced planning and other information in this chapter, as well as in the rest of this book, you will have the tools to:

- make staying on a *Candida* control and/or rotational diet easier.
- develop meals that will properly nourish your body.
- add diversity to your diet.
- make your mealtimes colorful, relaxing, and fun.
- develop a shopping list and system that enables you to:
    - purchase what you need.
    - decrease impulse buying of nonessential or improper foods.

If you feel you are not a person who can organize or plan, attempt to make the planning and organizing aspect of this diet a game or a challenge for you. Use advanced planning to save yourself preparation time in the kitchen and give yourself more time for other things. I think of planning as prayer. Christians pray before making decisions. Prayer makes life bearable and easier to handle and following God's answers to prayer smoothes your path and often saves you time.

Where to Begin

As a first step to meal planning, look at the list of foods eaten on each day. The lists are found at the beginning of each day's chapter: Day 1 on page 97, Day 2 on page 147, Day 3 on page 197, and Day 4 on page 237. Or see pages 342–343 for a facing-page listing of the foods for all four days. Read through each list and note, on a piece of paper or in the margins of this book, the foods on each day that you can incorporate in your diet. This will depend upon your food allergies and other dietary restrictions. Then you can evaluate whether there are enough foods on each day to form a balanced diet. Look for a cross section of proteins, carbohydrate starches, vegetables, and fruits (once you can add fruits to your diet).

After you have looked through the food lists and have decided that you **do have enough foods that you can eat on each day**:

- Look through the recipes. Pay particular attention to the recipe ingredients and choose those that you can eat or that you can modify slightly to fit your requirements.
- Make a list of or indicate in each day's Recipe Table of Contents the recipes that encourage you and that will allow you to follow your dietary restrictions. This list will help you as you begin actual meal planning and preparation.

If you do not have enough foods to eat on each day, your first task would be to modify the list of foods for each day according to your dietary restrictions. Help for this is found in Chapter 3—Rotational Diet. If you need help beyond the scope of this chapter, refer to Appendix D: Recommended Reading for other reference material on rotation. If you prefer to receive personalized help, refer to Section 3: Resources for Personalized Assistance for Food Allergies and Rotational Diet Planning in Appendix C: Resources. After making a list of food changes—either by yourself or with assistance—to develop a 4-day rotational diet personalized for your needs, you may require assistance with recipes and meal planning. If you need more help beyond the information contained in this book, see Appendix G: Canary Connect on how to receive my assistance.

Ingredient Substitutions within Recipes:

A few of the recipes list a substitution option. While many recipes do not specifically give an option, a substitution can often be incorporated into them. Many times the reason an option is not given is that it would break the rotation set up in this cookbook.

Vegetables, grains/nongrains, and/or meats are usually items you can substitute in each of the recipes. You may wish to consider length of cooking time and/or color when making substitutions. For example, if you make a vegetable, grain/nongrain, and/or meat substitution, note that the cooking time for the recipe may need to be adjusted depending upon the needed cooking time for the substitute food(s).

Chapter 6—Helpful Hints will help you if you want or need to develop a substitution. Begin by reading the various substitution listings in Chapter 6 which include substitutions for flours, starches, eggs, milk, sugar, and leavening agents. Following are some additional common substitution situations.

- The cereal recipes on each day do not have to include the nut milk listed. You may substitute additional water for the nut milk amount when preparing them.
- The "Mayo" recipes found on each day use a nut or seed for a base with the addition of a starch for thickening. Each of the base ingredients and/or starches in these recipes could

be substituted for those in other recipes. I have used this option many times when I did not have a particular starch on hand or was temporarily moving a particular food to another day to experiment with more recipes.

- To produce a standard product, a starch or other binder is necessary when baking with gluten-free, nongrain flours. Arrowroot is used on Day 2 with amaranth, tapioca starch on Day 3 with quinoa, and guar gum on Day 4 with buckwheat. Arrowroot and tapioca can easily be exchanged in the amaranth and quinoa recipes, but guar gum is not an equivalent exchange with a starch.
- Oils can be substituted in any of the recipes. However, be sure to check the nut, seed, or vegetable source family with regard to the possible need to move other members of the food family.

"Plain Food" Meals

When I first began eating on a rotational diet, I was encouraged by books and others to eat "plain food" meals. "Plain food" meals usually have three components—meat, starch, and vegetables—which are cooked separately. When implementing a major change in diet, it can seem simplest to cook the individual allowed foods in this manner—i.e., warm up tuna, cook brown rice, and steam broccoli. While these meals are often easy to plan and prepare, they can become very boring and tasteless when eaten for extended periods. In addition, they add to the clean-up process since each component is prepared separately requiring three separate cooking utensils—sauce pans, skillets, dishes, etc.—which cannot be washed until after the meal.

While "plain food" meals can be useful when doing your meal planning, you should remember that not only is preparation and cooking time a factor, but clean up should be considered as well. It is possible to prepare a "plain food" meal without using a large number of cooking utensils or having a sink full of dishes waiting for you after your meal. By preparing casseroles you not only streamline your clean up process, but you introduce new tastes and variety to your diet. Combining individual foods in a casserole format allows them to complement the flavors of the foods they are cooked with creating a new flavor in the process. Using complementary-flavor foods can also help eliminate the need to use condiments and sauces such as catsup which might otherwise be used on plain food dishes. The appearance of the foods is also often enhanced when the different colors and textures are combined.

While casseroles do not always mean that less cooking utensils are used, they do have an advantage in that while the casserole is cooking in the oven you are able to wash up the preparation pans and dishes. When your meal is finished the only clean up remaining is the casserole dish, the table dishes, and any flatware or drinking containers used. This makes after-meal clean up much quicker, easier, and relaxing. Also, since most casseroles take up to 1 hour to cook, you can often clean up the kitchen and still have some time to relax before your meal. Some casseroles—such as Chicken or Tuna Noodle or Rice Casseroles—expand this advantage even further because they can be prepared earlier in the day and put in the refrigerator until it is time to bake them.

The best examples of time-saving "plain food" meals are the following meals which can be prepared in one cooking utensil resulting in a very tasty meal with a minimum of clean up.

- Day 1—Tuna Rice Dinner
- Day 3—Salmon Millet Dinner
- Day 4—Easy Meal Banquet

Meal Planning Ideas

At the beginning of the chapter for each day, there is a section on meal planning ideas that was developed to help you choose food and recipe combinations for complete meals, the preparation time available, and the type of meal you will be serving. Many times an individual recipe is a complete meal and will not need other foods or recipes to complement it. Meal planning ideas are divided into several categories.

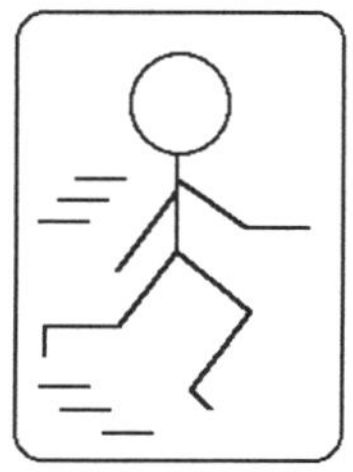

- Quick & Easy Meals—These are meals that can be prepared from start to finish in approximately 30 minutes. The actual time will depend somewhat on the size of recipe you are preparing because vegetable preparation usually takes the most time.
- Quick & Easy with Advanced Planning—Using some advanced planning, preparation, and/or *plan*overs (planned leftovers) makes these recipes quick and easy additions to your meal plans. When you look through the meal planning sections in each Day's chapter, notice how using advanced planning greatly increases the list of Quick and Easy Meals.
- Easy Meals—These recipes do take longer from start to finish, but the actual preparation time you spend in the kitchen is very short. The longer time for completion is usually due to the cooking style and the required cooking time (e.g., oven, slow cooker, etc.).

  EZ
- Lower Carbohydrate Meals—These meals are not just cave man diet suggestions, but are meals that have a lower carbohydrate level. [The cave man diet is a regimen having a very restricted carbohydrate level (60–80 grams per day) which may be needed by some during the early weeks of a *Candida* control diet. If knowing the carbohydrate levels of the foods you eat is important for your personal diet, see Appendix D: Recommended Reading which contains a list of resources that give carbohydrate levels for different foods.] Often casserole, soup, or salad recipes will give you better control over the amount of carbohydrates in your meal because the individual foods are measured rather than being guesstimated as when serving grains as a side dish.
- Breakfast Ideas—For each day there is a selection of foods such as cereals that can be prepared in the slow cooker or on top of the stove, some pancakes, or muffins that make excellent breakfast choices. On Day 2 there is not as wide a selection of breakfast foods because amaranth is a little more difficult to cook with, but often I will have a boiled potato or a leftover item from the freezer. I really love having a half serving of Low Carbohydrate Lasagna for breakfast. This gets extra vegetables into my day. Adding vegetables or a protein source to your breakfast is a good idea. By doing so, you add variety to your morning meal and help balance your diet by eating more than just carbohydrates at the start of the day. Everyone's metabolism is different, as is the way each individual body deals with the overgrowth of *Candida*, and you will need to adjust what you prepare for breakfast depending on your own system's needs. I often eat leftover meat or vegetables from the evening before for breakfast.
- Snack Ideas—Snack ideas for those times between meals when you need a little something to carry you through.
- Meals Away from Home—This section includes ideas that work well for those times you need to be away from home during mealtimes. Meals away from home, such as lunch at work, would vary depending upon what the workplace lunchroom facility has available or what your management will allow you to do. If I worked away from home on a regular basis, I would encourage my management:
  - to allow me and others to store food in a refrigerator or at least in my cooler in the coolest area of the building.

* to add a microwave to the lunchroom for all to use.
* to allow me to bring my lunch in a 1-quart size slow cooker all ready to plug in and cook or reheat (one of my Meals Away from Home ideas requires this but you can experiment other ideas).

I would even go to the point of a bribe—not money, just delicious homemade natural food occasionally shared with management. In fact, if my management was not cooperative about my needs due to allergies, I would probably be bold and work with them in a nice way using the disability law to my favor or find somewhere else to work where they appreciated me. Since I do not currently work away from home, I cannot say specifically what I would do, but I welcome any suggestions from my readers to share in Canary Connect News newsletter, see Appendix G.

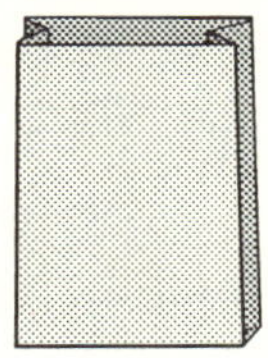

- Special Occasion Meals—Some recipe and meal ideas for those special times, including brunches, potlucks, and when company comes for dinner. Rotation does not have to be tossed out the window for guests. Many of these suggestions are meal ideas that take more preparation time. However, careful planning so that many things can be done in advance will allow you to be relaxed when company arrives.

For example, one of my favorite company meals is Shrimp Tofu Lasagna, Carob Cake Brownies, and Dacopa beverage (a Day 4 Special Meal). I prefer this recipe made with asparagus. It is much tastier and has a better appearance than the green bean variation. To prepare this meal and still allow myself time to relax and be ready for guests, I use the following schedule.

* Before lunch, prepare the brownies and the icing. While the brownies are baking, clean up the kitchen and prepare the Soy Lasagna Noodles. Place the noodles in the refrigerator or freezer as described in the recipe.
* Sometime after lunch, plan some relaxation time as a break from the standing time involved in the brownie and noodle preparation.
* Sometime in the afternoon, begin the lasagna preparation by making the sauce, which is the most time-consuming stage.
* Approximately 75 minutes (1 hour and 15 minutes) before the anticipated serving time, do steps 4, 5, and 6 from the recipe. This allows approximately 15 minutes to layer the lasagna in the pan and 60 minutes to bake it.
* Have your guests arrive approximately 15–30 minutes before the anticipated serving time. This will allow 30 minutes or longer after placing the lasagna in the oven to set the table and have a few minutes of relaxation time.

As a special note, realize that this recipe can be prepared with uncooked whole-wheat or spelt noodles in place of the soy noodles. If you do not have enough time to prepare Soy Lasagna Noodles for everyone, prepare just enough Soy Lasagna Noodles for yourself and assemble the lasagna in a Corning 10-inch square casserole dish by using Soy Lasagna Noodles for one portion and using the spelt or whole-wheat noodles for the other three portions. Be careful to mark which corner has the soy noodles so that you can be sure to get that portion on your plate when serving. My guests have eaten the Soy Lasagna Noodles and have not noticed any lack of flavor in comparison with other foods that they would eat and I have had very good compliments on this company meal.

Dacopa beverage is a coffee substitute made from dahlia tubers. It is a nice decaffeinated beverage to offer with a dessert for company. It looks like instant coffee and is very easily prepared by dissolving it in boiling water. Each guest can then mix their own beverage to the strength they prefer in their individual mug or coffee cup. My guests have enjoyed this drink hot or cold.

This is just one example of a company meal where you can do all of the preparation earlier in the day. This gives you a chance to relax throughout the day so you can be well rested when your company arrives and enjoy your visit with them.

Planning Ahead

I know that with all of our busy lifestyles, we are continually searching for something quick and easy to prepare for mealtime. Several recipes in this cookbook are quick and easy and can be prepared from start to finish in as little as 30 minutes. A working person may decide to prepare Quick and Easy meals on Monday through Friday and prepare more difficult or time-consuming meals and recipes on the weekend when more time is available to spend in the kitchen.

However, most of the time required to complete a recipe involves the vegetable preparation and the cooking time. In some instances, you can cut preparation time by choosing to use vegetables that you have frozen yourself ahead of time—such as green peppers, onions, zucchini, and eggplant—or purchase frozen vegetables. You can learn more about creating your own supply of organic foods in Chapter 12—Organics—The Only Way to Go! which includes tips and information on canning and freezing (page 290).

In order to supply yourself with easily accessible breads (muffins, hamburger buns, crackers, tortillas) and desserts (once you can tolerate fruits and/or alternative sweeteners), you will need to plan time when you can be in the kitchen for extended periods. By preparing breads and/or desserts and freezing them in individual portions, adding breads and desserts to your meals becomes as easy as using commercially prepared food products.

Also, when you are preparing a meal (perhaps even a quick and easy meal) prepare an additional amount of the recipe to be used at a later time. This "*plan*over" (planned leftover) food can be put in the freezer to use for the next rotation—four, eight, or more days later. Or use the *plan*overs for your lunch the following day if you are following a dinner/breakfast/lunch "day" rotation.

For example, on Day 1 you make Oven Fried Chicken for your dinner. You may cut up a whole chicken fryer and bake all the pieces or choose to cook the bonier pieces separately (see Chicken Broth, page 124). The broth may be used in a casserole or soup for the next day's lunch or frozen for later use. The cooked meat removed from these pieces may be made into a salad, a casserole, or a soup for the next day's lunch or frozen for later use. Also, when you are cutting up vegetables for dinner, such as for stir-fry vegetables, cut up extra amounts to be used in soup or to put into a salad for the next day's lunch. If you are going to make a salad for the next day's lunch, prepare the "Mayo" or salad dressing while your chicken is cooking. The next day while you are fixing breakfast you can combine the prepared salad ingredients or cook the soup. Pack the salad in a cooler or the soup in a thermos and you are ready to go. This same principle can be used with several meals on all four days.

The above example would be used by persons who follow a dinner/breakfast/lunch "day" plan (see page 28 for explanation). If you are using either the breakfast/lunch/dinner plan (as I usually do) or the lunch/dinner/breakfast plan (as I occasionally do), you may find, the following tips helpful. To shorten my kitchen preparation time, I figure out all the recipes I will fix on a particular day and determine how many cups of each of the vegetables I will need. Then I use one slot of time to prepare all of them, such as:

- during the cooking time for the evening meal the night before,
- while breakfast is cooking,
- sometime during the morning,
- or while preparing lunch.

Doing all of the vegetable preparation at one time assists me in preparing meals faster for that day.

Another technique I use is to prepare the same meal for lunch and dinner. When preparing lunch, I make three servings of the recipe and put two servings in the refrigerator to be reheated for my husband and myself for dinner.

Your freezer can be an important tool in helping to make meal preparation quicker and easier. Keep some cooked rice, millet, quinoa, buckwheat, and beans frozen ready to pull out and add to a recipe. If you look through the recipes, you will note several that list using these previously cooked ingredients. Also, many of the casseroles and soups use a broth of the day. When you are roasting a chicken or turkey or making a beef, buffalo, pork, or venison roast, you can save the broth and the leftover meat to use in future meals.

The list of helpful *plan*overs can go on and on. You can help determine the list of foods you want to have handy in the freezer by looking through the recipes that you have chosen to prepare. Check to see if the recipes use foods such as cooked meat or cooked grains or nongrains (e.g., cooked chicken, cooked rice). Another good indicator is when the recipe lists another recipe title with a page location. If so, more than likely the referenced recipe is something you can have stored in the freezer or that you need to make in advance. You could make the needed food just before making the recipe which uses it, but it is much easier and faster to have the already-prepared food in the freezer to be pulled out and used.

Reheating

While having *plan*overs (planned leftovers) in the freezer to use for future meals is a great help, it can sometimes be a challenge to thaw and reheat them. Here are some basic tips which I use.

First of all, I do use a microwave oven to thaw or reheat several casseroles. But if you do not have or cannot use a microwave oven, you can reheat foods using the following methods.

- To reheat tortillas, muffins, or other bread products, start with a pan of water. A skillet or very wide-topped pan works best. You do not need to have a large amount of water in the pan, but you will want enough so that it can be brought to a steaming state and kept steaming for the thawing and reheating time period. Place a splatter screen (page 60) over the top of the pan. The baked good should be in a closed cellophane bag—quite often I fold the top over and use tape to close the bag. Place the bag on the splatter screen over the steaming water. Turn the bag often enough so that the baked goods are thawed and heated evenly. I usually freeze baked goods in individual portions in cellophane bags sealed closed with tape so they are easy to remove from the freezer, thaw, and reheat.
- Since muffins are larger, they really need to have some thawing time at room temperature before being placed on a splatter screen over steaming water. It is best if they are thawed first and you are just warming them so they taste more like fresh baked.
- When reheating casseroles I love to use my steamer pan. Quite often I will freeze casserole *plan*overs in glass jars or Grab-It bowls. If frozen in a glass jar, thaw the casserole enough to remove it from the jar and transfer it to a Grab-It bowl. Purchase a steamer pan that is large enough for a Grab-It bowl to set down inside the steamer insert. Fill the bottom of the steamer pan with water to about 1/2 inch from the bottom of steamer insert. Heat water to boiling. Put the glass lid on the Grab-It bowl and set it in the steamer insert. Then put the lid on the steamer pan. You should open up both lids (the steamer pan and the Grab-It bowl) to stir your casserole often. The pan and the Grab-It bowl will be hot so remember to use hot pads when you handle them. For casseroles that should not be stirred, such as lasagna, it is best to use a slow oven (300°F.) for thawing and reheating.
- Pizza can also be reheated in a slow oven (300°F.) To facilitate this process, begin with the following tips on freezing *plan*over pizza. Cut the pizza into slices, loosen it from the bottom of the pan with a spatula, and separate the slices. Place the pizza pan in the freezer to individually freeze the slices (around 30–60 minutes). After the slices are

frozen, they are solid and easier to handle and package. Transfer the number of pizza slices you will want for a serving to a cellophane bag and close with a piece of tape or a twist-tie. Mark the bag with a self-adhesive label listing the type of pizza and the date. Be careful to store the pizza in the freezer where it will not be "knocked around" and damaged. The pizza slices should be removed from the freezer and thawed in the refrigerator during the day or overnight. Place the pieces on a stainless steel baking sheet (does not have to be oiled). Place the baking sheet in a slow oven (300°F.—do not preheat). Check the pizza occasionally to see if it is ready. If you have a microwave and can use one, you may thaw the pizza and even start it reheating in the microwave. But be aware that using the microwave will cause the dough to become very soggy—especially the amaranth dough. The best option is to thaw the pizza in the refrigerator and reheat it in the oven. For reheating individual servings, a toaster oven might be a nice addition to your kitchen. It is more efficient than heating up the whole big oven for just one or two pieces of pizza.

- If you have frozen soups, such as Minestrone Soup or Turkey Parsnip Soup, in glass jars and need to thaw them quickly, but you do not have or cannot use a microwave, you can use warm water. Set the jar(s) into a container of warm water so that the water covers as much of the jar sides as possible without "floating" the jar or reaching the lid. Change the water as it cools. As the soup begins to thaw, chip away the thawed portion and pour it into the pan you will use to reheat it. Continue this process until soup is thawed enough to remove the entire jar contents to the reheating pan. (Special Note: Freezing in wide-mouth jars with straight sides aids in the thawing process.)

All of the alternative thawing options listed above can be avoided if you learn to plan your meals for the following day and to pull the needed item from the freezer so they can thaw in the refrigerator. Do not thaw foods at room temperature except for a brief period of time. Thawing at room temperature can lead to the possibility of food-born illness and it is much safer and easier to develop habits that will make refrigerator thawing your standard method.

Creating a Shopping List

While developing and maintaining a food storehouse (a stored supply of nonperishable food staples) can seem a monumental task at first, you will soon have a valuable resource to help you in your journey toward better health. The process is not a "snap," but it is an accomplishable challenge. If possible for your situation, you may be able to build your storehouse in stages.

The lists of food staples on pages 94–95, which are divided by days, give you a starting point for stocking your storehouse. You can customize these lists to your individual needs by making photocopies of the lists. Cross off the food items you need to eliminate because of food allergies and add other items that you will use in your rotation. Keep these customized lists in a file folder or 3-ring binder along with pages where you keep notes on the resources you have used, the dates and amounts ordered, item order numbers, and/or other information that will aid you in stocking your storehouse.

By using photocopies of these lists, you can keep the originals to recopy later should you need to modify your customized list if/when your dietary needs change.

Start your shopping list with the following food items that you may need on all four days.

- baking soda
- vitamin C crystals
- flaxseed oil
- flaxseed
- Pau D'Arco tea
- Dacopa beverage
- sparkling mineral water
- spring water

To complete your shopping list, check the recipes you plan to prepare to learn which perishable food items you need—e.g., fresh or frozen vegetables and fruits, meats, eggs, yogurt, or tofu.

Getting Started

If you have taken time to read all the preceding chapters, you have the tools and the armor to move forward into meal planning and preparation. Many of you may still have one more question—"How do I begin?"

Begin at the Beginning

Take a few minutes to glance ahead at the separate chapters for each day. At the beginning of each one you will find:

- a list of the foods assigned to that day,
- the Recipe Table of Contents for the chapter, and
- a set of meal planning ideas. (These are only ideas to help you get started. You will be able to develop more as you become acquainted with this rotation.)

In the Meal Planning section, the first listing is Quick and Easy Meals. These are meals that can be prepared in 30 minutes or less and are the best place to start as you begin your rotation. Look at these meals and set up a plan for your first four days of rotation. You may want to set up two rotations (8 days) at this point to save time later. Choose a Quick and Easy meal that you feel you can accomplish for each meal that you need to prepare for that set of days. Add your breakfast idea for each day. Remember, some of your Quick and Easy Meals may be used for both lunch and dinner or for dinner and the next day's lunch, depending on which plan you are following. Using one recipe for two meals would cut down on the number of Quick and Easy Meals that you need at the start.

Purchase Your Supplies and Take the Plunge

Using your meal plan outline, look at the recipes and make a list of the ingredients needed. Decide where you need to purchase them. If you have a local health-food store that can provide all of them, shop there or, if you are chemically sensitive and cannot go yourself, send someone there to purchase them for you. Or use Appendix C: Resources to order the needed foods. Once you have all the foods on hand, set your day and say "I'm starting with Day 1 today." Put a smile on your face and be ready to go.

If you only planned for four days, on Day 3 of your rotation you will need to set up your plan for the next four days. Choose another set of Quick and Easy Meals that you can prepare for the next four days and purchase the needed foods. Do realize that if you ordered all of your foods by mail, you will need to plan a little further in advance to keep your storehouse stocked. Then you can keep going on your rotation without waiting for your food supplies.

Expand Your Horizon

As you plan the second set of four days using the Quick and Easy Meals, start thinking even further ahead as to what you can prepare to make the Quick and Easy Meals with Advanced Planning. This may involve such steps as cooking some extra Basic Buckwheat Groats to put in the freezer. Then you can prepare another quick and easy delicious meal such as my favorite, Stir-Fry Buckwheat and Vegetables.

When you are planning the third set of four days, plan some time when you can do some of the Easy Meal ideas—the ones that are quick as far as preparation time, but which require some advanced planning on your part. This may involve washing beans or starting

(continued on page 96)

Day 1 Staples

Animal Protein
Chuck's Seafood tuna
Northwest Natural Halibut Medallions

Grains
basmati rice, brown and/or white
brown rice, long-, medium-, or short-grain
Kamut® grain
spelt grain

Flours and Starches
Kamut® flour
rice flour
spelt flour
teff flour

Cereals
Arrowhead Mills® organic Puffed Kamut®
Arrowhead Mills Rice & Shine cereal
Erewhon Kamut® Flakes (breakfast cereal)
Lundberg Family Farms Creamy Rice™ Cereal
Lundberg Family Farms organic Brown Rice Crunchies
rice cakes
rice, Kamut®, spelt flakes (cooked cereal)

Pasta
Kamut® pastas
rice pastas
Vita-Spelt® spelt pastas

Oil
almond oil
sesame oil

Sweeteners
Lundberg Family Farms Sweet Dreams Organic Brown Rice Syrup

Herbs and Spices
cumin
dill weed
dry mustard
parsley

Nuts and Seeds
almonds
Jaffe Brothers organic almond butter
pecans
sesame seeds

Other
pear juice

Day 2 Staples

Animal Protein
Seafarer's Choice medium peeled & deveined shrimp (available from Schwan's Sales, see Appendix C: Resources)

Nongrains
whole amaranth

Flours and Starches
amaranth flour
arrowroot starch
garbanzo bean flour
potato starch

Cereals
puffed amaranth

Beans
garbanzo beans (chickpeas)

Oil
butter or ghee (clarified butter)
olive oil
sunflower oil

Sweeteners

Herbs and Spices
garlic powder
dehydrated minced garlic
whole fresh garlic
basil
cayenne (red) pepper–ground or leaf
chili powder
leaf oregano
marjoram
rosemary
summer savory

Nuts and Seeds
sunflower seed

Other
Mountain Sun Organic Lemonade
Muir Glen organic tomato paste
Muir Glen organic tomato puree

Day 3 Staples

Animal Protein
Chuck's Seafood salmon

Grains and Nongrains
hulled millet
oatbran
rolled oats
whole quinoa
wild rice

Flours and Starches
barley flour
cream of tartar
oat flour
quinoa flour
tapioca starch

Cereals
Arrowhead Mills Bits of Barley cereal
puffed millet

Pasta
Oak Creek 100% Rye Pasta
Oak Creek 100% Wild Rice Pasta
quinoa pasta (wheat-free)

Oil
canola oil
walnut oil

Sweeteners
FOS
100% pure maple granules

Herbs and Spices
bay leaf
caraway seed
cinnamon

Nuts and Seeds
filberts (hazelnuts)
walnuts

Other
apple juice
Santa Cruz Natural Organic Applesauce

Day 4 Staples

Animal Protein

Nongrains
buckwheat groats

Flours and Starches
carob powder
Jerusalem artichoke flour
kudzu (kuzu) starch
navy bean flour
soy flour
white buckwheat flour (or prepare your own)

Cereals
Cream of Buckwheat Cereal (or prepare your own)

Pastas or Beans
100% Buckwheat Soba Noodles
adzuki beans
black turtle beans
kidney beans
lentils
navy beans
pinto beans
split peas

Oil
soy oil
safflower oil

Sweeteners
honey
stevia

Herbs and Spices
tarragon
Watkins Salsa Seasoning Blend or other Mexican blend spices

Nuts and Seeds
cashews
macadamia nuts
roasted soy beans

Other
carob chunks
kombu (seaweed)
R.W. Knudsen 100% Just Cranberry Juice

your breakfast cereal the night before. Or cut up the vegetables the evening before so in the morning you can start Easy Steak Stew in the slow cooker. As you look at the Easy Meal ideas, you will find many more examples that can add variety to your diet. Make plans to schedule a little time earlier in the morning to start something in the slow cooker for dinner.

Congratulations, You Did It!

Now see, you are well on your way. You have completed 12 days of the rotational diet. You may have had to change your plans a little along the way, but you have started. Build from there. Maybe repeat some of the same meals that you chose earlier. After all, think about it. How many times did you really have that much of a variety before? What was your previous standard breakfast—cold cereal or hot cereal every morning? Or maybe you had an English muffin. Now you have a much greater variety in your diet. Even if you choose the same thing for each Day 1, 2, 3, or 4 on your rotation, you are having at least four different things for breakfast. For instance, perhaps you prepare Teff Pancakes every Day 1, Amaranth Cereal each Day 2, Creamy Millet Cereal (or better yet, Millet Pudding which is delicious for breakfast) on Day 3, and lentils or, my favorite, Buckwheat Pancakes on Day 4. If you only chose these four breakfast items and repeated them every four days, you still may have more variety in your breakfasts than the "normal" person has or that you once had.

As you continue using the rotational diet, you will become accustomed to the process that works for you in planning your meals and keeping your storehouse stocked. You will learn the techniques that will smooth out the process for you and make your life easier and full of wonderful, nourishing, and varied meals. And best of all, you will know that you are an essential part of the process in improving your health and your life. Believe in yourself and keep up the good work! You can do it!

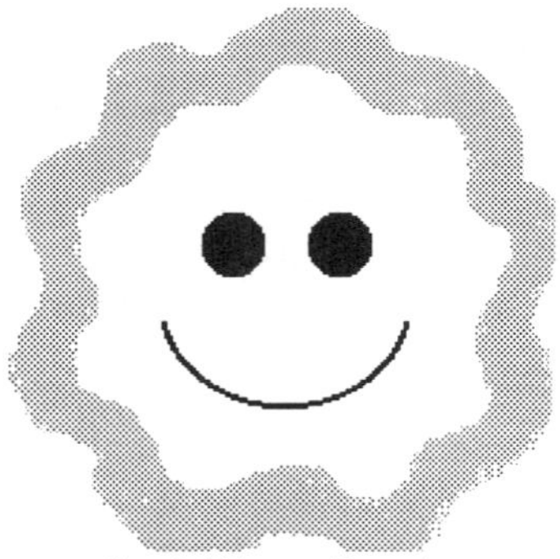

Seek Warm Fuzzies

The man who removes a mountain
begins by carrying away small stones.
–Chinese Proverb

If you don't know where you're going,
you'll end up somewhere else.

Failures are more commonly
caused by having made no decisions
than by making wrong ones.

8. FOODS, MEAL PLANNING, AND RECIPES FOR DAY 1

Foods for Day 1

Animal Protein		Foods That Float Between Days 1 & 3	
88	catfish		
98	tuna		
103	halibut, sole		
124	chicken, chicken egg, Cornish hen, pheasant, quail		
Vegetables			
6	bamboo shoots		
7	Chinese water chestnut		
28	beets, chard		
36	broccoli, cabbage, radish, turnip, collards		
65	celery	65	parsley
Grains, Flours, and Baking Foods			
6	Kamut®*, rice, spelt*, teff, wheat*		
Fruit			
40a	pear		
40b	apricot, peach, nectarine		
40c	raspberry		
Sweeteners			
6	rice syrup		
40a	pear		
Oils			
40b	almond oil		
75	sesame oil		
Herbs and Spices			
36	dill, dry mustard	34	cinnamon
65	cumin		
Seeds and Nuts			
22	pecan		
40b	almond		
75	sesame seeds		

* See page 29 for Rule 4 in Chapter 3—Rotational Diet and pages 37–38 and 40–41 for the Kamut and Spelt sections in Chapter 4—Specialty Foods for more information on including these grains in your rotational diet.

Recipe Table of Contents for Day 1

Biscuits, Crackers & Etc. Bread

Cereals, Grains, & NonGrains

Muffins and Pancakes

Protein Dishes

Protein Dishes (continued)

Vegetables, Salads, & Salad Dressings

Desserts

Miscellaneous

Meal Planning for Day 1

Quick & Easy Meals

- Tuna Broccoli Chowder
- Stir-Fry Chicken with your choice of pasta
- Grilled Fish for Day 1
  Cream of Broccoli Soup
- Pasta Primavera
- Chuck's Seafood tuna
  your choice of pasta with flaxseed oil and dill
  stir-fry or steamed vegetables

Quick & Easy Meals with Advanced Planning

- Sesame Goulash
- Chicken Spaghetti
- Chicken Broccoli Chowder
  Teff Crackers
- Chicken Broccoli Soup
  Kamut® Muffin
- Chicken Rice Soup
  with steamed collards
- Chicken Vegetable Salad
  with your choice of crackers
- Chicken or Tuna Salad with chard on your choice of tortillas
  celery sticks

Easy Meals

Oven Fried Chicken
Basic Brown Rice
Coleslaw

Tuna Rice Dinner
celery sticks

Chicken Rice, Spelt, or Kamut® Loaf
Basic Kamut® or Spelt Stir-Fry Vegetables

Easy Chicken Meal or Soup

Tuna Noodle or Rice Casserole
radishes

Chicken Noodle or Rice Casserole
radishes

Baked Fish for Day 1
Basic Brown Rice
Steamed Broccoli

Roast Chicken
"Stove Top" Dill Stuffing
steamed collards

Lower Carbohydrate Meals

Chicken or Tuna Broccoli Chowder

Chicken Broccoli Soup with or without crackers

Chicken Loaf (Choice of three varieties)
Stir-Fry Vegetables for Day 1
OR a steamed Day 1 vegetable

Easy Chicken Meal or Soup

Grilled Fish for Day 1
celery sticks with almond butter
Cream of Broccoli Soup

Tuna or Chicken Vegetable salad with or without the pasta or grain

Breakfast Ideas

your choice of muffins, pancakes, French toast, biscuits, or cooked cereals (see Recipe Table of Contents for Day 1)

Arrowhead Mills Rice & Shine cereal

Lundberg Family Farms Creamy Rice™ cereal

Erewhon Kamut® flakes or puffed Kamut® cold cereal with almond milk

fresh fruit

rice cake with almond butter

any *plan*over Day 1 vegetable, fish, casserole, or soup

chicken eggs cooked your favorite way

Snack Ideas

broccoli buds
celery stick with almond butter
rice cake with tahini
Teff, Kamut®, or Spelt Muffins
Teff, Kamut®, or Spelt Crackers
Puffed Kamut®
Raspberry Rice Granola
Almond-Sesame Granola Bars
Amazing Sugarless Cookies
almonds or pecans
fresh fruit

Meals Away from Home

Chicken Turnip Soup
with crackers or muffin

Tortilla sandwich with Egg,
Tuna, or Chicken Salad
celery sticks

Tortilla sandwich with *plan*over
Roast Chicken and fresh collards
fresh broccoli or Coleslaw

Easy Chicken Meal—take to work in a
1-quart slow cooker ready to plug in
and cook for 4 hours

Tuna or Chicken Vegetable Salad
with crackers or muffin

Any *plan*over casserole if you have
a microwave available to reheat it

Special Occasion Meals

Brunch–
Breakfast Brunch Squares
celery stuffed with almond butter
Dacopa

Company–
Oven Fried Chicken
Wild & Brown Rice with Herbs
steamed broccoli and/or Coleslaw
Pear Custard
Dacopa

Company–
Tuna or Chicken Cabbage Rolls
Kamut® or Spelt Dinner Rolls
celery sticks
iced Pau D'Arco tea
Teff Pear Cake

Potluck–
Cold Oven Fried Chicken
Coleslaw
sparkling mineral water

Recipes for Day 1

Teff Cereal I

1/2 cup	brown whole teff grain
1/4 teaspoon	sea salt
1 3/4 cups	water (room temperature)
1/4 cup	Almond Milk (page 104) OR additional water

Teff Cereal II

1/3 cup	brown whole teff grain
2 tablespoons	brown teff flour
1/4 teaspoon	sea salt
1 3/4 cups	water (room temperature)
1/4 cup	Almond Milk (page 104) OR additional water

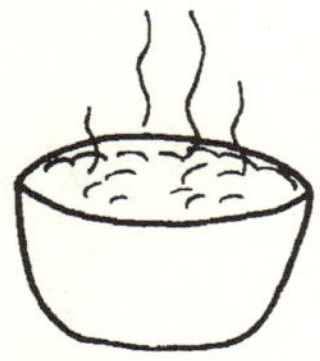

1. Combine your choice of the above ingredients in a 1-quart size slow cooker.* Cook overnight and awake to enjoy this ready-to-eat, mouth-watering cereal.

2. Stir before serving. Enjoy this cereal plain or with a tablespoon of raspberries or Pear Sauce (page 144).

Special Note: I have attempted to cook teff cereal on top of the stove but with no real success.

Recipe idea for Teff Cereal I is from Mastering Food Allergies newsletter, July-August 1989.

Yield: 2 cups

Cream of Kamut® or Spelt Cereal

2/3 cup	Kamut® or spelt grain
1/4 teaspoon	sea salt
1 3/4 cups	water (room temperature)
1/4 cup	Almond Milk (page 104) OR additional water

1. Grind grain in a blender just long enough to prepare a coarse meal.

2. Follow steps 1 and 2 as above in Teff Cereal recipe.

Yield: 2 cups

*These recipes are too small to cook in a standard-sized slow cooker, but they can be easily doubled or tripled if desired. Cook on low if slow cooker has two settings. Also, see page 61 for more information on slow cooker.

Recipe idea from Mastering Food Allergies newsletter, December-January 1992.

Raspberry Rice Granola

2 cups	rice flakes
1/4 cup	chopped almonds or pecans
2 tablespoons	hulled sesame seeds
1/2 teaspoon	sea salt
1/4 cup	brown rice syrup
1/4 cup	raspberry juice*
2 tablespoons	almond or sesame oil
1 teaspoon	alcohol-free almond extract (optional)

1. Preheat oven to 350ºF.
2. Combine rice flakes, nuts, sesame seeds, and salt in mixing bowl. Toss to distribute ingredients evenly.
3. Measure rice syrup in a 1-cup glass measure. Add juice, oil and extract. Mix. Pour this syrup mixture evenly over flake mixture. Mix thoroughly with rubber spatula. Transfer to 9x13-inch baking dish. Spread evenly.
4. Bake for 45 minutes until crispy. Remove from oven after the first 15 minutes and every 10 minutes thereafter to stir. Cool completely. As the granola cools it will become crispier.
5. Serve as a cereal with rice or almond milk, as topping for Vanilla Rice Dream**, or plain as a crunchy snack or dessert. Store in glass jar in the freezer.

Yield: approximately 3 cups

*Special Note: When I prepare raspberry muffins or pancakes, I save and freeze the raspberry juice so it will be handy to thaw and use in this recipe.

**Realize that some ingredients in Vanilla Rice Dream breaks rotation.

Almond Milk

1/4 cup	almonds
1 cup	water

1. Blend almonds in blender on highest speed until they become a fine powder, approximately 1–2 minutes. Stop once or twice to scrape sides and bottom of blender jar.

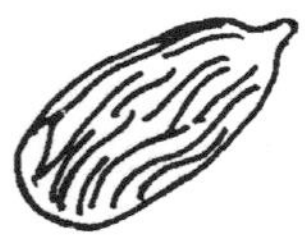

2. Add water and blend on highest speed approximately 1 minute until well blended. Stop at least once to scrape sides and bottom of blender jar. Chill. Add salt and/or brown rice syrup if desired. Stir before serving. I love the rich flavor that Almond Milk adds to Day 1 cereals.
3. Since I do not desire to make this nut milk each time I serve hot or cold cereal, I usually prepare 1 or 2 cups at a time. After blending, pour immediately into ice cube trays. After frozen, remove the milk cubes and transfer to cellophane bags.

Yield: slightly more than 1 cup

French Toast*

1	egg, beaten
	OR 1 egg yolk, beaten with 1 tablespoon water
1/8 teaspoon	sea salt
dash	cinnamon (optional)
2 slices	your choice of bread:
	French Meadow brand yeast-free, organic, 100% spelt bread
	Kamut® or Spelt Yeast-Free Bread (page 110)
	"Ener-G" brand yeast-free, brown rice bread*

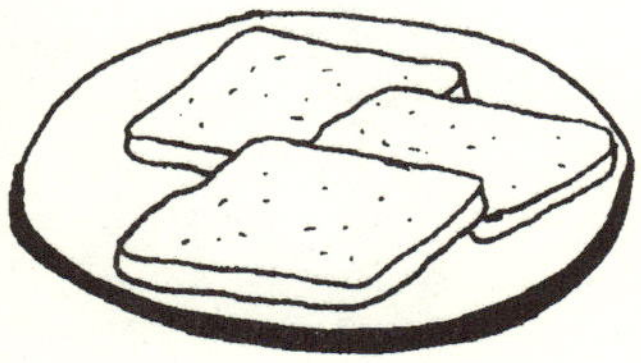

1. Preheat griddle. I use a well-seasoned cast-iron griddle (see How to Season Cast Iron on page 63). Griddle is hot enough when water dances when sprinkled on the griddle. Lightly oil griddle after preheating.
2. Beat egg (or yolk and water) with salt and cinnamon in shallow flat-bottom bowl. Dip bread slices into egg mixture to coat them on both sides. Cook approximately 2 minutes on each side.
3. Serve plain with flaxseed oil, almond butter, all-fruit jam, or heated Pear Sauce (page 144).

*Realize that the rice bread has a few ingredients that break rotation. I usually do not concern myself with this break since I only have this occasionally.

Spelt or Kamut® Biscuits

1 1/4 cups	spelt or Kamut® flour
1/4 teaspoon	sea salt
1 teaspoon	baking soda
1/4 teaspoon	unbuffered, corn-free vitamin C crystals
3/8 to 1/2 cup	water
	use 3/8 cup for spelt (3/8 cup = 1/4 cup + 2 tablespoons)
	use 1/2 cup for Kamut®
3 tablespoons	sesame oil
2–3 tablespoons	flour to knead and roll out biscuits

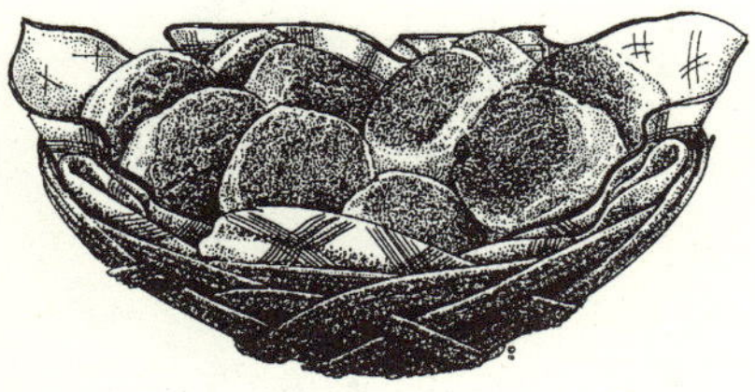

1. Preheat oven to 400°F.
2. In mixing bowl, whisk together dry ingredients starting with only 1 1/4 cups of flour. Make "well" in center.
3. Add water and oil. Stir with rubber spatula or fork until dough clumps into a ball and flour is well mixed.
4. Knead dough lightly on a floured board using 1–2 tablespoons of flour. Pat out to 1/2 inch thick using more flour if needed.
5. Cut with biscuit cutter or drinking glass with a diameter of approximately 2 1/4 inches. Cut 4 spelt or 5 Kamut® biscuits. Form together the scraps of dough, pat out, and cut 2 more biscuits. Repeat and cut 1 more biscuit. If there is enough dough remaining, form it into another biscuit. Bake on ungreased stainless steel baking sheet for 15 minutes.

Yield: 7 to 8 Spelt Biscuits or 8 to 9 Kamut® Biscuits

Kamut® Pancakes

8 Dollar-size	24 Dollar-size	YIELD
1/2 cup	1 1/2 cups	Kamut® flour
1/2 teaspoon	1 1/2 teaspoons	baking soda
3 pinches	scant 1/4 teaspoon	sea salt
1/4 teaspoon	1/2 teaspoon	unbuffered, corn-free vitamin C crystals
1/2 cup	1 1/2 cups	water
2 teaspoons	2 tablespoons	sesame oil

1. Preheat griddle. I use a well-seasoned cast-iron griddle (see How to Season Cast Iron on page 63). Griddle is hot enough when water dances when sprinkled on the griddle. Spread 1 teaspoon of oil on griddle after preheating.
2. In mixing bowl, whisk together dry ingredients. Add water and oil. Stir with whisk for 15 seconds. Allow batter to set up to 30 seconds to thicken. Stir again.
3. Dip batter onto the griddle using tablespoon. Cook on first side until pancake is golden brown, approximately 1 1/2 minutes. Turn. Cook until golden brown on second side, approximately 1 minute. If your batter thickens, you may desire to stir in very small amounts of additional water. Also, you may need to add additional oil to griddle as you cook repeated batches.
4. Serve plain or with flaxseed oil, almond butter, all-fruit jam, and/or heated Pear Sauce (page 144).

Teff Pancakes

8–9 Dollar-size	YIELD
1/2 cup	brown teff flour
1/2 teaspoon	baking soda
2 pinches	sea salt
1/4 teaspoon	unbuffered, corn-free vitamin C crystals
1/2 cup	water
2 teaspoons	sesame oil

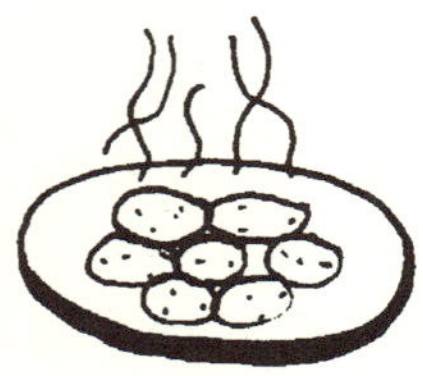

Prepare steps 1–2 the same as Kamut® Pancakes (recipe above).

3. Dip batter onto the griddle using tablespoon. Cook on first side about 2 minutes until pancake bubbles and is slightly dry around edges. Turn. Cook 1 1/2 minutes until dry on second side.
4. Serve plain or with flaxseed oil and/or heated Pear Sauce (page 144).

Raspberry Teff Pancakes

<u>Add to above recipe:</u>
1/3 cup raspberries, fresh or frozen

Just before dipping batter onto the griddle, fold in thawed, drained raspberries. Cook as above.

Spelt Pancakes

10 Dollar-size	30 Dollar size	YIELD
2/3 cup	2 cups	spelt flour
1/2 teaspoon	1 1/2 teaspoons	baking soda
3 pinches	scant 1/4 teaspoon	sea salt
1/4 teaspoon	1/2 teaspoon	unbuffered, corn-free vitamin C crystals
1/2 cup	1 1/2 cups	water
2 teaspoons	2 tablespoons	sesame oil

Prepare steps 1–2 the same as Kamut® Pancakes (page 106). However spelt batter will be a little thicker. In fact, you may need to shake the spoon some to remove the batter.

3. Dip batter onto the griddle using tablespoon or larger spoon. Cook on first side until pancake bubbles, then smoothes out, and is slightly dry around edges, approximately 2 minutes. Turn. Cook until dry on second side, approximately 1 1/2 minutes. If your batter thickens, you may desire to stir in very small amounts of additional water. Also, you may need to add additional oil to griddle as you cook repeated batches.

4. Serve plain or with flaxseed oil, almond butter, all-fruit jam, and/or heated Pear Sauce (page 144).

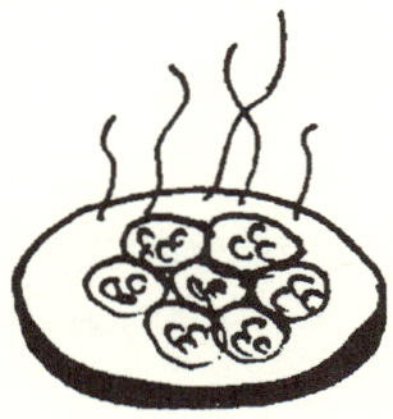

Raspberry Kamut® or Spelt Pancakes

<u>Add to your choice of either Kamut® or Spelt Pancake recipes</u>:

8 Kamut® OR 10 Spelt Dollar-size	24 Kamut® OR 30 Spelt Dollar-size	YIELD
1/3 cup	1 cup	raspberries, fresh or frozen

Just before dipping batter on the griddle, fold in thawed, drained raspberries. Cook as above.

Basmati Rice Cereal/Dessert

3/4 cup	cooked Basmati rice (page 117)
1/2 cup	Almond Milk (page 104)
1 teaspoon	brown rice syrup
as desired	chopped almonds

In small saucepan, combine all ingredients and heat to serving temperature. Stir occasionally to prevent scorching. If desired, add a dash of cinnamon and more rice syrup. Serve for quick breakfast or for dessert.

Special Note: This recipe can be prepared with other cooked rice, but I believe Basmati rice is far superior in flavor.

Kamut® or Spelt Muffins

6 Muffins	12 Muffins	YIELD
1 1/4 cups	2 1/2 cups	Kamut® or spelt flour
1 teaspoon	2 teaspoons	baking soda
1/8 teaspoon	1/4 teaspoon	sea salt
1/4 teaspoon	1/2 teaspoon	unbuffered, corn-free vitamin C crystals
2 tablespoons	1/4 cup	sesame oil
For Kamut®:		
1 cup – 1 tablespoon	1 7/8 cups	pear juice (7/8 cup = 3/4 cup + 2 tablespoons)
For Spelt:		
3/4 cup	1 1/2 cups	pear juice

1. Preheat oven to 350ºF.
2. Oil and flour the bottom and sides of muffin cups.
3. In a mixing bowl, whisk together dry ingredients.
4. Add pear juice and oil. Stir just to moisten the dry ingredients. Gently smash larger lumps against side of bowl. Smaller lumps will bake out.
5. Equally portion batter into prepared muffin cups, slightly more than 1/4 cup of batter each. Bake 20–25 minutes.
6. Cool muffins in the pan(s) on wire rack for 5 minutes. Then turn muffins out of pan(s). Sometimes you need to take a sharp, thin knife around the edges of the muffins to loosen them from the side. Muffins are best when served warm. They freeze and reheat well in the microwave.

Raspberry Muffins

Add to your choice of Kamut® or Spelt Muffins:

6 Muffins	12 Muffins	YIELD
1/2 cup	1 cup	raspberries, fresh or frozen

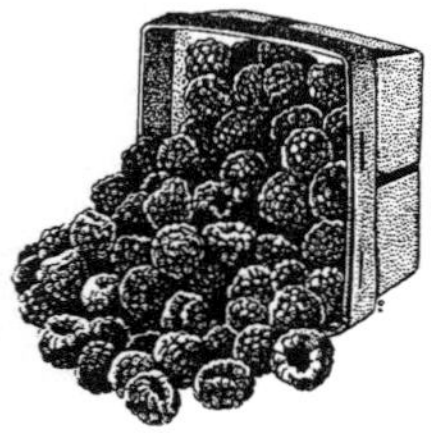

Just before portioning batter into muffin cups, fold in thawed, drained raspberries. Portion almost 1/3 cup of batter per muffin cup. Bake as above except usually the raspberry muffins will take 25–27 minutes to bake. Also, with this variation, you may substitute water for the pear juice.

Teff Muffins

1 cup	brown teff flour
1 teaspoon	baking soda
1/4 teaspoon	sea salt
1/4 teaspoon	unbuffered, corn-free vitamin C crystals
3/4 cup	water
2 tablespoons	sesame oil
1	egg (optional)
	OR 1 tablespoon ground flaxseed and 1/4 cup water

1. Preheat oven to 400ºF.
2. If using the flaxseed for egg substitute, whisk flaxseed with 1/4 cup of water in a small saucepan. Bring to boil, reduce heat to medium high, and boil for 1–2 minutes until you have the consistency of egg white (however, color will not be like egg white). While boiling the mixture, stir with a whisk almost continuously. Set aside to cool.

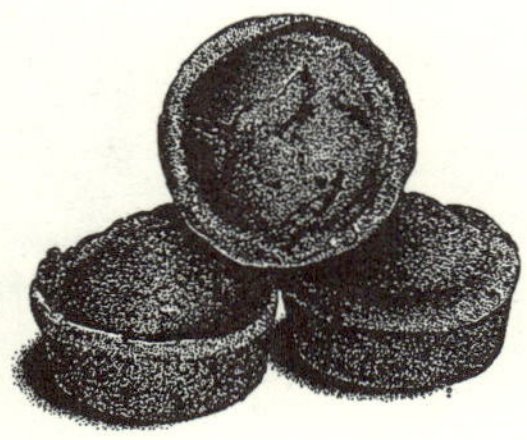

3. Oil and flour the bottom and sides of 6 muffin cups.
4. In a mixing bowl, whisk together dry ingredients.
5. Add water, oil, and egg (or egg substitute). Stir just to moisten the dry ingredients. Batter will have some lumps but they will bake out.
6. Equally portion batter into prepared muffin cups, slightly more than 1/4 cup of batter each. Bake 20 minutes.
7. Cool muffins in the pan(s) on wire rack for 5 minutes. Then turn muffins out of pan(s). Sometimes you need to take a sharp, thin knife around the edges of the muffins to loosen them from the side. Muffins are best when served warm. They freeze and reheat well in the microwave.

Special Note: I cannot tell any difference in taste between teff muffins without egg, with egg, or with flaxseed. However, the muffins without egg seem to crumble when frozen and reheated. The flax variation crumbles a little less than those without egg. Also, flax and egg variations raise more when baking.

Yield: 6 muffins

Raspberry Pear Jam

2 cups	frozen raspberries
2 cups	Pear Sauce (page 144)
	OR 1 1/3 cups Pear Sauce Sweetener (page 145)
2 tablespoons	flour—brown rice, spelt, or Kamut®

Combine fruits and flour in a deep saucepan. Cook on medium-high for 5–10 minutes until thickened. Stir almost constantly with whisk to prevent burning. Freeze leftovers in small wide mouth jar or in ice cube trays 1/2 tablespoon per cube. After jam has frozen, remove from the trays and keep frozen in a cellophane bag until ready to use.

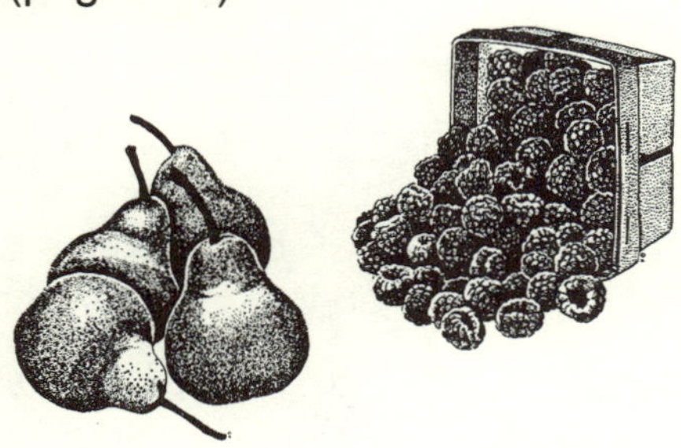

Yield: 1 1/3 cups

Kamut® Yeast-Free Bread, "Hamburger" Buns, and Dinner Rolls

3 cups	Kamut® flour
3/4 teaspoon	sea salt
1 1/2 cups	water
3/8 cup	sesame oil (3/8 cup = 1/4 cup + 2 tablespoons)
1/2 cup	Kamut® flour
1 1/2 teaspoons	baking soda
1/2 teaspoon	unbuffered, corn-free vitamin C crystals

Spelt Yeast-Free Bread, "Hamburger" Buns, and Dinner Rolls

3 cups	spelt flour
3/4 teaspoon	sea salt
1 1/4 cups	water
3/8 cup	sesame oil (3/8 cup = 1/4 cup + 2 tablespoons)
5/8 cup	spelt flour (5/8 cup = 1/2 cup + 2 tablespoons)
1 1/2 teaspoons	baking soda
1/2 teaspoon	unbuffered, corn-free vitamin C crystals

1. Preheat oven to 350°F.
2. Oil and flour baking dish(es)—stainless steel does not need to be floured.

For Bread	9x5-inch loaf pan
For "Hamburger" Buns	3 8-inch square pans OR 2 baking sheets
For Dinner Rolls	8-inch square pan

3. In large mixer bowl, whisk together first measurement of flour and salt. Set aside.
4. Measure amount of water and oil in separate containers ready for use. In small bowl, whisk together second measurement of flour, baking soda, and vitamin C. Set aside.
5. Set up mixer with dough hooks.* To the large bowl of flour mixture, add water. Mix on low speed (stir speed) to moisten flour. Scrape sides with rubber spatula to assist in moistening the flour. Then beat mixture on medium speed (mix speed) for 3 minutes. Scrape sides of bowl with rubber spatula throughout mixing process. The dough will become cohesive and climb up the dough hooks.
6. Without stopping mixer, add oil to dough. Continue to mix on medium to mix the oil into the dough. Scrape sides to assist working the oil into the batter.
7. Again without stopping mixer, add second measurement of flour, soda, and vitamin C mixture. Continue to mix on medium speed or a little lower until all flour is moistened, scraping sides. Then beat for 30 seconds on medium.
8. For bread: Transfer dough to prepared loaf pan. Lightly coat hands with oil and shape dough evenly in pan and smooth on top.

   For "hamburger" buns: Lightly oil hands. Divide dough as equally as possible into 12 portions. Shape each portion into flat dough portions approximately 3 1/2–4 inches in diameter. Place in baking pans or on baking sheets with smooth side up. To accomplish this you will need to reoil your hands often.

   For dinner rolls: Lightly oil hands. Pinch off an approximately 2-inch portion of dough. Shape into roll. Place in square pan with smooth side up. Repeat to prepare 16 rolls. Reoil hands as needed.

continued on next page

Kamut® or Spelt Yeast-Free Bread, "Hamburger" Buns, and Dinner Rolls (continued)

9. Bake according to time table below or until toothpick comes out clean when inserted into center:

	Spelt	Kamut®
For Bread	50–55 minutes	55–60 minutes
For Hamburger Buns	15–17 minutes	18–20 minutes
For Dinner Rolls	20 minutes	25 minutes

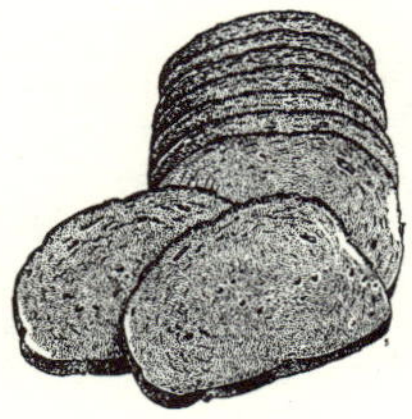

10. For Bread and Buns: Immediately or at least within 5 minutes after baking, loosen bread and buns from sides of dish(es) and remove to cool on wire rack. Using a serrated knife, slice bread into approximately 1/2-inch slices and slice buns in half horizontally when they are either slightly or completely cooled.

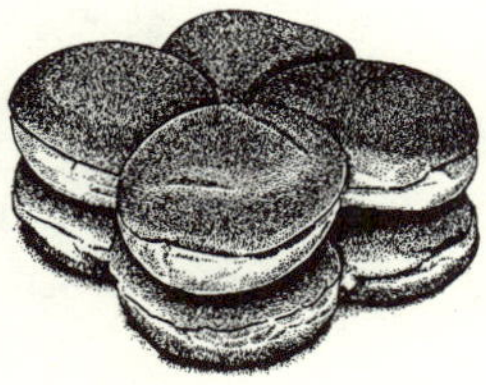

For Dinner Rolls: Cut rolls along divisions. Finish by removing from pan, pulling them apart, and placing them in a towel-lined basket to serve warm.

11. Leftovers may be frozen. I prefer to freeze bread with sheets of cellophane between the slices. Wax paper should also work if you can tolerate it.

Yield: 1 loaf of bread, 12 "hamburger" buns, or 16 dinner rolls

*If you do not have a mixer with dough hooks you will need to change the directions slightly. For step 3 use 1/2 cup less flour in the first measurement. This 1/2 cup of flour becomes a third measurement that you will need to knead in by hand after step 7.

Recipe idea for Spelt Bread & Buns are from Allergy Cooking With Ease by Nicolette M. Dumke, p.47.

Cheerfulness is what greases
the axles of the world.
Don't go through life creaking.
H. W. Byles

Laughter is by definition healthy.
Doris Lessing

Spelt or Kamut® Crackers

1 1/4 cup	spelt or Kamut® flour
1/2 teaspoon	baking soda
1/4 teaspoon	sea salt
1/4 teaspoon	unbuffered, corn-free vitamin C crystals
1/3 to 1/2 cup	water
	use 1/3 cup for Spelt Crackers
	use 1/2 cup for Kamut® Crackers
3 tablespoons	sesame oil

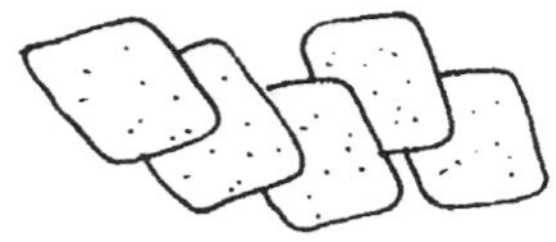

Teff Crackers

1 1/8 cups	brown teff flour (1/8 cup = 2 tablespoons)
1 teaspoon	baking soda
1/4 teaspoon	sea salt
1/4 teaspoon	unbuffered, corn-free vitamin C crystals
2 tablespoons	hulled sesame seeds
1/2 cup	water
3 tablespoons	sesame oil

1. Preheat oven to 350°F.
2. Place 1 teaspoon of oil on a 14 x 10-inch stainless steel baking sheet and set aside. (This amount of oil is in addition to the amount listed above.)
3. In large mixing bowl, whisk together your choice of dry ingredients (and sesame seeds for Teff Crackers). Make "well" in center.
4. Add water and oil. Stir with rubber spatula or fork until dough clumps into a ball and flour is well mixed.
5. Spread oil on baking sheet with fingers to within one inch of edge. As the dough is rolled out, it will push the oil to the edge of the baking sheet. In addition, using your fingers to spread the oil will lightly coat them and aid in working with the dough.
6. Transfer dough to center of the baking sheet. Use your hands to form dough so it has no rough edges. Press dough out evenly in all four directions until it cannot be spread further with your hands, making sure to maintain rectangular shape.
7. If your baking sheet has sides on it, be sure the rolling pin will fit all the way down onto surface on both the width and length of the sheet and that its handles clear the edges.
8. Lightly dust rolling pin with flour and roll dough out from center to edges. Be sure to press in all four directions and to keep dough at a uniform thickness. Occasionally run your hand across top of dough to feel if there are any thick areas that need to be evened out.
9. As the dough gets thinner, use the dull back side of a table knife to press edges of dough to maintain rectangular shape. Continue rolling and shaping until dough is about 1/8–1/4 inch thick and fills baking sheet. To help reduce possibility of extra-thin dough edge, use back side of a table knife to gently push all four edges of dough to make edge thickness uniform with remaining dough.

continued on next page

Spelt, Kamut®, and Teff Crackers (continued)

10. Using a pizza cutter, cut dough into squares as follows. (For Teff Crackers, be sure to move pizza cutter slowly and with a back and forth motion to help avoid tearing dough if cutter goes directly across a sesame seed.) Cut rectangle in half along dough length (see number 1 on diagram). Cut each half in half (see number 2), then cut each fourth in thirds (see number 3). This will create 12 strips.

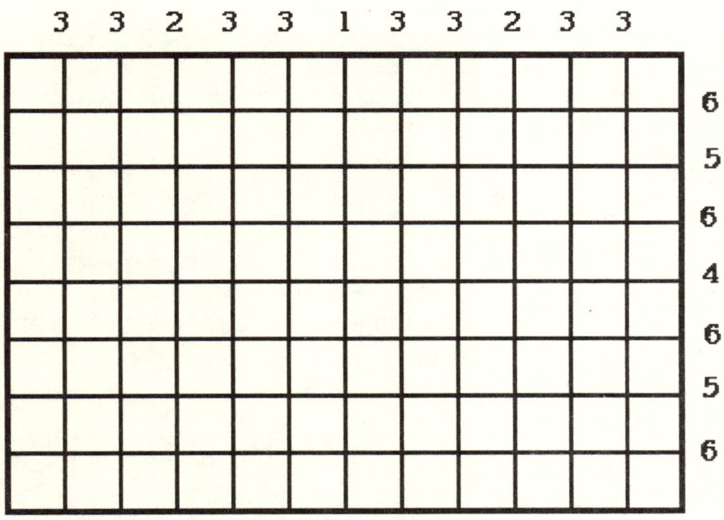

11. Next cut rectangle in half along dough width (see number 4). Cut each half in half (see number 5) and each fourth in half (see number 6). This will create 8 sections and 96 individual crackers. Next use a sharp knife to be sure each cut on the outer edge of the rectangle is completely separated.

12. Prick holes in each square with fork. If you wish, you can salt the tops of the crackers with sea salt before baking.

13. Bake crackers for first baking time listed below. Remove baking sheet from oven and carefully remove outer circle of crackers if they are crispy. Return remaining crackers to oven for second baking time listed below. To crisp crackers further, carefully loosen crackers from baking sheet and return them to oven for the third baking time listed below with oven turned off. Some Teff Crackers will crack but for the most part they hold together.

	1st	2nd	3rd
Spelt	20 minutes	5 minutes	10 minutes
Kamut®	25 minutes	5 minutes	10 minutes
Teff	20 minutes	5 minutes	20 minutes

14. Cool crackers on cooling rack by either leaving them on the baking sheet or removing and placing them directly on the cooling rack. After cool, store in the freezer. I prefer to use a wide-mouth quart jar. No need to thaw, eat straight from the freezer.

Yield: 96 crackers, almost a full quart for Spelt and 3/4 quart for Kamut® or Teff

Kamut® Tortillas

1 1/8 cups	Kamut® flour (amount needed to start) (1/8 cup = 2 tablespoons)
1/2 teaspoon	sea salt
1/2 cup	water
1/2 cup	Kamut® flour (amount needed for kneading and rolling)

Spelt Tortillas

1 1/4 cups	spelt flour (amount needed to start)
1/2 teaspoon	sea salt
1/2 cup	water
1/2 cup	spelt flour (amount needed for kneading and rolling)

Teff Tortillas

1/2 cup	brown teff flour (amount needed to start)
1/4 teaspoon	sea salt
1/4 cup	water
1/2 teaspoon	sesame oil
1/2 cup	brown teff flour (amount needed for kneading and rolling)

Special Note: Before starting your tortilla preparation, I suggest you read Helpful Hints on Tortilla Preparation starting on page 79.

1. Preheat nonstick, unoiled griddle or skillet. I use a well-seasoned cast-iron griddle (see How to Season Cast Iron on page 63). Griddle is hot enough when water dances when sprinkled on the griddle.
2. In a curved-sided bowl, whisk together first measurement of flour (amount needed to start) and salt. Make a "well" in the center.
3. Add water. Stir with rubber spatula or fork until dough clumps together into a moist ball.
4. Scatter flour on rolling surface (see amount in chart below). Transfer dough to floured rolling surface and knead to work in as much of this additional flour as possible. Dough texture should resemble Play Doh. Add more flour if needed. Form dough into ball and cut into equal portions (see chart below). Flour the cut surfaces of each dough portion with remaining flour.

	Kamut®	Spelt	Teff
flour on rolling surface	1 tablespoon	1–2 tablespoons	1 tablespoon
divide dough into portions	8 portions	8 portions	4 portions

5. Lightly flour rolling pin. Pat dough portion into circular shape, then roll out tortilla by pressing evenly from the center out in all directions and working to keep tortilla as round as possible. Keep dough well floured on both sides (see chart on next page for approximate amount of flour needed per tortilla). Turn dough over often by loosening with a spatula before flipping. Feel dough surface occasionally to be sure it is evenly thin. Finished tortilla will be very thin. See chart on next page for final diameter of each tortilla. Using a pastry brush, gently brush both sides of tortilla or with the Kamut® or Spelt Tortillas you may gently toss tortilla from hand to hand to remove excess flour.

continued on next page

Kamut®, Spelt, or Teff Tortillas (continued)

	Kamut®	Spelt	Teff
flour needed per tortilla	3/4 tablespoon	3/4 tablespoon	1 tablespoon
final diameter of each tortilla	7–8 inches	7–8 inches	6 inches

6. Cook each side of each tortilla on preheated, unoiled griddle for cooking time indicated in chart below. Cool each tortilla on cooling rack as indicated in chart below. Place the slightly cooled tortillas between two layers of a clean cotton towel.

	Kamut®	Spelt	Teff
cooking time on each side	40 seconds	45 seconds	45 seconds
cooling time on cooling rack	1 minute	1–2 minutes	1 minute

7. Serve either whole or cut in half. Use your imagination to create a simple deli-like sandwich—for example: chicken, Swiss chard, Almond "Mayo," and/or diced celery are all good for Day 1. Also, use for egg, chicken, or tuna salad sandwich as well as Chicken Fajitas. Leftover tortillas may be frozen flat in a cellophane or plastic bag for future meals.

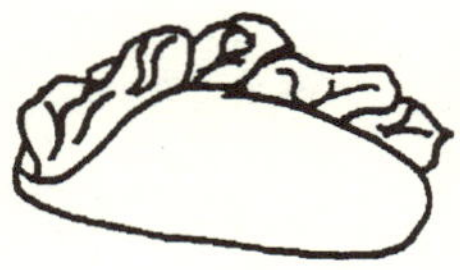

Yield: 8 Kamut® or Spelt Tortillas; 4 Teff Tortillas

Happiness is found along the way—not at the end of the road.

Sol Gordon

Keep your face to the sunshine and you cannot see the shadow.

Helen Keller

Homemade Kamut® or Spelt Noodles

1	egg, medium, large, or extra large size OR 1/4 cup water OR 3 tablespoons water and 1 tablespoon ground flax seed
1/4 teaspoon	sea salt
3/4 to 1 cup	Kamut® or spelt flour, depending on egg size and choice of flour
3 cups	Chicken Broth (page 124)

1. Lightly beat egg and salt in a medium-size bowl with curved sides.
2. Add 1/4 cup flour and mix with rubber spatula or fork. Continue to add flour (1–2 tablespoons at a time) and mix until you cannot mix any more with the rubber spatula or fork.
3. Also, attempt to get all the dry dough crumbs that tend to form worked into the large ball of dough. At this point I usually have used a total of 1/2 cup of flour, but the trick is to work as much flour as possible into the dough.
4. Now, sprinkle 2 tablespoons of flour on rolling surface (for more information on rolling out dough or rolling surfaces, read Helpful Hints on Tortilla Preparation starting on page 79). Knead until dough is no longer sticky.
5. Lightly flour your rolling pin. Roll dough out to approximately 1/16 inch thick and into a 12–14 inch circle. Keep adding flour to any sticky dough area. Also, turn dough over often to flour the underneath side. If you are inexperienced, the rule of thumb is to roll dough from the center out evenly in all directions. However it is not necessary for noodles to be in a perfect circle (and believe me, mine usually are not). Also, for more ease in rolling and handling the dough, you may desire to divide the dough in half before you start with step four and roll out 2 circles of approximately 9–10 inches in diameter.
6. For ease in cutting, allow dough to dry for 30 minutes. Then turn dough over and flour any sticky areas. Allow dough to dry another 15–30 minutes (Kamut® noodles require less drying time than spelt). If you do not allow the dough to dry before cutting it into noodles, it will drastically increase the cutting time (7 fold). However, do not over dry.
7. Before you cut the noodles, transfer the dry dough circle(s) onto a cutting board. Cut the noodles with a sharp knife by first cutting the circle into strips (1 1/2–2 inches wide). Next, cut each strip along the narrow end to make 1/4–3/8 inch wide noodles. If you have allowed your noodles to dry, you should be able to stack 2 or 3 layers of the narrow strips on top of each other to cut. Toss noodles with 1 to 2 teaspoons of flour.
8. In large saucepan, heat Chicken Broth to boiling. Add noodles a little at a time while stirring the boiling broth. After all noodles are added, cook Kamut® noodles for approximately 12 minutes and spelt noodle for 15 to 20 minutes or until tender. Stir occasionally. Add more broth or water if needed. Also, add salt to taste.

Yield: approximately 1 1/4 cups (4–5 ounces) uncooked; 2 1/2–3 cups cooked

Special Note: Save yourself time and prepare 2 or 3 eggs at one time and freeze the extra uncooked noodles in a cellophane bag.

Basic Brown Rice

1 cup	brown rice—long-grain, short-grain, or Basmati
2 1/4 cups	water
1/2 teaspoon	sea salt

1. Wash rice (page 36). Combine rice, water and salt in 2 1/2 quart sauce pan. Bring to boil on high. Cover. Reduce heat to between low and medium to allow the rice to simmer. Simmer 35–40 minutes.

2. Turn heat off but do not remove pan from burner. Allow pan to set 5–10 minutes. Stir to fluff.

Yield: 3 cups

Special Note: For best results, rice should not be stirred or uncovered during the cooking process. If it is necessary to check the progress of the rice during the cooking time, do so quickly to minimize the loss of steam. Do not stir the rice as this will disrupt the even cooking of the grain. If tasting for doneness, use a fork to gently remove a small amount from the surface of the rice. Different stoves and different pans may require adjustment in time, temperature, and amount of liquid used.

Wild & Brown Rice with Herbs*

1 cup	brown rice—long-grain, short-grain, or Basmati
1/4 cup	wild rice*
2 1/2 cups	water
1/4 teaspoon	sea salt
1/4 teaspoon each	marjoram, rosemary, tarragon*
as desired	broken pecans or chopped almonds

Prepare same as Basic Brown Rice (recipe above). Add spices with the salt. Add nuts at step 2. Stir before serving.

*Wild rice is usually eaten on Day 3, so you need to avoid eating it on your Day 3 just before and after eating this recipe on Day 1. Also, realize these spices do break rotation but sometimes you need some spice in your life, especially during Iowa's gray winters. HA!! Also, you may omit tarragon from this recipe and omit the spices in the Mint Family (number 73—see Herb and Spice listing on Day 2) on Days 2 and 4 before and after eating this recipe on Day 1.

Special Note: My family and I dearly love brown Basmati rice. The cooking fragrance is, "Mmmm! Who is cooking popcorn?" The cooked rice is sticky similar to that served in Chinese restaurants. Also, occasionally I prepare white Basmati rice when I am in a hurry because it cooks in 15 minutes.

Basic Kamut® or Spelt

1 cup	Kamut® or spelt grain kernels
3 cups	cooking water
1/4 teaspoon	sea salt

Prepare the same as Basic Brown Rice (recipe above) except you need to simmer for 2 1/2 hours.

Yield: 3 cups

Stuffing*

	neck and giblets from 1 roasting hen
2 1/2 cups	water
1/2 teaspoon	sea salt
4 cups	your choice of bread, cubed, slightly dried
	French Meadow brand yeast-free, organic, 100% spelt bread
	Spelt Yeast-Free Bread (page 110)
	Kamut® Yeast-Free Bread (page 110)
	"Ener-G" brand yeast-free, brown rice bread*
1 1/4 cup	celery, diced (also include celery leaves)
1/2 cup	onion, diced*
1/2 cup	sesame oil
	OR 1/2 cup unsalted butter, melted (1 stick)*
1/4 teaspoon	sea salt
1 teaspoon	sage leaves, crushed*
1/2 teaspoon	thyme leaves*

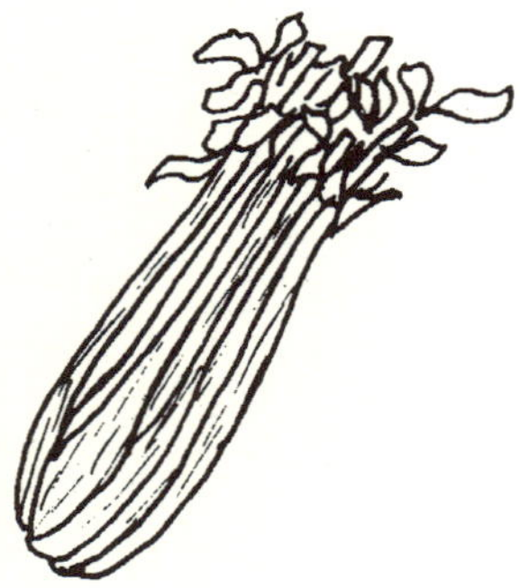

1. Remove any fat and skin on neck and giblets. Bring first 3 ingredients to boil in large saucepan, reduce heat, cover, and simmer 45 minutes to 1 hour or until tender.
2. Remove chicken meat from broth and allow to cool just enough to touch the meat without burning yourself. Remove gristle from gizzard and meat from neck bone and dice. This should yield approximately 3/4 cup of diced chicken. Measure out broth and add water to yield 1 cup.
3. In a large mixing bowl, combine diced bread, celery, onion, diced chicken, and seasonings. Mix to evenly distribute the spices. Pour broth and oil or melted butter evenly over the bread mixture and stir to moisten the bread. Then I prefer to use my hands to actually smash the bread with my fingers to break up the bread cubes into small crumbs. There may be some extra liquid at this point but it will be soaked up during the baking process.
4. Pour into an 8-inch square baking dish. Bake at 350°F. for 35–40 minutes.

Yield: 4–6 servings

Special Notes: Stuffing may be cooked in microwave on full power, for 15 to 25 minutes, turning pan one quarter turn every 5 minutes. Time depends on wattage of your microwave. Be careful not to dry the stuffing too much.

Also, stuffing can be placed inside the cavity of a roasting hen or turkey. Allow at least 1/2 hour more roasting time. Roast stuffed bird until internal temperature of stuffing is 180°F.

*Realize that this recipe breaks rotation so you need to plan ahead and make modifications within your rotation to temporarily move onions, sage, thyme, and butter from Day 2 to Day 1. Also the rice bread has a few ingredients that break rotation. I usually do not concern myself with the break in rotation, since I usually only have this recipe occasionally, especially to compliment holiday meals.

Dill "Stove-Top" Stuffing

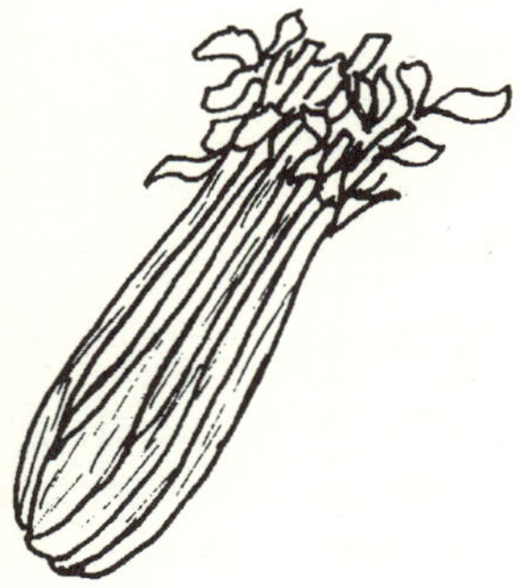

2 tablespoons	sesame oil
1 cup	celery, diced OR 1 1/2 cups cabbage, finely chopped OR 1/2 cup celery, diced and 3/4 cup cabbage, finely chopped
1 teaspoon	sea salt
1 teaspoon	dill weed
1/4 cup	pecan pieces
2 cups	quick cooking Kamut® or spelt flakes*
1 cup	Chicken Broth (page 124)
1 cup	water

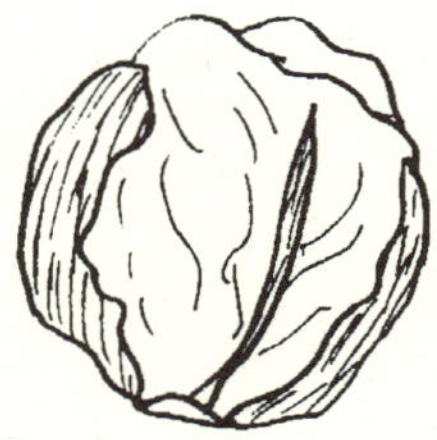

1. In skillet over medium heat, sauté celery in oil until celery is just tender. Stir often to prevent burning. (Omit this stage if only using cabbage.)
2. Add salt, dill weed, and pecans and stir to evenly distribute spices.
3. Add flakes. Toast flakes over medium heat for approximately 5 minutes. Stir often.
4. Add Chicken Broth and water all at once. If using cabbage, add now. Stir. Cover. Allow stuffing to cook on medium heat for 5 minutes or until flakes are done and the liquid is all absorbed. Stir and serve.

Yield: 4 cups However you can easily divide this recipe in half or fourths.

*This recipe was developed using the quicker-cooking brands of spelt or Kamut® flakes, e.g., Country Grown brand.

Dare to be wise; begin!
He who postpones the hour of living rightly
is like the rustic who waits for the river
to run out before he crosses.

Horace

Easy Chicken Meal or Soup

1 serving	chicken breast, skin removed
as desired	dill weed (optional)
1 cup	celery, thick sliced
1 cup	cabbage, chopped in large pieces
1/4 teaspoon	sea salt
1 1/2 cups	water

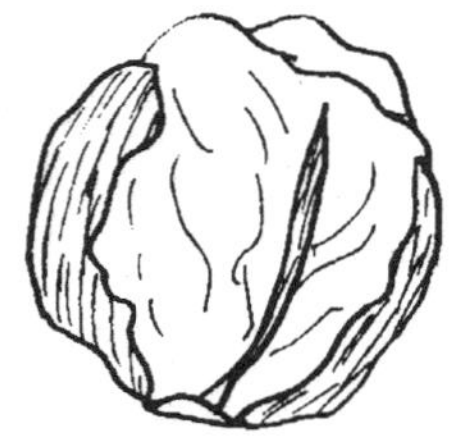

To Serve as a Meal:

1. Sprinkle chicken breast with 1/2 of the amount of salt and dill weed. Layer chicken breast, celery, and cabbage in a 1-quart size slow cooker.* Sprinkle with remaining amount of salt and dill weed. Add water. Note that some of the cabbage will not be completely covered with the water.
2. Cook for 4 hours on low.
3. Serve without broth as a meal. After the meal, boil the broth to make 1/2 cup. Freeze for later use. After you have prepared this meal twice, you have enough delicious chicken vegetable broth to prepare other recipes for Day 1 that use celery and cabbage such as my favorite, Chicken Spaghetti (page 129).

To Serve as a Chunky Soup:

1. Debone and cut the raw chicken meat into bite-size pieces. Partially frozen chicken is easier to debone. Layer the chicken bone, raw chicken meat, and the rest of the ingredients as above. You need to cook the chicken bone with the vegetables for more flavor.
2. Cook for 4 hours on low.
3. Remove the rest of the cooked meat from the bone and add it to the soup. Serve ingredients and broth together as a soup.

Yield: a delicious, simple meal for 1

*This recipe is designed for cooking in a 1-quart size slow cooker. However, you can easily double, triple, or quadruple this recipe and cook in a standard-size slow cooker. Cook on low if slow cooker has two settings. Also, see page 61 for more information on slow cooker.

Chicken Broccoli Soup

1 cup	Chicken Broth (page 124)
1/2 cup	water
1/2 cup	cooked chicken, diced
1 cup	broccoli cuts, fresh or frozen
1/8 teaspoon	sea salt
1/8 teaspoon	dill weed

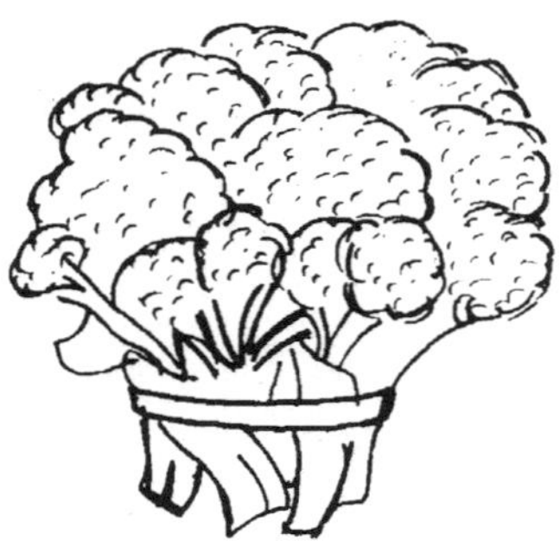

Combine all ingredients except broccoli in saucepan, bring to boil. Reduce heat, add broccoli, cover, and simmer 5 minutes or until broccoli is just barely tender. Serve immediately.

Yield: 2 1/4 cups

Cream of Broccoli Soup*

1 cup	water
3/8 teaspoon	sea salt
2 cups	broccoli cuts, fresh or frozen
1/4 cup	chopped macadamia or Brazil nuts*
2 tablespoons	flour—rice, Kamut®, or spelt
1 cup	water
1/4 teaspoon	dill weed

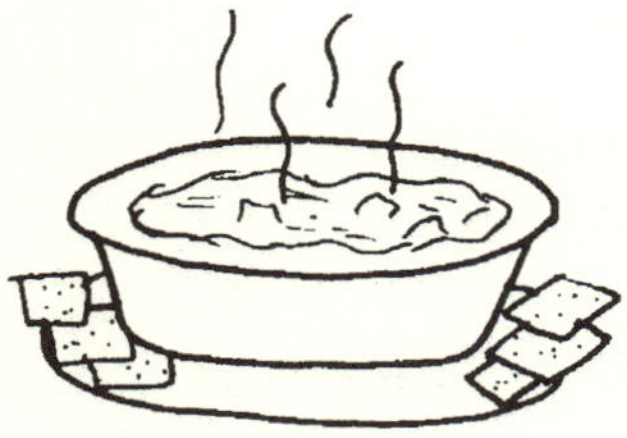

1. In saucepan, bring water and salt to boil, reduce heat. Add broccoli, cover, and simmer 5 minutes.
2. While broccoli is cooking, combine flour, nuts and approximately 1/3 cup of water in blender. Blend on highest speed for 1–2 minutes until well blended. Stop at least once to scrape sides and bottom of blender jar. Add the rest of the remaining water and approximately 1/2 of the cooked broccoli mixture to blender. Blend about 20 seconds on low speed.
3. Pour blended mixture into saucepan. Add dill weed. Heat just to serving temperature and to thicken. Stir almost constantly. Serve with crackers, biscuit, or muffin for a quick light lunch or as side dish with meal.

Yield: 2 3/4 cups

Tuna Broccoli Chowder*

Prepare same as Cream of Broccoli Soup except add 1 (one) 7 1/2 oz. jar of Chunk's Seafood tuna with dill weed. Also you may desire to increase salt to at least 1/2 teaspoon.

Yield: 3 2/3 cups

Chicken Broccoli Chowder*

2 cups	Chicken Broth (page 124), separated
1/4 teaspoon	sea salt
2 cups	broccoli cuts, fresh or frozen
2 tablespoons	flour—rice, Kamut®, or spelt
1/4 cup	chopped macadamia or Brazil nuts*
1 cup	cooked chicken, diced
1/4 teaspoon	dill weed

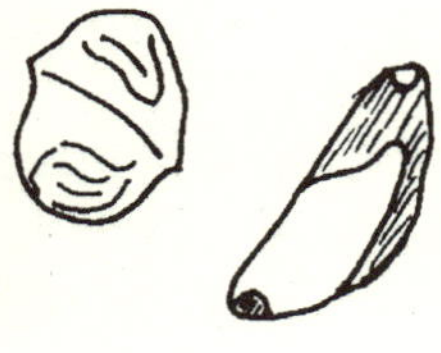

Prepare same as Cream of Broccoli Soup except replace water with broth and add chicken with dill weed. Serve with crackers or muffin for complete light lunch.

Yield: 3 cups

*Brazil and macadamia nuts are unassigned "Fun Foods" in this rotational diet, see explanation on pages 30–31.

Chicken Rice or Turnip Soup

2 cups	Chicken Broth (page 124)
1/2 cup	cooked brown rice OR turnips, peeled and diced
1/2 cup	celery, diced
1/2 cup	cooked chicken, diced
1/8 teaspoon	sea salt
1/8 teaspoon	dill weed

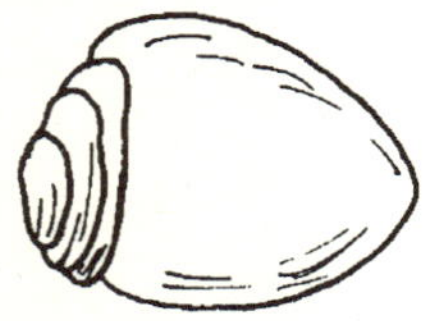

Combine all ingredients in saucepan. Bring to boil, reduce heat, cover and simmer 10–15 minutes or until vegetables are tender.

Yield: 2 cups

Chicken Fajita

2	Kamut®, Spelt, or Teff Tortillas (page 114)
1/2 cup	deboned chicken breast, cut into thin strips (a split chicken breast is usually enough)
3/4 cup	cabbage, thinly sliced or shredded
1/2 cup	celery, sliced thin
1 teaspoon	sesame oil
as desired	sea salt

1. Prepare or thaw tortillas.
2. Preheat well-seasoned cast-iron skillet on medium (see How to Season Cast Iron on page 63) or electric skillet to 300°F.
3. Prepare chicken and vegetables as described above. Chicken will cut into strips easier if partially frozen.
4. Add oil to preheated skillet. Stir fry chicken, stirring often to brown evenly. When not stirring, cover with splatter screen (information on page 60).
5. Add vegetables and sprinkle with salt. Stir often to cook chicken and vegetables evenly. I prefer my vegetables crunchy.
6. Serve immediately. I have found the easiest way to serve fajitas is to begin with the tortilla on your plate. Spread approximately 3/4 cup of filling in the center of the tortilla lengthwise but about 1 inch from one side as Diagram A shows. Fold the 1-inch edge side over first, then fold the 1/3 side edges over the filling as Diagram B shows. Lift and hold with both hands. Eat and enjoy.

Yield: approximately 1 1/2 cups of filling, ample amount for 2 tortillas

Diagram A

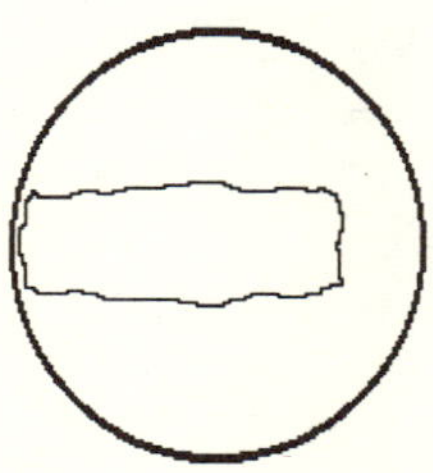

Diagram B

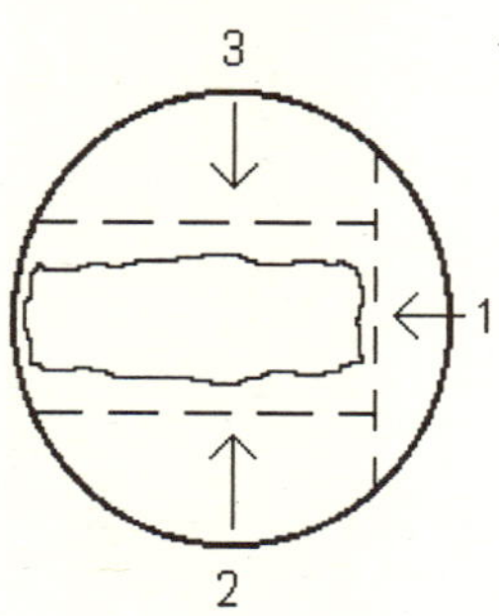

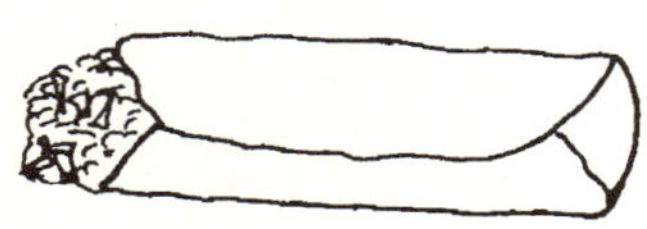

Pasta Primavera

1 ounce	spaghetti—Kamut®, rice, or spelt OR Kamut® angel hair
1 teaspoon	sesame or almond oil or 1/2 teaspoon of each
1	chicken breast
3 1/2 cups	your choice of fresh Day 1 vegetables I prefer: 1 1/2 cups cabbage, chopped 1 1/2 cups broccoli cuts, fresh 1/2 cup celery, thick sliced slant cup
as desired	almonds (optional)
as needed	sea salt

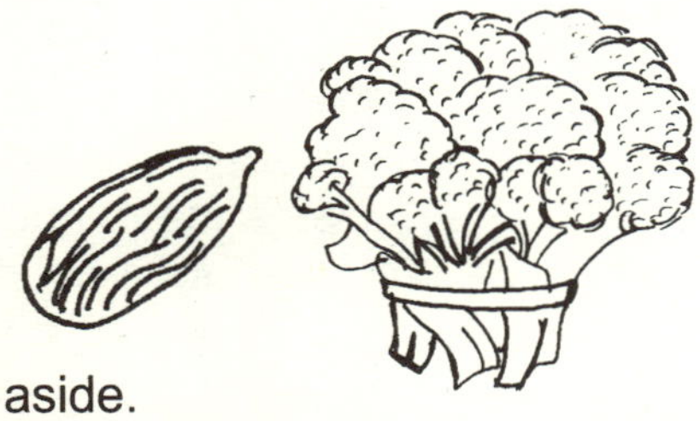

Method 1—Dry

1. Preheat electric skillet or wok to 350°F.
2. Remove the skin and bone from the chicken breast. Cut the chicken meat into thin bite-size strips and set aside. This works best if the meat is slightly frozen. Prepare fresh vegetables and set aside.
3. In large saucepan, cook broken spaghetti or angel hair in salted, boiling water for 10 minutes until tender. See directions on package. Stir occasionally to prevent sticking. When done, drain and set aside until finished with step 4.
4. While spaghetti is cooking, add oil and chicken to preheated skillet and cook, stirring almost continuously. Add prepared vegetables and almonds. Season as desired with salt. Stir almost continuously until vegetables are cooked to your liking. I prefer mine hot yet crunchy.
5. Add cooked, drained spaghetti. Stir constantly until spaghetti is mixed into vegetables and has returned to serving temperature. Serve immediately. The amount and choice of vegetables may be changed to fit your taste.

Method 2—With Sauce

Additional ingredients:	1/2 cup	water
	1 tablespoon	hulled sesame seeds
	1 tablespoon	flour—rice, spelt, or Kamut®

Follow Method 1, steps 1–4.

5. Combine approximately 1/4 cup of water, sesame seeds, and flour in blender. Blend on highest speed for 1–2 minutes until well blended. Stop at least once to scrape sides. Add rest of water and blend a couple of seconds more.
6. Add cooked, drained spaghetti and sesame mixture to cooked vegetables and chicken. Stir constantly until sauce has thickened and coated all ingredients. Serve immediately.

Yield: 2 1/2–3 cups

Roast Chicken and Broth

1	7–8 pound roasting hen or 3–4 pound chicken fryer
1–2 teaspoons	sea salt
1–2 cups	water

There are many ways to roast a hen or chicken. I prefer to use a covered stainless steel roasting pan or Reynolds Oven Cooking Bag.

1. Wash your bird inside and out. Remove any pin feathers from the skin. Rub the inside and outside of bird with salt. Tuck wings under back of bird and tie legs together with heavy cotton string.
2. Place bird on roasting rack inside roasting pan. Add water. Cover and roast at 325–350°F. Allow approximately 1 3/4 to 2 hours for fryer and 2 1/2 to 3 hours for roasting hen. Use a meat thermometer and roast until the internal temperature reaches 180°F. Be sure thermometer is inserted into the thickest part of the meat and is not touching a bone. If chicken is not browning to your liking, roast uncovered for the last 15–30 minutes.

   OR

   Insert bird into appropriate size Reynolds Oven Roasting Bag. I follow the directions that come with the bags except I do not shake flour in the empty bag but I do add 1–2 cups of water. Do not forget to make six 1/2-inch slits in top of bag.
3. After the meal, strain leftover broth through fine-meshed strainer and chill. After chilling, remove the fat that is solid on the top. Also, after the meal, I usually remove remaining cooked meat from the bones. Then simmer the carcass in a small amount of salted water until excess chicken is so tender that it falls off the bones. Add this broth to the broth that you got from roasting. Measure broth and add more water if needed to yield 3 cups of broth for a 3–4 pound fryer and 6–7 cups of broth for roasting hen. Finally, measure out and freeze broth in 1 cup servings. This way the chicken broth is all ready for most recipes in this cookbook.

Chicken Broth

1. Simmer the neck, wings, and back pieces of a chicken fryer in 2 1/2 cups of water, 1/2 teaspoon of sea salt, and 1/4 teaspoon of vitamin C crystals (optional). Cook until chicken is tender and the water has reduced to approximately 1 cup of broth.
2. Chill the broth and cooked chicken separately. As the broth chills the fat will solidify on the top. Remove this fat and freeze the broth. Remove the cooked meat from bones and freeze in packages of 1/2 cup each so they are ready to use in several recipes in this cookbook.
3. Chicken broth can be used in many chicken recipes in this cookbook. The recipes using chicken broth are based on a yield of 1 cup of chicken broth for this recipe.

Country Fried Chicken and Rice Gravy

1	whole chicken fryer, 3–4 pound
1/2 cup	brown rice flour
1 tablespoon	sesame oil
to season	sea salt

Ingredients for the gravy:

2 cups	water
2 tablespoons	brown rice flour
1/4 teaspoon	sea salt

1. Cut up chicken and remove the skin.
2. Preheat electric skillet to 350°F. Add oil. This recipe was developed using a stainless steel electric skillet; others may require more oil.
3. Pat the chicken pieces dry and roll each piece in the flour. Place the chicken in hot skillet with the meaty side down. Sprinkle with salt as desired. Cover with a splatter screen (information on page 60). Brown the chicken for 8–10 minutes—the browner the chicken, the browner the gravy—but be careful not to dry the chicken out or burn it. Turn the chicken using tongs or spatula. A fork pierces the meat and allows the natural juices to escape. Cover with splatter screen and brown for another 8–10 minutes.
4. While the second side is browning, combine the gravy ingredients and blend with small whip or fork. After chicken is browned, add the gravy mixture to skillet. Loosen any stuck chicken pieces with a spatula. Cover with lid. Reduce heat to between simmer and 200°F. Simmer the chicken and gravy for 20–25 minutes. Check occasionally for cooking progress and to loosen any chicken that is sticking to pan.

Yield: 4 servings

Pheasant and Gravy

Prepare the same as Country Fried Chicken and Rice Gravy except in step 4. Transfer browned pheasant to shallow covered casserole dish(es). Add gravy mixture. Cover and bake at 350°F. for at least 1 hour or until tender. Also, I suggest you soak pheasant several hours or overnight in salt water to remove most of the wild game taste.

Chicken and Noodles

Prepare 2 recipes of Homemade Kamut® or Spelt Noodles (page 116). When cooking the noodles (step 7), add 1 pound of cooked ground chicken or 2 cups of cooked diced chicken which may be leftover from roasting a chicken.

Yield: approximately 6–7 cups

Kamut® Pizza Crust

Ingredients	5-inch	7-inch
Kamut® flour	1/4 cup	1/2 cup
baking soda	1/8 teaspoon	1/4 teaspoon
vitamin C crystals	1/16 rounded teaspoon	1/8 rounded teaspoon
sea salt	2 pinches	scant 1/8 teaspoon
water	scant 2 tablespoons	3 tablespoons + 1 teaspoon
sesame oil	1 1/2 teaspoons	1 tablespoon
pizza sauce	1/2 cup	3/4 cup

Ingredients	12-inch	10 x 14-inch
Kamut® flour	1 1/4 cups	1 1/2 cups
baking soda	5/8 teaspoon	3/4 teaspoon
vitamin C crystals	3/8 teaspoon	1/2 teaspoon
sea salt	scant 1/4 teaspoon	1/4 teaspoon
water	1/2 cup	2/3 cup
sesame oil	2 tablespoons + 1 1/2 teaspoons	3 tablespoons
pizza sauce	2 cups	2 1/2 cups

Spelt Pizza Crust

Ingredients	5-inch	7-inch
spelt flour	1/4 cup	1/2 cup
baking soda	1/8 teaspoon	1/4 teaspoon
vitamin C crystals	1/16 rounded teaspoon	1/8 rounded teaspoon
sea salt	2 pinches	scant 1/8 teaspoon
sesame oil	1 1/2 teaspoons	1 tablespoon
pizza sauce	1/2 cup	3/4 cup

Ingredients	12-inch	10 x 14-inch
spelt flour	1 1/4 cups	1 1/2 cups
baking soda	5/8 teaspoon	3/4 teaspoon
vitamin C crystals	3/8 teaspoon	1/2 teaspoon
sea salt	scant 1/4 teaspoon	1/4 teaspoon
water	1/3 cup + 1 tablespoon	1/2 cup
sesame oil	2 tablespoons + 1 1/2 teaspoons	3 tablespoons
pizza sauce	2 cups	2 1/2 cups

Combine the 5- and 7-inch pizza crust recipes to yield approximately a 10-inch pizza crust. 10 x 14-inch recipe can also be made into six 5-inch crusts.

1. Have your pizza sauce completely ready and warm.
2. Preheat oven to 350ºF.
3. Measure and place oil in center of stainless steel pizza pan or baking sheet. Set aside.

1/2 teaspoon for 5-inch
3/4 teaspoon for 7-inch
1 teaspoon for 10- and 12-inch
1 1/4 teaspoons for 10 x 14-inch

continued on next page

Kamut® and Spelt Pizza Crust(continued)

4. In mixing bowl, whisk together dry ingredients. Make a "well" in the center.
5. Add water and oil. Stir with rubber spatula, making sure all dry ingredients are moistened.
6. Using fingers, spread oil on pizza pan to within one inch of edge. Make sure hands are lightly coated with oil before beginning next step.
7. With your lightly oil coated fingers, touch dough. If dough seems a little too soft and is sticky to your fingers, you have probably added too much liquid, which is easy to do especially if making the small sizes. I suggest that you mix between 1 teaspoon and 1 tablespoon more flour into your dough before proceeding with the next step.
8. Transfer dough to pizza pan or baking sheet. Press dough out in a circular shape, maintaining even thickness and pressing out from the center in all directions. Push outer edge of dough circle up on outer edge of pizza pan to form crust edge, or create an edge if forming on flat surface. Dough should be about 3/8 inch thick. If dough appears thin in spots, press surrounding dough toward thin area to remedy.
9. Wash oil off of hands. Pour warm Chicken White Sauce for Pizza (page 128) onto crust and spread out to cover crust surface.

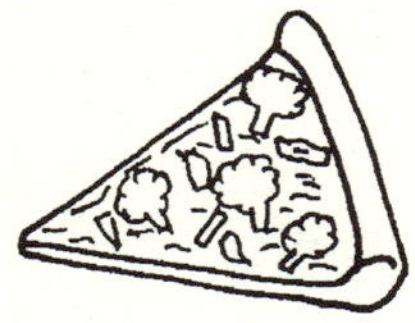

10. Bake at 350°F. for 20-25 minutes (see chart):

20 minutes for 5-inch or 7-inch pizza
25 minutes for 10-inch, 12-inch, or 10 x 14-inch pizza

Special Note: Be aware when measuring a tablespoon of water that it may tend to "round up" on the measuring spoon. Be sure to check that your tablespoon of water is a LEVEL tablespoon.

Recipe idea for Spelt Pizza Crust is from Mastering Food Allergies newsletter, May 1991.

> *For anything worth having*
> *one must pay the price;*
> *and the price is always*
> *work, patience, love, and*
> *self-sacrifice.*
>
> *John Burroughs*

Chicken White Sauce for Pizza*

2 cloves	garlic, minced*
1/2 teaspoon	sesame oil
1/2 pound	ground chicken or 1 1/4 cups of cooked diced chicken
2 1/2 cups	diced celery, chopped green cabbage, and/or broccoli cuts
1 cup	Chicken Broth, separated (page 124)
1/2 teaspoon	sea salt
1/2 teaspoon	basil*
3/4 teaspoon	leaf oregano*
1 tablespoon	hulled sesame seeds
3 tablespoons	flour—spelt or Kamut®

1. Sauté garlic in oil until soft in the same saucepan that you will use to prepare the sauce. Set aside until step 3.
2. In skillet, cook ground chicken. Stir often to chop meat and brown evenly. If needed, drain off fat.
3. While chicken is cooking, add to sautéed garlic the prepared vegetables, 3/4 cup of Chicken Broth, and seasonings. Steam for 3 minutes.
4. Combine 1/4 cup of Chicken Broth, sesame seeds, and flour in a blender. Blend on the highest speed for 1–2 minutes until well blended. Stop at least once to scrape sides. Add to cooked vegetable mixture and cook 1–2 minutes on medium to medium high until thickened. Stir almost constantly to prevent sticking.
5. Add cooked chicken and stir. Set aside to keep warm.
6. Pour and spread the warm sauce onto prepared crust. Bake according to crust recipe.

Yield: approximately 2 3/4 cups of sauce

*Realize these spices do break rotation but sometimes you need a little spice.

Baked Fish for Day 1

Your choice of Day 1 fish fillets	halibut, sole, fresh tuna
Your choice of Day 1 seasonings	dill weed, ground cumin
Your choice of Day 1 foods	sliced celery, sliced water chestnuts, bamboo shoots, almonds, pecans, and/or sesame seeds
Your choice of Day 1 oil	sesame or almond oil

Place fish fillets in covered casserole dish. Sprinkle with salt and seasonings. Garnish with your choice of other foods. Drizzle with approximately 1/2 teaspoon of oil per serving. Also, I usually add 1–2 tablespoons of water to casserole dish. Cover and bake for 45 minutes at 350°F. until fish is flaky. Time will depend on thickness of fillet, whether fillet is frozen or thawed, and amount of other foods used. Garnish with fresh parsley and serve.

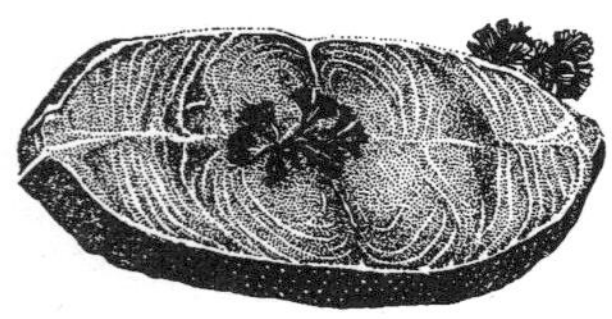

Yield: 1 pound of fish equals 3–4 servings

Grilled Fish for Day 1

Day 1 fish fillet for grilling	fresh tuna steak, halibut steak
Your choice of Day 1 seasonings	dill weed, ground cumin
Oil for Day 1	sesame oil

Baste both sides of fish fillet with small amount of oil. Sprinkle both sides of fish fillet with salt and your choice of seasonings. Cook on small electric grill. Turn often to prevent burning. I use a grill which has a thermostat control for better temperature regulation which is especially needed for fish. Grill until fish is flaky. Garnish with fresh parsley and serve.

Yield: 1 pound of fish equals 3–4 servings

Chicken Spaghetti*

2 cloves	garlic, minced*
1/2 teaspoon	sesame oil
2 1/2 cups	your choice of Day 1 vegetables I prefer: 1 cup cabbage, chopped 1 cup broccoli cuts, fresh or frozen 1/2 cup celery, diced
as desired	spaghetti—Kamut®, rice, or spelt OR Kamut® angel hair
1/2 cup	cooked chicken, diced
1 cup	Chicken Broth (page 124)
1/4 teaspoon	sea salt
1/4 teaspoon	basil*
1/2 teaspoon	leaf oregano*
1/4 cup	water
1 tablespoon	hulled sesame seeds
2 tablespoons	flour—spelt, rice, or Kamut®

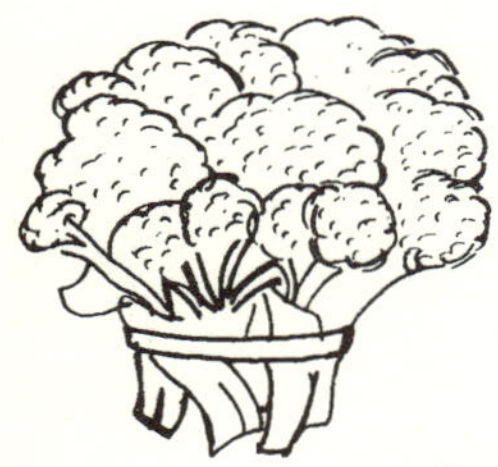

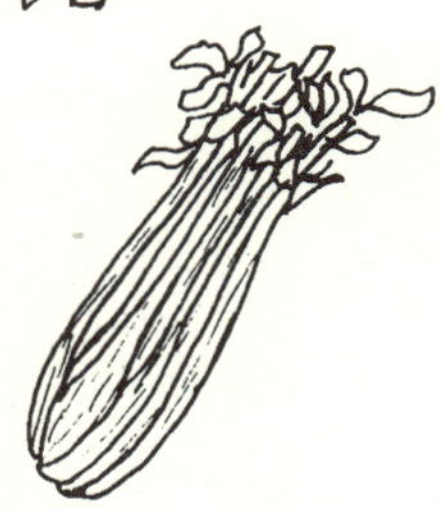

1. Sauté garlic in oil until soft. I prefer to use the same saucepan that I will be using to prepare the sauce. Set aside until ready for step 4.
2. In large saucepan, cook broken spaghetti or angel hair in salted, boiling water for 8–10 minutes until tender. See directions on package. Stir occasionally to prevent sticking.
3. While spaghetti is cooking, add to the sautéed garlic the prepared vegetables, chicken, broth, salt, and seasonings. Steam for 3–5 minutes. I prefer my vegetables a little crisp but do note that you will be cooking them a little more in step 4.
4. Combine water, sesame seeds, and flour in blender. Blend on highest speed for 1–2 minutes until well blended. Stop at least once to scrape sides. Add to cooked vegetable mixture and cook 1–2 minutes on medium to medium high until thickened and vegetables are cooked as you prefer them. Stir almost constantly to prevent sticking.
5. Drain tender spaghetti and serve immediately, pouring sauce over cooked spaghetti.

Yield: approximately 2 1/2 cups of sauce

*Realize these spices do break rotation but sometimes you need a little spice in your life.

Chicken Rice Loaf

1 pound	ground chicken
2/3 cup	cooked brown rice
1/2 cup	celery, chopped
1/4 cup	water
1/2 teaspoon	sea salt

Chicken Kamut® or Spelt Loaf

1 pound	ground chicken
1/2 cup	Kamut® or spelt flakes
1/2 cup	celery, chopped
1/2 cup	water
1/2 teaspoon	sea salt

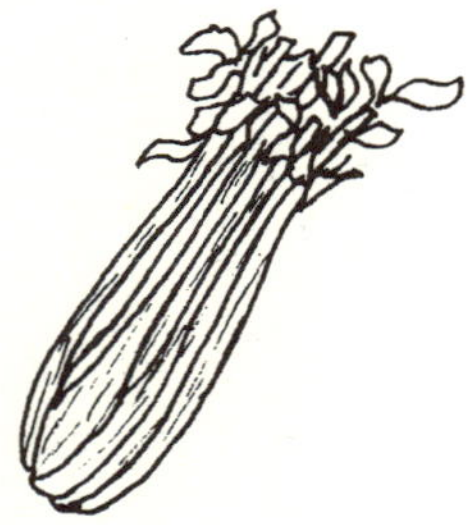

1. In large mixing bowl, combine your choice of ingredients thoroughly. I prefer to mix with my hands while wearing disposable plastic gloves.
2. Shape meat mixture in 9 x 5-inch loaf pan, 9 muffin cups (1/3 cup of meat mixture per muffin cup), or 6 custard cups (1/2 cup of meat mixture per custard cup).
3. Bake at 350°F. for 50–60 minutes in loaf pan, 20–25 minutes in muffin pans, or 35–45 minutes in custard cups.

If you wish, ingredients may be mixed early in the day and stored in refrigerator to be cooked for evening meal.

Yield: 4 servings

Chicken Noodle Casseroles

(Three Variations)

	With More Vegetables	With Extra Vegetables	
2	2	2	SERVINGS
3 cups	4 cups	5 1/2 cups	YIELD
1/2 pound	1/2 pound	1/2 pound	ground chicken
1/4 teaspoon	1/4 teaspoon	1/4 teaspoon	sea salt
1 1/3 cups	1 1/3 cups	1 1/3 cups	Vita-Spelt dry noodles, loosely packed OR Kamut® rotini, loosely packed
1/2 cup	2 cups	4 cups	total measure of vegetables: your choice of diced celery (leaves may be included), fresh or frozen broccoli cuts, and/or chopped cabbage
none	5/8 cup	1 1/4 cups	water (5/8 cup = 1/2 cup + 2 Tbsp.)
1 cup	1 cup	1 cup	Chicken Broth (page 124)
2 tablespoons	3 tablespoons	1/4 cup	hulled sesame seeds
2 tablespoons	3 tablespoons	1/4 cup	flour—spelt or Kamut®
1/4 teaspoon	3/8 teaspoon	1/2 teaspoon	sea salt (3/8 tsp. = 1/4 tsp. + 1/8 tsp.)

continued on next page

Chicken Noodle Casseroles (continued)

1. Oven temperature—350°F. Preheating not necessary.
2. Combine ground chicken with first measurement of salt in a skillet. Cook until meat is done, stir often to chop meat and brown evenly. If needed, drain off fat. Transfer to covered casserole dish(es).
3. In a saucepan of boiling salted water, cook noodles for only 4 minutes or Kamut® rotini for only 8 minutes. Stir occasionally. Drain and add to casserole dish(es).
4. Add vegetables to casserole dish(es), stir gently.
5. Combine approximately 1/4 cup of liquid, sesame seeds, flour, and salt in blender. Blend on highest speed for 1–2 minutes until well blended. Stop at least once to scrape sides. Add rest of the liquids and blend a couple of seconds more.
6. Pour liquid mixture over ingredients in casserole dish(es). Lightly push any floating ingredients down into the mixture. Cover. Bake 45–60 minutes or until vegetables are tender. Casserole may be mixed earlier in the day and refrigerated until baking time.

Chicken Rice Casseroles

(Three Variations)

	With More Vegetables	With Extra Vegetables	
2	2	2	SERVINGS
3 cups	4 cups	5 1/2 cups	YIELD
1/2 pound	1/2 pound	1/2 pound	ground chicken
1/4 teaspoon	1/4 teaspoon	1/4 teaspoon	sea salt
1 cup	1 cup	1 cup	cooked rice
1/2 cup	2 cups	4 cups	total measure of vegetables: your choice of diced celery (leaves may be included), fresh or frozen broccoli cuts, and/or chopped cabbage
none	5/8 cup	1 1/4 cups	water (5/8 cup = 1/2 cup + 2 Tbsp.)
1 cup	1 cup	1 cup	Chicken Broth (page 124)
2 tablespoons	3 tablespoons	1/4 cup	hulled sesame seeds
2 tablespoons	3 tablespoons	1/4 cup	brown rice flour
1/4 teaspoon	3/8 teaspoon	1/2 teaspoon	sea salt (3/8 tsp. = 1/4 tsp. + 1/8 tsp.)

1. Oven temperature—350°F. Preheating not necessary.
2. Combine ground chicken with first measurement of salt in a skillet. Cook until meat is done, stir often to chop meat and brown evenly. If needed, drain off fat. Transfer to covered casserole dish(es).
3. Add rice and vegetables to casserole dish(es), stir gently.
4. Combine approximately 1/4 cup of liquid, sesame seeds, flour, and salt in blender. Blend on highest speed for 1–2 minutes until well blended. Stop at least once to scrape sides. Add rest of the liquids and blend a couple of seconds more.
5. Pour liquid mixture over ingredients in casserole dish(es). Lightly push any floating ingredients down into the mixture. Cover. Bake 45–60 minutes or until vegetables are tender. Casserole may be mixed earlier in the day and refrigerated until baking time.

Oven Fried Chicken
(Several Variations)

Flour Breaded Chicken

1/4 cup	flour—brown teff, brown rice, Kamut®, or spelt
1/2 teaspoon	sea salt
1/4 teaspoon	dill weed (optional)
8 pieces	chicken, skin removed
as needed	sesame oil

Cracker Breaded Chicken

3/4 cup	Kamut® or Spelt Cracker crumbs (page 112)
3/8 teaspoon	sea salt
1/4 teaspoon	dill weed (optional)
8 pieces	chicken, skin removed

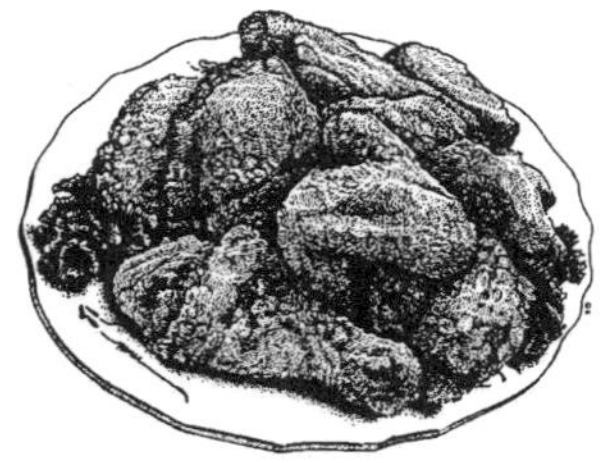

1. Preheat oven to 450°F.
2. Oil baking dish(es). I prefer an uncovered stainless steel roasting pan with flat rack. However, a 9x13-inch baking dish will do fine.
3. Cut up chicken and remove skin. Rinse. Drain and pat dry leaving the chicken a little moist.
4. In a bowl, combine your choice of flour or cracker crumbs and seasonings. Add a small amount (approximately 1–2 tablespoons) to a small bowl with a lid that seals, such as a Tupperware bowl.
5. Add 1 piece of chicken to bowl. Seal. Shake to coat. Place in baking dish bone side down. Repeat for each piece. Add more flour or cracker mixture to bowl as needed.
6. Put into oven and reduce heat to 400°F. Bake for approximately 50 minutes until internal temperature is 180°F.

Special Note: The chicken will be crispier on all sides if you cook the chicken on a wire rack. If you choose this method, you may desire to baste a small about of oil (1/4 teaspoon or less per piece of chicken) on flour breaded chicken variation midway through the baking time. When using a wire rack you do not need to oil the pan as described in step 2. In addition, for crispier chicken increase oven temperature to 450°F. for final 10 minutes of baking time.

Batter Fried Chicken

1 1/3 cups	flour—spelt, Kamut®, brown rice, or brown teff (some variations may need more flour, see step 4)
1 teaspoon	sea salt
1/2 teaspoon	dill weed (optional)
1 cup	cold water
1/4 cup	sesame oil
8 pieces	chicken (cold), skin removed

Follow steps 1–3 from flour and cracker breaded chicken recipe except dry chicken pieces thoroughly.

4. Combine your choice of flour, salt, and dill weed in a chilled glass bowl. Add cold water and oil. Mix to make a thick batter. If needed, add more flour in small amounts and mix after each addition. The key is to make the batter cohesive (stick to itself) rather than adhesive (stick to the bowl).

continued on next page

Oven Fried Chicken (continued)

5. Dip each chicken piece into batter. Place in prepared baking dish bone side down. Attempt to do this quickly and to touch the chicken as little as possible. The batter and chicken needs to stay cold in order for the batter to stick to the chicken.

6. Put into oven and reduce heat to 400°F. Bake for approximately 50 minutes until internal temperature is 180°F.

Yield: 8 pieces of chicken

Special Note: The taller the sides on the baking dish the less likely the chicken is to splatter in oven. I also remove the top rack in oven. For easier clean up, soak pan in warm, soapy water while eating.

My favorite of all these variations is brown teff flour breaded chicken which is also one of the easiest to prepare. If you desire to prepare less than 8 pieces of chicken, simply use the amount of flour or cracker mixture that you need and freeze the rest for the next time.

Laughter is the sun that drives winter from the human face.
Victor Hugo

True enjoyment comes from activity of the mind and exercise of the body; the two are ever united.
Humboldt

Chicken Cabbage Rolls

1/2 pound	ground chicken
1 cup	celery, diced
1/4 teaspoon	sea salt
1 cup	cooked brown rice
2 cups	Chicken Broth (page 124)
2 tablespoons	hulled sesame seeds
1/4 cup	brown rice flour
1/4 teaspoon	sea salt
4–6	medium-size cabbage leaves

Oven temperature—350°F. Preheating not necessary. Since this recipe takes so long to prepare and you may do this recipe in separate stages during the day as I do. I suggest that you turn on the oven when you are ready to bake the cabbage rolls.

1. Combine ground chicken, celery, and salt in skillet. Cook until meat is done, stir often to chop meat and brown evenly. If needed, drain off fat. Add cooked rice, stir, and set aside.

2. While meat and celery are cooking, boil 2 cups of Chicken Broth to make a concentrated broth of 1 1/2 cups. Then combine approximately 1/4 cup of the concentrated Chicken Broth, sesame seeds, flour and the second measure of salt in a blender. Blend on highest speed for 1–2 minutes until well blended. Stop at least once to scrap sides. Add the remainder of concentrated Chicken Broth and blend a couple of seconds more. Pour mixture into saucepan that you used to boil the broth. Heat slowly on low until thickened, stirring often. (I prefer to stir with a whisk to keep the mixture smooth.)

3. When finished with steps 1 and 2, remove both from heat. Add 2/3 cup of thickened white sauce to meat mixture, stir, and set aside. This amount of sauce should be enough just to moisten and help hold the meat mixture together. The meat mixture yields approximately 2 1/4 cups. Reserve the rest of the thickened sauce for later.

4. Heat a large kettle of salted water until boiling.

5. Remove cabbage leaves from head. I have found the easiest way to do this is to cut each leaf, one at a time, from the center core and carefully remove leaf beginning from core end. You may need to loosen parts of each leaf from other leaves. Wash leaves and remove any bad places. The amount of leaves needed will vary depending on the size of the leaves. I usually need at least 4–6 medium-size leaves.

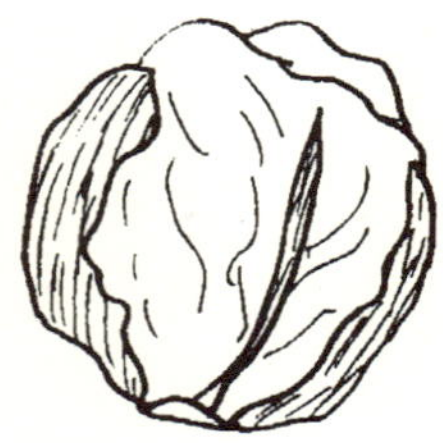

6. Add cabbage leaves to the boiling water and boil for 3–4 minutes to slightly cook leaves and to soften the core. I usually turn the range down to medium high to cook the leaves.

7. Remove leaves from water by grasping core end with tongs and allowing leaf to drip slightly before placing in colander to drain. Cool at least long enough that leaves can be handled. I usually leave my water in the pan and keep it hot just in case I need to boil more leaves.

continued on next page

Chicken Cabbage Rolls (continued)

8. To stuff each leaf, lay cooled cabbage leaf on a large plate so that the curled edges are up and the core end is toward you. Spoon desired amount of thickened meat mixture (1/3–1/2 cup) onto the cabbage leaf at least 1 inch from core or near the widest part of leaf. Spread mixture in an even log shape across center of leaf. Fold core on top of meat mixture then roll away from you to edge of leaf. Repeat stuffing process to use all of the meat mixture.

9. Lay each stuffed leaf in a shallow baking dish which has a lid. I use my 10-inch square Corning casserole dish. You may place the cabbage rolls close together.

10. Pour reserved thickened white sauce evenly over all cabbage rolls. Cover. Bake for 20–25 minutes until sauce bubbles and begins to turn golden brown around edges. (If ingredients are room temperature or colder at start, you may need to allow the casserole to bake for 30–35 minutes.) Serve immediately, use 2 metal spatulas to lift and remove cabbage rolls from dish to individual plates.

Special Note: Although this dish does take a while to prepare and you need to plan in advance to have leftover cooked rice and chicken broth, the wonderful flavor is well worth the effort. In addition, double this recipe for an excellent meal for company since you can prepare the entire dish up to the baking stage and then refrigerate. Another advantage is that you can wash up the pans and clean up your kitchen so you only have a little cleanup after the meal. Also, I have frozen this meal for a later quick meal. To freeze and reheat, I suggest that you freeze the stuffed cabbage rolls on a baking sheet until frozen solid, then transfer the frozen rolls to a cellophane bag. Freeze the extra prepared white sauce in a separate glass container. Thaw the cabbage rolls in the baking dish, spread with the thawed white sauce and bake as before. What a wonderful meal to enjoy on a lazy day!

Yield: makes a complete meal for two

*There are two ways
of meeting difficulties:
you alter the difficulties
or you alter yourself
meeting them.*
Phyllis Bottome

Tuna Noodle Casseroles
(Three Variations)

	With More Vegetables	With Extra Vegetables	
2	2	2	SERVINGS
3 cups	4 cups	5 1/2 cups	YIELD
1 1/3 cups	1 1/3 cups	1 1/3 cups	Vita-Spelt dry noodles, loosely packed OR Kamut® rotini, loosely packed
1/2 cup	2 cups	4 cups	total measure of vegetables: your choice of diced celery (leaves may be included), fresh or frozen broccoli cuts, and/or chopped cabbage
1 jar	1 jar	1 jar	Chuck's Seafood tuna, flaked (7 1/2 oz.)
1 cup	1 5/8 cups	2 1/4 cups	water (5/8 cup = 1/2 cup + 2 Tbsp.)
2 tablespoons	3 tablespoons	1/4 cup	hulled sesame seeds
2 tablespoons	3 tablespoons	1/4 cup	flour—spelt or Kamut®
1/4 teaspoon	3/8 teaspoon	1/2 teaspoon	sea salt (3/8 tsp. = 1/4 tsp. + 1/8 tsp.)

1. Oven temperature—350°F. Preheating not necessary.
2. In a saucepan of boiling salted water, cook noodles for only 4 minutes or Kamut® rotini for only 8 minutes. Stir occasionally. Drain and add to casserole dish(es).
3. Add vegetables and tuna to casserole dish(es), stir gently.
4. Combine approximately 1/4 cup of water, sesame seeds, flour, and salt in blender. Blend on highest speed for 1–2 minutes until well blended. Stop at least once to scrape sides. Add rest of water and blend a couple of seconds more.
5. Pour liquid mixture over ingredients in casserole dish(es). Lightly push any floating ingredients down into the mixture. Cover. Bake 40–60 minutes or until vegetables are tender. Casserole may be mixed earlier in the day and refrigerated until baking time.

Tuna Rice Casseroles
(Three Variations)

	With More Vegetables	With Extra Vegetables	
2	2	2	SERVINGS
3 cups	4 cups	5 1/2 cups	YIELD
1 cup	1 cup	1 cup	cooked rice
1/2 cup	2 cups	4 cups	total measure of vegetables: your choice of diced celery (leaves may be included), fresh or frozen broccoli cuts, and/or chopped cabbage
1 jar	1 jar	1 jar	Chuck's Seafood tuna, flaked (7 1/2 oz.)
1 cup	1 5/8 cups	2 1/4 cups	water (5/8 cup = 1/2 cup + 2 Tbsp.)
2 tablespoons	3 tablespoons	1/4 cup	hulled sesame seeds
2 tablespoons	3 tablespoons	1/4 cup	brown rice flour
3/8 teaspoon	1/2 teaspoon	3/4 teaspoon	sea salt (3/8 tsp. = 1/4 tsp. + 1/8 tsp.)

continued on next page

Tuna Rice Casseroles (continued)

1. Oven temperature—350°F. Preheating not necessary.
2. Combine rice, vegetables, and tuna in covered casserole dish(es).
3. Combine approximately 1/4 cup of water, sesame seeds, flour, and salt in blender. Blend on highest speed for 1–2 minutes until well blended. Stop at least once to scrape sides. Add the rest of the water and blend a couple of seconds more.
4. Pour liquid mixture over ingredients in casserole dish(es). Lightly push any floating ingredients down into the mixture. Cover. Bake 45–60 minutes or until vegetables are tender. Casserole may be mixed earlier in the day and refrigerated until baking time.

Tuna Cabbage Rolls

1 jar	Chuck's Seafood albacore tuna, flaked (7 1/2 ounces)
1 cup	celery, diced
1 cup	cooked brown rice
1/8 teaspoon	sea salt
1 1/2 cups	liquid (tuna broth, celery broth, and water)
2 tablespoons	sesame seeds
1/4 cup	brown rice flour
1/4 teaspoon	sea salt
4–6	medium-size cabbage leaves

1. Drain tuna, reserving the broth in a 2-cup liquid measure. Steam celery in medium-size saucepan for 3–5 minutes, only to partially cook. Drain over the 2-cup liquid measure to reserve the broth.
2. Add water to reserved tuna and celery broth to yield 1 1/2 cups. Combine 1/4 cup of this liquid, sesame seeds, rice flour, and the second measure of salt in blender. Blend on highest speed for 1–2 minutes until well blended. Stop at least once to scrape sides. Add remainder of the liquid and blend a couple of seconds more. Pour mixture into saucepan that you used to steam celery. Heat slowly on low until thickened, stirring often. (I prefer to stir with a whisk to keep the mixture smooth.) Remove from heat.
3. Remove 7/8 cup (2 tablespoons less than 1 cup) of white sauce from saucepan and reserve for later. Add tuna (flake it as you add it), celery, rice, and the first measure of salt to saucepan, stir, and set aside. Tuna mixture yields approximately 2 1/2 cups.

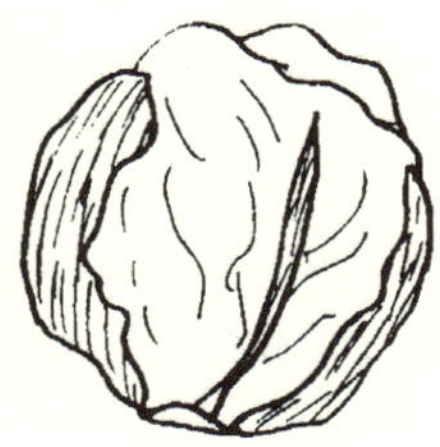

Continue recipe the same as Chicken Cabbage Rolls (page 134) starting with step 4. However, allow 30–35 minutes baking time since the filling is not hot.

Tuna Rice Dinner

1/2 cup	brown rice, long-grain, short-grain, or basmati
1 1/2 cups	water
1/2 teaspoon	sea salt
1 jar	Chuck's Seafood Tuna, flaked, 7 1/2 ounce
4 cups	Day 1 vegetables I prefer 2 cups each broccoli and cabbage.

1. Wash rice (page 36). Add rice, salt, and tuna to a 2 1/2 quart saucepan. Do not stir. Cover. Bring to boil. Reduce heat to allow food to simmer for 35 minutes or until rice is almost tender. Do not peek during cooking time.
2. Carefully add vegetables so as not to disturb the steam pockets formed by the cooking rice. Continue to cook for approximately 15 minutes until vegetables and rice are tender. Stir and serve.

Yield: 5 cups

Breakfast Brunch Squares*

2 3/4 cups	your choice of bread, cubed
	French Meadow brand yeast-free, organic, 100% spelt bread
	Spelt Yeast-Free Bread (page 110)
	Kamut® Yeast-Free Bread (page 110)
	"Ener-G" brand yeast-free, brown rice bread*
2 cups	broccoli cuts, fresh or frozen
1/4 cup	hulled sesame seeds
1/4 cup	brown rice flour
3/4 teaspoon	sea salt
1 cup	water
4	eggs

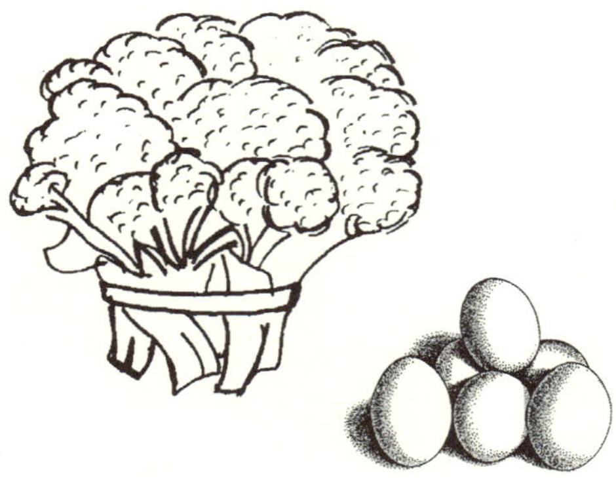

1. Preheat oven to 350°F.
2. Oil the bottom and sides of an 8-inch stainless steel square baking pan with approximately 1 teaspoon of sesame oil. I do not recommend glass because this dish tends to stick in a glass baking dish.
3. Evenly layer cubed bread and broccoli cuts in the prepared pan.
4. Combine sesame seeds, flour, and salt with approximately 1/3 cup of the water in a blender. Blend on highest speed for 1–2 minutes until well blended. Stop at least once to scrap sides. Add the remaining water and eggs and blend on low speed only a couple of seconds more. Pour liquid mixture evenly over broccoli and bread cubes. Lightly push any floating broccoli or bread cubes down into the mixture.
5. Bake for 45–50 minutes or until egg mixture is set. Cut into squares and remove from pan with stiff metal spatula.

Yield: 4 servings

*Realize that the rice bread has a few ingredients that break rotation. I usually do not concern myself with this break since I only have this occasionally.

Sesame Goulash

1 pound	ground chicken
1/2 teaspoon	sea salt
1 cup	elbow macaroni—Kamut®, spelt, or rice
2 cups	cabbage, shredded
1 cup	celery, diced
1 cup	Chicken Broth (page 124)
1 2/3 cups	water
1/4 teaspoon	ground cumin
1/2 teaspoon	sea salt
1/4 cup	flour—Kamut®, spelt, or rice
1/4 cup	hulled sesame seeds
1/3 cup	water

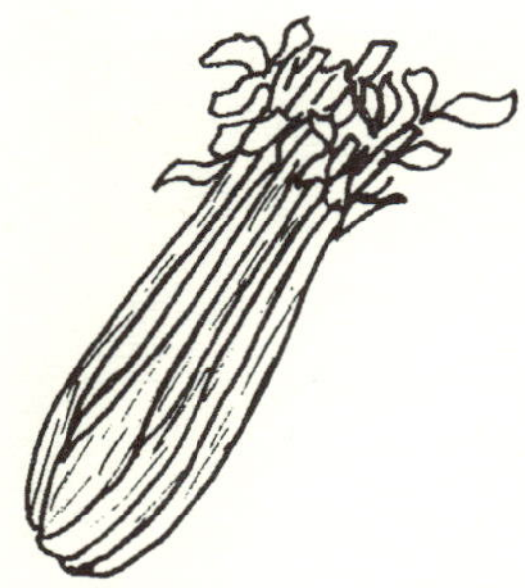

1. Combine ground chicken with first measurement of salt in a skillet. Cook until meat is done, stir often to chop meat and brown evenly. If needed, drain off fat.
2. Add macaroni, vegetables, broth, 1 2/3 cups of water, cumin, and second measurement of salt. Bring to boil. Reduce heat. Cover. Simmer 10–12 minutes or until macaroni and vegetables are tender.
3. While casserole is cooking, combine flour, sesame seeds, and 1/3 cup of water in blender. Blend on highest speed for 1–2 minutes until well blended. Stop at least once to scrape sides. Add to skillet and cook, stirring constantly until mixture thickens.

Yield: 6 cups, 4 servings

Stir-Fry Chicken

deboned chicken breast, cut into thin strips
broccoli cuts
cabbage, thinly sliced or shredded
celery, slant cut
sliced water chestnuts and/or bamboo shoots
almonds or pecans
sesame and/or almond oil
sea salt
dill weed

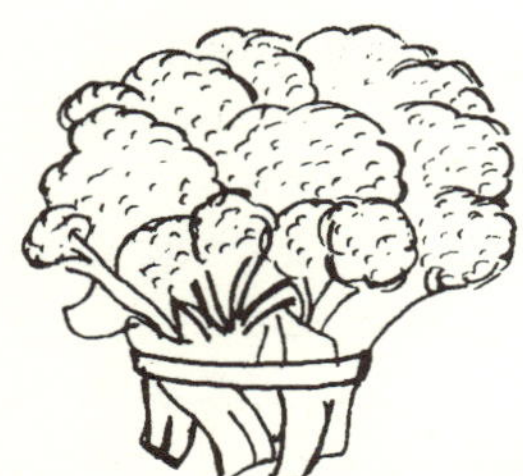

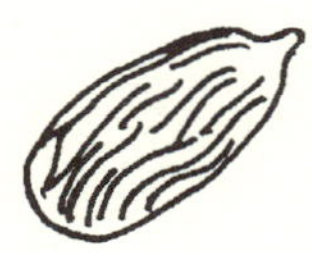

1. Preheat well-seasoned cast-iron skillet on medium (see How to Season Cast Iron on page 63) or electric skillet to 300°F. Add oil after preheating.
2. Prepare chicken and vegetables in amounts desired. Chicken will cut into strips easier if partially frozen.
3. Stir fry chicken, stirring often to brown evenly. When not stirring, cover with splatter screen (information on page 60).
4. Add vegetables and nuts. Sprinkle with seasonings. Stir often to cook chicken and vegetables evenly. I prefer my vegetables crunchy. Serve immediately with Basic Rice (page 117).

Yield: I usually allow 3 ounces of chicken, 2 cups of vegetables, and 1 teaspoon of oil per serving.

Almond "Mayo"

1/2 cup	raw, whole almonds
1 cup	water
1 teaspoon	unbuffered, corn-free vitamin C crystals
1 tablespoon	flour—Kamut®, spelt, or rice
1/4 teaspoon	sea salt
1/2 teaspoon	dry mustard (optional)

1. Blend almonds in blender on highest speed until they become a fine powder, approximately 1–2 minutes, stopping once or twice to scrape sides and bottom of blender jar. Be careful not to create an almond butter.
2. Add rest of the ingredients. Blend on highest speed for a minute longer, stopping once or twice to scrape sides and bottom of blender jar.
3. Pour mixture into small saucepan. Cook over medium heat, stirring constantly until mixture thickens. I prefer to stir with a whisk to keep mixture smooth.
4. Chill. If necessary, you may store in glass jar in refrigerator for a week. If too thick, you may add a tablespoon more water. Taste and add more dry mustard if you desire.

Yield: 1 1/3 cups

Recipe idea is from The Yeast Connection Cookbook by Crook and Jones, page 208.

Chicken or Tuna Vegetable Salad

1/2 cup	cooked macaroni—Kamut®, rice, or spelt OR cooked rice
1/2 cup	celery, diced
1 cup	broccoli, fresh, small bite-size cuts
1/2 jar	Chuck's Seafood albacore tuna, flaked (3 3/4 ounces) OR 1/2 cup of cooked chicken, diced
1/4 teaspoon	sea salt
few sprigs	fresh parsley, torn or cut into small pieces (optional)
1/2 cup	Almond "Mayo" (recipe above) OR 1/3 cup Cabbage-Sesame Salad Dressing (page 142)
as desired	Swiss chard

1. Cook macaroni in salted water until tender. Drain, rinse, and chill.
2. Prepare vegetables and dressing. In bowl, gently toss all ingredients except dressing and chard. Add dressing and mix to coat all ingredients. Chill.
3. Serve on a bed of Swiss chard leaves or tear leaves and mix into salad along with more dressing just before serving. Makes a complete meal, but I also enjoy the salad with crackers.

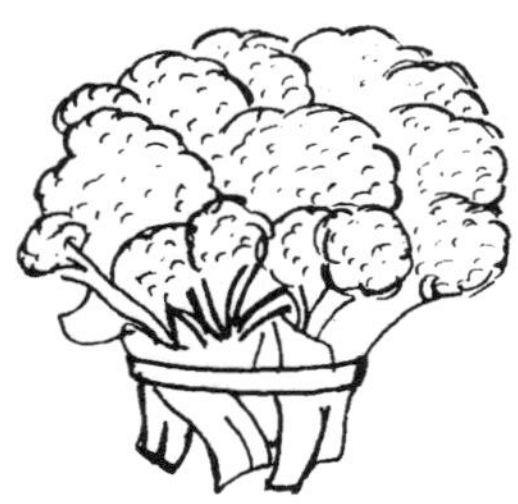

Special Note: Rice macaroni does not have as much flavor as the other listed pasta, so I usually add a little extra dry mustard to Almond "Mayo" before adding to salad.

Yield: 3 cups, serves 1

Coleslaw

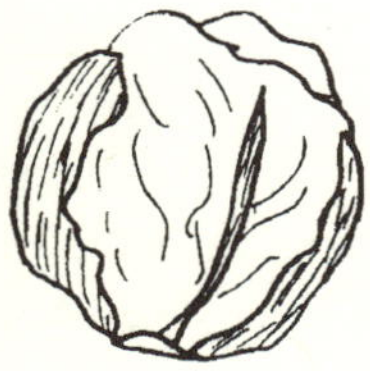

1 cup	cabbage, shredded or finely chopped
1/4 cup	celery, diced
1/4 cup	Almond "Mayo" (page 140)
as desired	sea salt

Combine and chill.

Yield: 1 cup

Tuna Salad

1/2 jar	Chuck's Seafood albacore tuna, flaked. (3 3/4 ounces)
1/3 cup	celery, diced
few sprigs	fresh parsley, torn or cut into small pieces (optional)
3 tablespoons	Almond "Mayo" (page 140)
to taste	sea salt

Combine and chill. Serve on bed of Swiss chard as a salad or as my favorite, a sandwich on a Day 1 tortilla with Swiss chard. Makes enough for 2 tortillas.

Yield: 3/4 cup

Tuna/Egg Salad

Add to the above recipe: 1 diced hard boiled egg and an extra tablespoon of dressing. Serve as above.

Yield: 1 cup

Egg Salad

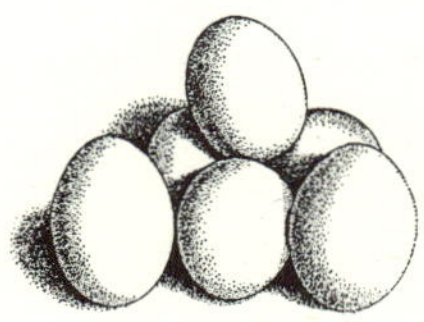

2	eggs, hard boiled, diced
1/3 cup	celery, diced
few sprigs	fresh parsley, torn or cut into small pieces (optional)
2 tablespoons	Almond "Mayo" (page 140)
to taste	sea salt

Prepare and serve as described in Tuna Salad (recipe above).

Yield: 1 cup

Chicken Salad

1/2 cup	cooked chicken, diced
1	egg, hard boiled, diced
1/3 cup	celery, diced
few sprigs	fresh parsley, torn or cut into small pieces (optional)
3 tablespoons	Almond "Mayo" (page 140)
to taste	sea salt

Prepare and serve as described in Tuna Salad (recipe above).

Yield: 1 cup

Cabbage-Sesame Salad Dressing

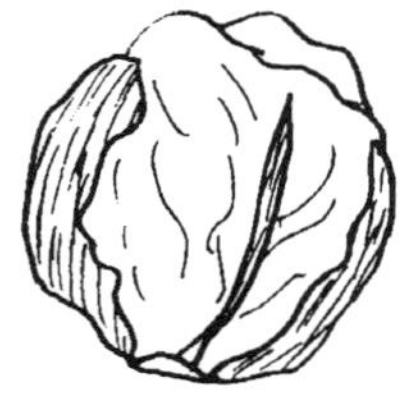

1/3 cup	cabbage, chopped small, packed
1/4 cup	water
1 1/2 teaspoons	sesame oil
1/4 teaspoon	unbuffered, corn-free vitamin C crystals
pinch	sea salt
1/4 teaspoon	dry mustard
1/2 teaspoon	hulled sesame seeds (optional)

1. Combine all ingredients, except sesame seeds, in blender. Blend on highest speed for 1–2 minutes until smooth, stopping once or twice to scrape sides and bottom of blender jar.
2. Add sesame seeds and stir. Chill. I do not prepare this dressing in advance because if it is stored longer than 1 day the taste turns sour.

Yield: 1/3 cup

Broccoli Cuts

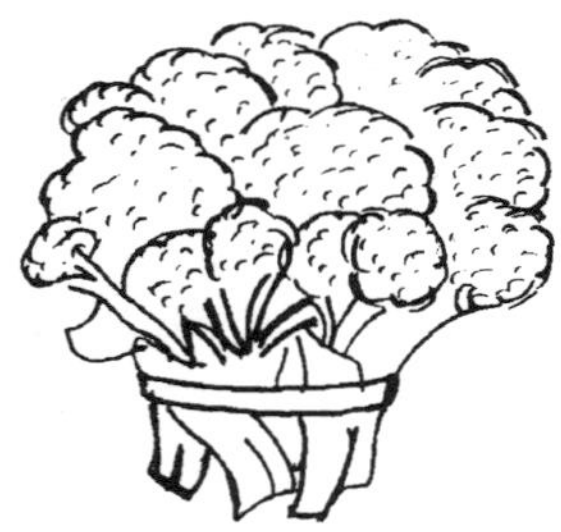

Use this method to prepare fresh broccoli cuts or spears for casseroles, stir fry, or as vegetable side dish.

Cut off florets part of broccoli. Remove leaves from stalk and floret portion. Peel stalk portion with vegetable peeler or paring knife to remove the fibrous outer bark. This outer bark is a little darker green and you can see the fibers in this woody covering. The inner tender stalk is lighter green and has a smooth, even texture. Cut stalk into medallion (disk) pieces. Cut floret portion into bite-size pieces. Soak pieces in salted water for 5 minutes to kill bugs. Drain, rinse again.

Broccoli Spears

Prepare as broccoli cuts except cut both stalk and floret portion into strips instead of medallion or bite-size pieces.

Stir-Fry Vegetables for Day 1

broccoli cuts
cabbage, thinly sliced or shredded
celery, slant cut
sliced water chestnuts and/or bamboo shoots
almonds or pecans
sesame and/or almond oil
sea salt
dill weed

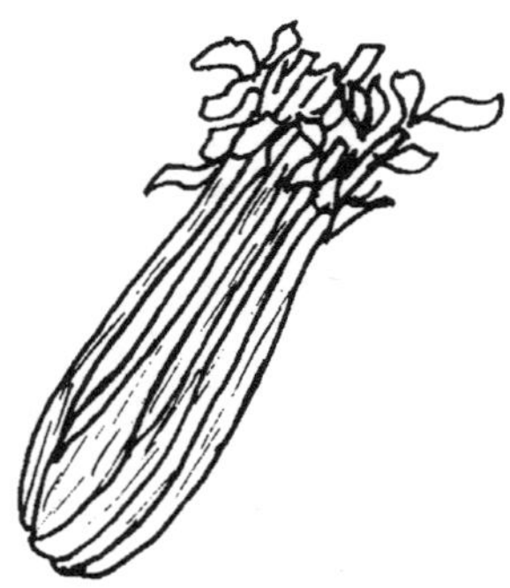

1. Preheat well-seasoned cast-iron skillet on medium (see How to Season Cast Iron on page 63) or electric skillet to 300°F.
2. Prepare vegetables in amounts desired.
3. Add oil to preheated skillet (cast-iron skillet will require less oil). Add vegetables and nuts. Sprinkle with seasonings. Stir often to cook vegetables evenly. I prefer my vegetables crunchy. Serve immediately.

Amazing Sugarless Cookies

1 cup	brown rice flour
1 teaspoon	baking soda
1/4 teaspoon	sea salt
1/4 teaspoon	unbuffered, corn-free vitamin C crystals
1 cup	whole raw almonds, chopped in food processor (optional)
1/3 cup	brown rice syrup
2 tablespoons	almond oil
1 teaspoon	alcohol-free almond extract (optional)
2/3 cup	almond butter*

1. Preheat oven to 350°F.
2. In a mixing bowl, whisk together dry ingredients and almonds.

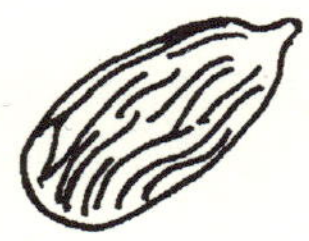

3. Measure out brown rice syrup in a glass measuring cup. Add oil and almond extract. Mix.
4. Add almond butter and rice syrup mixture to dry ingredients and mix thoroughly. Batter will be a little stiff and slightly sticky.
5. Roll dough into 1-inch balls. Place balls onto cookie sheet about 2 1/2 inches apart. Flatten each ball with a fork or the bottom of a drinking glass to approximately 1/4 inch thick and 2 inches in diameter. You will need to dip the fork or glass in water frequently to prevent cookies from sticking to it.
6. Bake cookies for 8–10 minutes. These cookies do not brown much except on the bottom. In fact, the baked cookie seems to be lighter in color than the raw batter. Cool cookies on cookie sheet just long enough to completely set up and successfully transfer easily to cooling rack. Leftover cookies freeze nicely in a wide-mouth pint glass canning jar.

Yield: 3 dozen (2 1/2 dozen if almonds are omitted)

Special Note: These have been named Amazing Sugarless Cookies because everyone who eats them is so amazed that they are sugar free. These cookies make a great hit at any social gathering.

*If you desire to use Almond Butter as prepared on page 146; you will need to add 2 tablespoons of water to rice syrup mixture. After mixing, if too much water seems to be added, you can stir in a little more flour.

Creamy Sweet Rice and Almonds*

1/2 cup	cooked rice
1/4 cup	Organic Original-Lite Rice Dream Beverage*
as desired	raw almonds, chopped

Combine in small saucepan, heat on low, stirring often. Serve warm for breakfast or dessert. Also, you may combine ingredients and just serve cold.

Yield: 1/2 cup

*Organic Original-Lite Rice Dream Beverage is made from organic brown rice with addition of safflower oil and sea salt. 1 cup has 130 calories. It may not be a good non-dairy beverage to consume in large amounts for people on a *Candida* control diet, especially those in the first 2–4 weeks of the diet. Also, the safflower oil does cause a break in rotation.

Teff Pear Cake

1 cup	brown teff flour
1 teaspoon	baking soda
1/4 teaspoon	sea salt
1/4 teaspoon	unbuffered, corn-free vitamin C crystals
1/2 cup	pear juice
1/4 cup	Pear Sauce (recipe below)
2 tablespoons	sesame oil

1. Preheat oven to 400ºF.
2. Oil and flour the bottom and sides of a 9-inch pie pan.
3. In mixing bowl, whisk together dry ingredients. Add pear juice and sauce and oil. Stir just to moisten the dry ingredients.
4. Transfer to prepared pan. Spread evenly. Bake 20 minutes. Cool slightly. Cut into 8 wedges. I prefer to serve this warm with additional heated Pear Sauce.

Yield: 8 servings

Pear Sauce Method 1

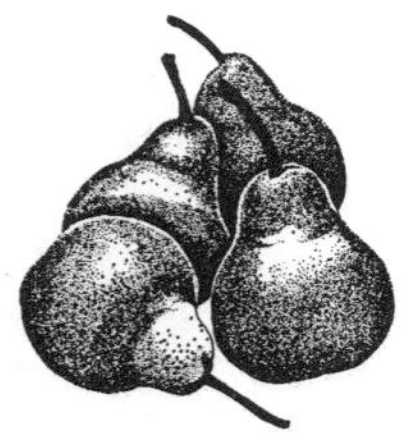

1. Wash fresh, ripe fruit (be careful not to over ripen). Peel, core, rinse, and drain.
2. Run fruit through Champion Juicer set up for homogenizing This will make the sauce very quickly.
3. To prevent fruit from darkening, add approximately 1/4 teaspoon unbuffered, corn-free vitamin C crystals to 8 cups of pear sauce. It is best to add the vitamin C before the fruit begins to darken. I find it works best to add the vitamin C crystals to about the first 2 cups of homogenized fruit. Then as you continue the process, stir after each addition. Add more vitamin C if needed.

Pear Sauce Method 2

1. Wash fresh, ripe fruit (be careful not to over ripen). Peel, core, rinse, and drain.
2. Transfer to a saucepan. To prevent fruit from darkening, add unbuffered, corn-free vitamin C crystals, approximately 1/2 teaspoon for 8–10 cups of pear quarters. It is best to add the vitamin C before the fruit begins to darken so I suggest that you stir in the crystals when you have about 2 cups of quarters ready to cook. Then as you continue the process, stir the pear quarters after each addition. Add more vitamin C crystals if needed. Cook on low until soft. Stir often to prevent sticking. It's not necessary to add additional water to the fruit before cooking since it will create its own juice as it cooks.
3. Blend in blender or press through a canning sieve or food mill.

Yield: 25 pounds of pears yields approximately 7 quarts of Pear Sauce

Tips on Freezing Pear Sauce

An easy way to freeze the sauce for later use is to freeze in ice cube trays, approximately 1 tablespoon per cube. After the sauce is frozen, remove from the trays and keep frozen in a cellophane bag until ready to use.

Pear Sauce Sweetener

After preparing Pear Sauce, transfer to saucepan, cover with splatter screen, and cook on medium to thicken. My recipes are developed with the ratio of 1 cup of Pear Sauce cooked down to yield 2/3 cup of Pear Sauce Sweetener. Stir often to prevent sticking, especially at the end of the process. Also, towards the end you will need to reduce the heat to at least low. I usually cook 16 cups of Pear Sauce in a large Dutch-oven kettle to yield 10 2/3 cups. Then I freeze the Pear Sauce Sweetener in glass jars in portions needed for my recipes. The sauce will darken a little as it becomes thicker.

Almond-Sesame Granola Bars

2 cups	quick-cooking spelt or Kamut® flakes*
1/4 cup	almonds or pecans
2 tablespoons	hulled sesame seeds
1/2 teaspoon	sea salt
2/3 cup	Pear Sauce Sweetener (recipe above)
2 tablespoons	almond or sesame oil
1 teaspoon	alcohol-free almond extract (optional)

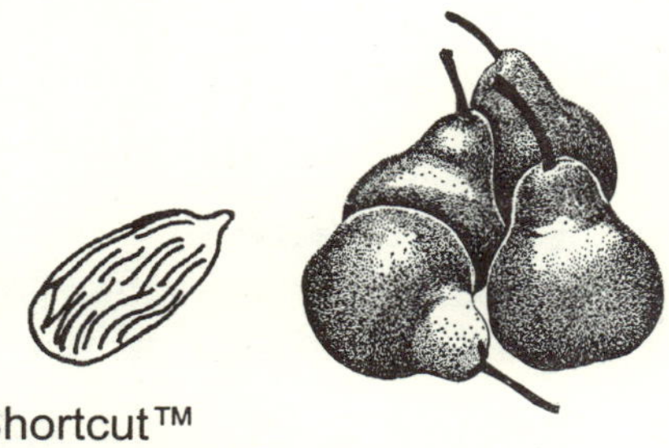

1. Preheat oven to 350°F.
2. Oil an 8-inch square baking pan with approximately 1/2 teaspoon oil.
3. Pour flakes into chopper cup of Black & Decker® Handy Shortcut™ food processor (the cup holds 2 cups). Chop for 10 seconds. Stop, stir with knife or handle of spoon. Chop for 5 seconds more. The flakes should be just coarsely chopped. Pour into mixing bowl.
4. Place nuts in chopper and chop for approximately 20 seconds or longer to desired size.
5. Add chopped nuts, salt, and sesame seeds to mixing bowl. Toss to distribute ingredients evenly.
6. Combine together Pear Sauce Sweetener, oil, and extract. Pour evenly over flake mixture. Mix thoroughly with rubber spatula to evenly coat flake mixture with liquids.
7. Transfer to prepared pan and spread evenly. Press mixture firmly in pan with metal spatula or with hands, pressing one on top of the other.
8. Bake 25 minutes. Cool completely. Cut 4x2. Enjoy for breakfast, dessert, or snack. Leftovers can be frozen. I individually bag them in cellophane bags. No need to thaw, you can just unwrap and enjoy. These granola bars do crumble a little, but for the most part they hold together.

Yield: 8 servings

*This recipe was developed using the quicker-cooking brands of spelt or Kamut® flakes, e.g., Country Grown brand.

Pear Custard*

1/4 cup	almonds
2/3 cup	water
2	eggs
1/4 teaspoon	sea salt
2/3 cup	pear juice
1/2 teaspoon	alcohol-free almond extract
sprinkle	cinnamon
sprinkle	nutmeg* (optional)

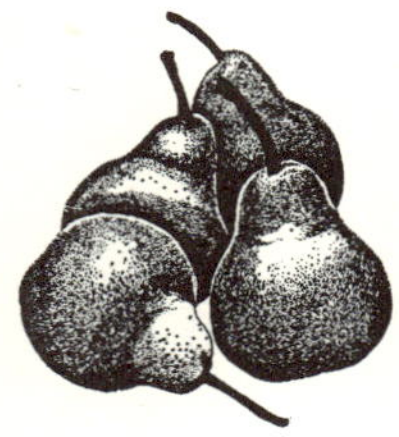

1. Preheat oven to 350ºF.
2. Blend almonds in blender on highest speed until they become a fine powder. Add small amount of water and blend on the highest speed for 1–2 minutes until well blended, stopping at least once to scrap sides and bottom of blender jar.
3. Beat egg in small bowl with whisk. Add rest of ingredients and nut milk. Stir.
4. Pour into 4 custard cups. Place cups in an 8-inch square glass baking dish. Add room temperature water to the baking dish so that water is 1 inch deep in pan.
5. Bake 40–45 minutes or until knife comes out clean when inserted in the center of custard. To cool slightly, remove baked custard dishes from water in baking dish. Serve warm or cold. I prefer warm.

Yield: 4 servings (1/2 cup each)

*Nutmeg is labeled an unassigned "Fun Food" on this rotational diet, see explanation on pages 30–31.

Almond Butter

3 cups whole raw almonds

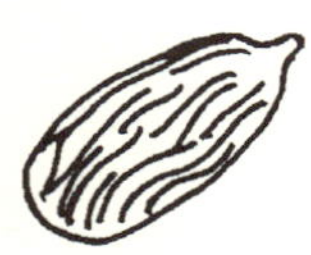

1. Chill almonds in freezer at least overnight. Leave almonds in the freezer until ready to process.
2. Assemble Champion Juicer for homogenizing. Use the funnel for easier insertion of the nuts.
3. Remove almonds from freezer and run through approximately 1/4–1/3 cup of almonds at a time. I prefer to push my nuts through fast so as to make crunchy almond butter. The Champion Juicer manufacturer recommends to discontinue making nut butter if the juicer body becomes excessively warm. I prefer to process only 3 cups of nuts, quit, and clean up the juicer.
4. Store in glass, wide-mouth pint jar. Spread on celery, crackers, or tortillas and use in recipes such as Amazing Sugarless Cookies (page 143).

Yield: almost 2 cups of nut butter

Special Note: This almond butter is not as spreadable as purchased almond butter. Now that I have found an excellent source for organic almond butter (see Appendix C: Resources), I rarely prepare this recipe.

9. FOODS, MEAL PLANNING, AND RECIPES FOR DAY 2

Foods for Day 2

Animal Protein

82	shrimp, crab, prawn, lobster
87	cod (scrod), pollack
129	rabbit
137	beef, buffalo, plain yogurt
	red snapper

Vegetables

11	onion
41	garbanzo (chickpea), lima beans
54	okra
74	potato, tomato, green pepper, eggplant
79	cucumber, pumpkin, spaghetti and zucchini squash
80	lettuce

Grains, Flours, and Baking Foods

19	arrowroot starch
30	amaranth
41	garbanzo bean flour (chickpea)
74	potato starch

Fruit

16	banana, plantain	56	kiwi
45	grapefruit, lemon	79	melons

Sweeteners

Currently recipes for Day 2 are developed using stevia or honey floated from Day 4.

Oils

69	olive oil
80	sunflower oil
137	butter, ghee (clarified butter)

Herbs and Spices

63	allspice, clove
73	basil, marjoram, rosemary, sage, savory, thyme
74	cayenne (red) pepper

Foods That Float Between Days 2 & 4

11	garlic
73	oregano
74	chili powder

Seeds and Nuts

79	pumpkin seeds
80	sunflower seeds

Recipe Table of Contents for Day 2

Biscuits, Crackers, & Bread

Cereals, Grains, & Nongrains

Protein Dishes

Protein Dishes (continued)

Vegetables, Salads, & Salad Dressing

Desserts

Miscellaneous

Meal Planning for Day 2

Quick & Easy Meals

Grilled Shrimp with lemon
boiled potatoes with Clarified Butter
Zucchini and Tomato

Minute Steak & Garbanzo Bean Gravy
Mashed Potatoes
lettuce with Zucchini Salad Dressing

Vegetable Shrimp Soup

ground meat patty
Creamed Potatoes
tomato and zucchini slices

Quick & Easy Meals with Advanced Planning

Chef Salad
Amaranth Crackers

Beef Stew

Hot Beef Sandwich
tomato slices

Garbanzo Bean & Potato Soup
green pepper strips

Vegetable or Nightshade Beef & Bean Soup
Amaranth Crackers

Vegetable or Nightshade Beef Soup
Amaranth Crackers

Tacos

Vegetable Shrimp and Bean Soup
Soy Bread

Easy Meals

Spicy Baked Fish
Garbanzo Beans and Broth
lettuce with Creamy Italian Dressing

Spaghetti Squash
with Spaghetti Meat Sauce
lettuce with Lemon/Oil Dressing

Easy Steak Dinner
boiled, diced potatoes
cucumber slices

Chili
green pepper strips

Minestrone Soup
Baked Fish for Day 2

Your choice of pizza
lettuce with Creamy Italian Dressing

Your choice of lasagna
lettuce with Lemon/Oil Dressing

Lower Carbohydrate Meals

Low Carbohydrate Lasagna
lettuce with Lemon/Oil Dressing

Easy Steak or Rabbit Dinner
cucumber slices

Chef Salad

Grilled Steak
Stir-Fry Vegetables for Day 2

Shrimp Vegetable Salad

Tossed Shrimp Salad

Breakfast Ideas

Amaranth Cereal

Amaranth Griddle Bread with Kiwi Sauce

fresh fruit

Yogurt Delights I, II, III, or IV

any *plan*over Day 2 vegetable, fish, casserole, or soup—especially my favorites:
- —steamed potato
- —Fried Potatoes with onions and green pepper
- —Low Carbohydrate Lasagna
- —Mixed Vegetable Salad

Snack Ideas

green pepper strips	sunflower seeds
cucumber slices	Amaranth Carob Cookies
zucchini slices	Lemon Pudding
sliced tomatoes	Yogurt Delight I, II, III, or IV
Amaranth Crackers	Grapefruit Spritzer
Soy Bread	fresh fruit

Meals Away from Home

Your choice of the many Day 2 soups with or without crackers

Amaranth Tortilla with Shrimp Salad and lettuce
cucumber slices

Amaranth Tortilla with *plan*over Roast Beef and tomato slices
green pepper strips

Your choice of the many Day 2 salads with or without crackers

Potato Salad with *plan*over roast beef

Any *plan*over spaghetti, lasagna, or stew, if you have a microwave available to reheat it

Special Occasion Meals

Company–
Grilled Steak
Baked Potato or Scalloped Potatoes
lettuce with Creamy Italian Dressing
Blueberry Tofu "Cheesecake" with Amaranth Crust (moved from Day 4)
Dacopa beverage

Company–
Tofu Lasagna
lettuce with Lemon/Oil Dressing
Carob Amaranth Cookies
iced Pau D'Arco tea

Picnic–
grilled hamburgers with Quick Catsup and Amaranth Bun
Potato Salad or Kidney Bean Salad
tossed greens, cucumber, and tomato with Creamy Italian Dressing
Zucchini Amaranth Cookies
sparkling mineral water

Recipes for Day 2

Amaranth Cereal I*

1/2 cup	amaranth whole seed
1/4 teaspoon	sea salt
1 3/4 cups	water (room temperature)
1/4 cup	Brazil Nut Milk* (page 154) OR additional water

Amaranth Cereal II*

1/3 cup	amaranth whole seed
2 tablespoons	amaranth flour
1/4 teaspoon	sea salt
1 3/4 cups	water (room temperature)
1/4 cup	Brazil Nut Milk* (page 154) OR additional water

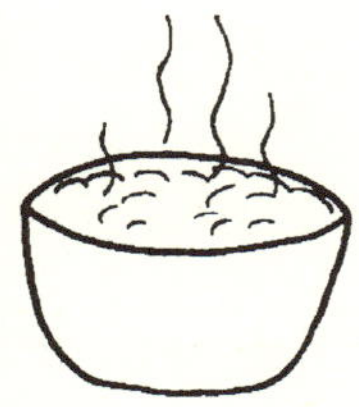

1. Combine your choice of the above ingredients in a 1-quart size slow cooker.** Cook overnight and awake to enjoy this ready-to-eat, mouth-watering cereal.
2. Stir before serving. Enjoy this cereal plain or with a tablespoon of Kiwi Sauce (page 191) or a teaspoon of flaxseed oil.

Yield: 2 cups

Special Note: I prefer a thinner consistency for my Amaranth Cereal I and use only 3 tablespoons of amaranth per 1 cup of water. Since I don't care for this cereal frozen and reheated, I only prepare the amount I know I will be eating.

**These recipes are too small to cook in a standard-sized slow cooker, but they can be easily doubled or tripled if desired. Cook on low if slow cooker has two settings. Also, see page 61 for more information on slow cookers.

Recipe idea for Amaranth Cereal I from Mastering Food Allergies newsletter, December-January 1988.

Amaranth Cereal III

1/2 cup	amaranth whole seed
1/4 teaspoon	sea salt
2 3/4 cups	water
1/4 cup	Brazil Nut Milk* (page 154) OR additional water

1. Bring water and salt to boil in saucepan.
2. Stir in amaranth. Reduce heat. Cover and simmer for 35–45 minutes. Stir occasionally. Add more water if needed. Serve as described above.

Yield: approximately 1 3/4 cups

*Brazil nuts is an unassigned "Fun Food" on this rotational diet, see explanation on pages 30–31.

Brazil or Macadamia Nut Milk*

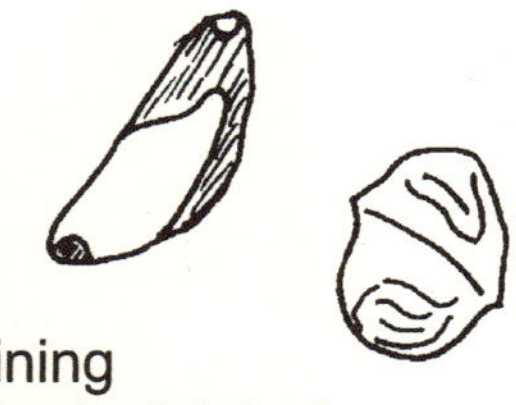

1/4 cup chopped Brazil or macadamia nuts*
1 cup water

1. Combine chopped nuts and small amount of water in blender. Blend on highest speed for 1–2 minutes until well blended. Stop at least once to scrape sides and bottom of blender jar. Add remaining water and blend a couple of seconds longer. Chill. Add salt if desired. Stir before serving. I love the rich flavor that 1–2 tablespoons adds to Amaranth Cereal.

2. Since I do not desire to make this nut milk each time I serve Amaranth Cereal, I prepare 1–2 cups at a time. After blending, pour immediately into ice cube trays. After frozen, transfer to cellophane bag. Thaw as needed.

Yield: slightly more than 1 cup

*Brazil and macadamia nuts are unassigned "Fun Foods" on this rotational diet, see explanation on pages 30–31.

Soy Bread*

1 cup	soy flour*
1/2 cup	arrowroot starch
2 1/4 teaspoons	Featherweight brand baking powder**
1/2 teaspoon	sea salt
2 tablespoons	soy oil*
1 cup	water

1. Preheat oven to 375°F.

2. Oil and flour the bottom and sides of an 8-inch square baking pan.

3. In mixing bowl, whisk together dry ingredients. Add water and oil. Mix thoroughly.

4. Transfer batter to prepared pan and spread evenly. Bake for 20 minutes. Bread is done when it sounds hollow when tapped on top surface.

5. Cool at least 5–10 minutes. I prefer to cut bread into 8 pieces (4x2). Serve for breakfast, with a meal, or as a snack. This is also a nice treat served with wheat-free gravy (see recipes on pages 166 and 168). Freeze leftover bread for later use.

Yield: 8 servings

*Soy is usually eaten on Day 4, so you need to avoid eating soy on your Day 4 just before and after eating this recipe on your Day 2.

**At publication date, I have not been successful in preparing this bread using vitamin C crystals and baking soda as the leavening agents. For those allergic to potatoes, do realize that Featherweight brand baking powder contains potato starch.

Recipe idea from Rotational Bon Appetité! by Hayes & Maynard, p. 38.

Amaranth Griddle Bread/Pancake

1/3 cup	water
1/4 cup	amaranth flour
2 pinches	sea salt
1 teaspoon	sunflower oil

1. Preheat a griddle that is at least 10 inches in diameter. I use a well-seasoned cast-iron griddle (see How to Season Cast Iron on page 63). Griddle is hot enough when water dances when sprinkled on the griddle.
2. Measure water in a glass 1-cup measure. Add the flour and salt. Whisk together.
3. Lightly oil preheated griddle with 1/2 teaspoon of the oil. A good way to spread the oil is to use the back of a wooden spoon or a metal spatula.
4. Stir the batter again and pour all at once onto the center of the griddle. With a skillet lid, cover the griddle or at least the batter. Cook covered for 2 minutes.
5. Uncover briefly and dribble another 1/2 teaspoon of oil over the surface of the bread. Use the back of a wooden spoon to spread oil around. Cover and cook another 4 minutes.
6. Turn bread over, cover, and cook 2 minutes. Then uncover and cook for 3 more minutes. This flat bread is a little crispy. Serve immediately with heated fruit sauce or gravy. I prefer to serve this as a flat pancake for breakfast with Kiwi Sauce (page 191).

Yield: approximately a 7-inch circle

Recipe idea from The Allergy Self-Help Cookbook by Jones.

Garbanzo Bean Griddle Bread

1/3 cup	water
1/4 cup	garbanzo bean flour
2 pinches	sea salt
1 teaspoon	sunflower oil

1. Follow steps 1–4 as in Amaranth Griddle Bread.
2. Uncover briefly and dribble another 1/2 teaspoon of oil over the surface of the bread. Use the back of a wooden spoon to spread it around. Cover and cook another 5 minutes.
3. Turn bread over, cover, and cook another 5 minutes. This flat bread is a little crispy. Serve immediately with heated fruit sauce or gravy. I prefer to serve this for dinner with gravy to make a Hot Beef Sandwich (page 166)

Yield: approximately a 7-inch circle

Recipe idea from The Allergy Self-Help Cookbook by Jones.

Yogurt Delights

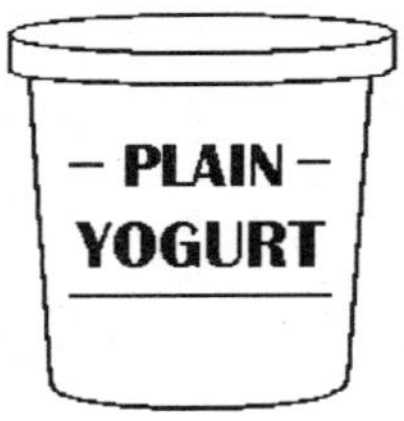

Choose one of the following to add to plain sugar-free yogurt. I love and fully recommend 7-Stars original plain Organic Yogurt.

Delight I

Add alcohol-free vanilla extract to plain yogurt.

Delight II

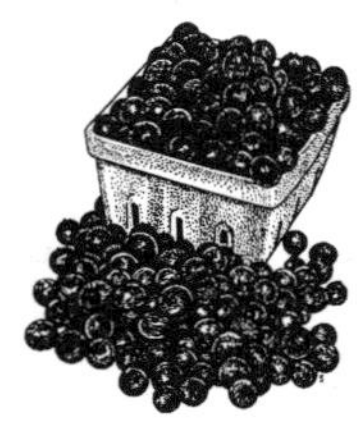

Avoid eating blueberries on your Day 4 just before and after your Day 2 to enjoy blueberries with yogurt. Simply thaw blueberries (do not drain) and add to yogurt and stir. I prefer to smash the blueberries before adding the fruit and juice to the yogurt.

Delight III

Simply stir desired amount of puffed amaranth into yogurt. Eat immediately.

Delight IV

Enjoy a combination of Delight I and III or II and III.

Amaranth Crackers

3/4 cup	amaranth flour
1/3 cup	arrowroot starch
1/4 cup	ground sunflower seeds (ground in food processor)
1 teaspoon	baking soda
1/4 teaspoon	sea salt
1/4 teaspoon	unbuffered, corn-free vitamin C crystals
1/3 cup	water
3 tablespoons	olive or sunflower oil

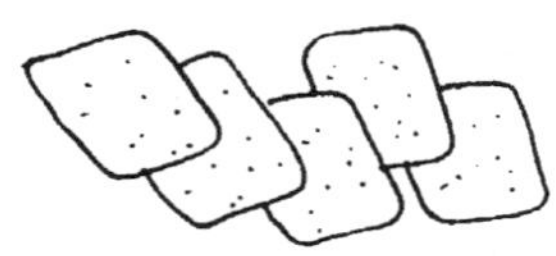

1. Preheat oven to 350°F.
2. Place 1 teaspoon of oil on a 14 x 10-inch stainless steel baking sheet and set aside. (This amount of oil is in addition to the amount listed above.)
3. In large mixing bowl, whisk together dry ingredients and ground sunflower seeds. Make "well" in the center.
4. Add water and oil. Stir with a rubber spatula or fork until dough clumps into a ball and flour is well mixed. Often the dough is rather sticky, so I gradually add up to 1 more tablespoon of flour. Mix after each small addition.
5. Spread oil on baking sheet with fingers to within one inch of edge. As the dough is rolled out, it will push the oil to the edge of the baking sheet. In addition, using your fingers to spread the oil will lightly coat them and aid in working with the dough.
6. Transfer dough to center of the baking sheet. Use your hands to form dough so it has no rough edges. Press dough out evenly in all four directions until it cannot be spread further with your hands, making sure to maintain rectangular shape.

continued on next page

Amaranth Crackers (continued)

7. If your baking sheet has sides on it, be sure the rolling pin will fit all the way down onto surface on both the width and length of the sheet and that the handles clear the edges.

8. Lightly dust rolling pin with flour and roll dough out from center to edges. Be sure to press in all four directions and to keep dough at a uniform thickness. Occasionally run your hand across top of dough to feel if there are any thick areas that need to be evened out.

9. As the dough gets thinner, use the dull back side of a table knife to press edges of dough to maintain rectangular shape. Continue rolling and shaping until dough is about 1/8–1/4 inch thick and fills baking sheet. To help reduce the possibility of extra-thin dough edge, use back side of a table knife to gently push all four edges of dough to make edge thickness uniform with remaining dough.

10. Using a pizza cutter, cut dough into squares as follows. Be sure to move pizza cutter slowly and with a back and forth motion to help avoid tearing dough if cutter goes directly across a sunflower seed. Cut rectangle in half along dough length (see number 1 in diagram). Cut each half in half (see number 2), then cut each fourth in thirds (see number 3). This will create 12 strips.

11. Next cut rectangle in half along dough width (see number 4). Cut each half in half (see number 5) and each fourth in half (see number 6). This will create 8 sections and 96 individual crackers. Next use a sharp knife to be sure each cut on the outer edge of the rectangle is completely separated.

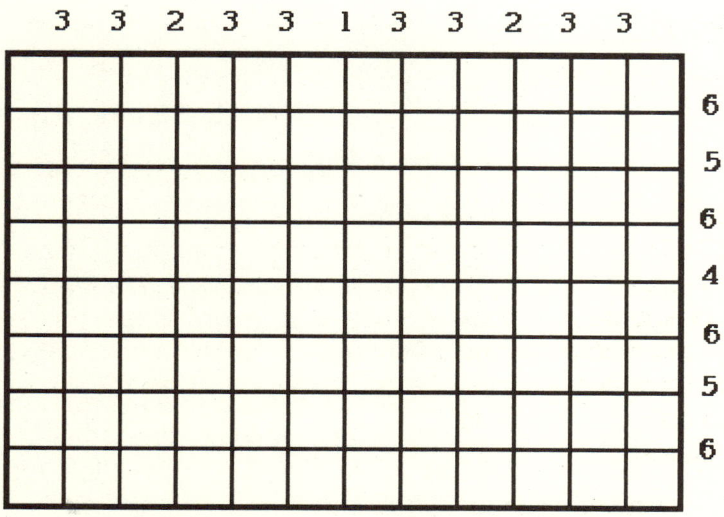

12. Prick holes in each square with fork. If you wish, you can salt the tops of the crackers with sea salt before baking.

13. Bake for 25 minutes. Remove baking sheet from oven and carefully remove outer circle of crackers if they are crispy. Return remaining crackers to oven for 5 minutes. To crisp crackers further, loosen crackers from baking sheet and return them to oven for at least 15 minutes with oven turned off.

14. Cool crackers on cooling rack by either leaving them on the baking sheet or removing and placing them directly on the cooling rack. After cool, store in the freezer. I prefer to use a wide-mouth quart jar. No need to thaw, eat straight from the freezer.

Yield: 96 crackers, approximately 3/4 quart

Variation: Omit sunflower seeds and substitute 2 additional tablespoons of amaranth flour. This variation is often used as breading, see recipes for delicious Fried Eggplant and Italian Eggplant with Amaranth Cracker Crumbs. One recipe of crackers equals 1 1/2 cups of crumbs.

Basic Amaranth

1 cup	amaranth whole seed
2 cups	water
1/4 teaspoon	sea salt

1. Wash amaranth (page 36). Combine ingredients in a 2 1/2 quart stainless steel saucepan. Bring to boil on high. Cover. Reduce heat to between low and medium to allow the amaranth to simmer. Simmer 30 minutes or until all the water is evaporated.
2. Stir and serve as side dish in place of potato with a meal or as cereal for breakfast. I also enjoy adding 1/4 teaspoon of FOS per serving, however do realize that adding FOS does break rotation.

Yield: approximately 2 1/4 cups

Special Note: For best results, amaranth should not be stirred or uncovered during the cooking process. If it is necessary to check the progress of the amaranth during the cooking time, do so quickly to minimize the loss of steam. Do not stir as this will disrupt the even cooking of the amaranth. If tasting for doneness, use a fork to gently remove a small amount from the surface of the cooked amaranth. Different stoves and different pans may require adjustment in time, temperature, and amount of liquid needed.

Roasted Basic Amaranth

Roasting amaranth intensifies the delicious earthy taste of the amaranth. Prepare as you do Basic Amaranth except dry roast the rinsed amaranth before cooking. To dry roast:

1. Transfer the rinsed and drained amaranth to a cold, heavy-bottomed pan. I prefer a well-seasoned cast-iron skillet (see How to Season Cast Iron on page 63). Place skillet on range. Turn burner to medium-high. Roast on medium-high, stirring almost constantly for approximately 6 minutes or until the amaranth has become rather dry.
2. Lower heat to medium-low and continue to roast, stirring constantly for approximately an additional 4 minutes or until you can smell the intense earthy aroma of the amaranth. Be careful not to burn the amaranth or allow it to become so hot that it pops and looks similar to Puffed Amaranth.
3. Transfer the roasted amaranth to the boiling salted water and continue to cook as described in Basic Amaranth (recipe above).

Amaranth Tortillas

5/8 cup	amaranth flour (amount needed to start) (5/8 cup = 1/2 cup + 2 tablespoons)
1/4 teaspoon	sea salt
1/4 cup	water
1/2 teaspoon	sunflower or olive oil
1/2 cup	amaranth flour (amount needed for kneading and rolling)

Special Note: Before starting your tortilla preparation, I suggest you read Helpful Hints on Tortilla Preparation starting on page 79.

1. Preheat nonstick, unoiled griddle or skillet. I use a well-seasoned cast-iron griddle (see How to Season Cast Iron on page 63). Griddle is hot enough when water dances when sprinkled on the griddle.

continued on next page

Amaranth Tortillas (continued)

2. In a curved-sided bowl, whisk together 5/8 cup (1/2 cup + 2 tablespoons) of flour and salt. Make a "well" in the center.

3. Add water and oil. Stir with rubber spatula or fork until dough clumps together into a moist ball. This dough ball is too sticky for kneading, so add 1 tablespoon more flour and stir in thoroughly with the rubber spatula or fork.

4. Scatter 1 tablespoon flour on rolling surface. Transfer dough to floured rolling surface and knead dough to work in as much of this additional flour as possible. Dough texture should resemble Play Doh. Add more flour if needed. You will usually need a total of 1–2 tablespoons of flour during this kneading process. Form dough into a ball and cut into fourths. Flour cut surfaces of the 4 dough portions with remaining flour.

5. Special Note: If you have difficulty working additional flour into the delicate amaranth dough, first cut the dough into the 4 portions. Then knead about 1/2 tablespoon or more of flour into each dough portion until the dough texture resembles Play Doh.

6. Lightly flour rolling pin. Pat dough portion into circular shape, then roll out tortilla by pressing evenly from the center out in all directions and working to keep tortilla as round as possible. Keep dough well floured on both sides (you will need approximately 1/2 tablespoon of flour per tortilla). Turn dough over often by loosening with a spatula before flipping. Feel dough surface occasionally to be sure it is evenly thin. Finished tortilla will be very thin and approximately 6–8 inches in diameter. Using a pastry brush, gently brush both sides of tortilla to remove excess flour.

7. Special Note: Amaranth Tortillas are very delicate and tear easily. If you have difficulty, I would suggest that you only roll the tortillas to be 6 inches in diameter or try preparing only three tortillas from this recipe. In this way, you end up with thicker tortillas and therefore they should not tear as easily.

8. Cook each tortilla on preheated, unoiled griddle approximately 45 seconds on each side. (The thicker tortillas mentioned in step 7 will need between 50–55 seconds cooking time on each side.) You will note that tiny air pockets form and cause a bubble or pebble effect on the surface of the amaranth tortillas when cooking them on the second side. Cool each tortilla 1–2 minutes on cooling rack. Place the slightly cooled tortillas between two layers of a clean cotton towel.

9. Serve either whole or cut in half. Use your imagination to create a simple deli-like sandwich—for example: roast beef, lettuce, sunflower "Mayo," sliced tomatoes, cucumbers, and zucchini are all good for Day 2. Also, use for Shrimp Salad Sandwich, Enchiladas, and Tacos, as well as Beef Fajita. Leftover tortillas may be frozen flat in a cellophane or plastic bag for future meals.

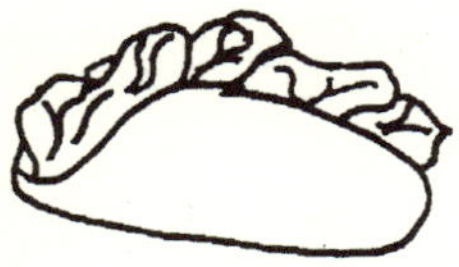

Yield: 3–4 tortillas, 6–8 inches in diameter

Special Note: For easier preparation of amaranth tortillas, you may add 1/2 teaspoon of guar gum to the above recipe starting with only 1/2 cup of flour. However, do realize that guar gum is a Day 4 food.

Recipe idea from The Yeast Connection Cookbook by Crook & Jones, p. 159.

Amaranth "Hamburger" Buns

1 3/4 cups	amaranth flour
1/2 cup	arrowroot starch
1 1/2 teaspoons	baking soda
3/8 teaspoon	unbuffered, corn-free vitamin C crystals
1/2 teaspoon	sea salt
3/4 cup	water
3 tablespoons	olive or sunflower oil

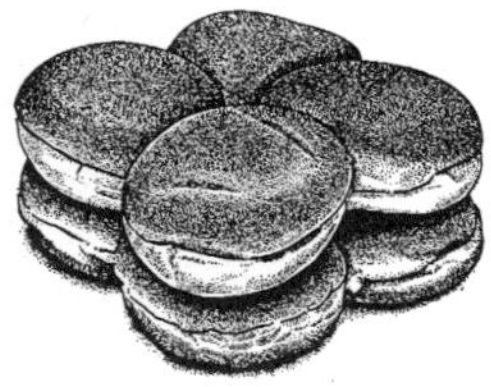

1. Preheat oven to 350°F.
2. Oil and flour desired dishes:
   3 Corning Grab-It bowls for Kaiser-size buns
   5 custard bowls for smaller size buns (I prefer this size)
3. In large bowl, whisk together dry ingredients. Make a "well" in the center.
4. In smaller bowl, whisk together water and oil for approximately 15 seconds. This will disperse the oil into the water, but not thoroughly mix them together. Immediately add this mixture to the dry ingredients. Mix thoroughly until dry ingredients are evenly moist (do not beat). Dough will be delicate and stiff but manageable.
5. Divide dough into equal portions (3 or 5). I find this easier if I press the dough evenly and firmly into the bottom of the mixing bowl. Then I take a table knife and cut the dough into equal portions.
6. Lightly oil hands. Patty and flatten each portion in shape of desired bowl. Place in prepared bowls. Bake 30 minutes or until toothpick comes out dry when inserted into the center of buns.
7. Within 5 minutes after baking, remove buns from baking dishes and allow to cool on a wire rack. Use serrated knife to slice each bun in half. Leftovers may be frozen for future meals. Thaw only at room temperature. Do not thaw under heat application such as microwave. Thawing using heat causes the buns to become doughy and to taste undone.

Yield: 3–5 buns

Recipe idea from Allergy Cooking with Ease by Nicolette M. Dumke, p. 48.

Garbanzo Bean Soup

1 cup	Garbanzo Beans and Broth (page 161)
1 tablespoon	green pepper, chopped
1/8 teaspoon	summer savory and/or basil

Combine ingredients in saucepan. Simmer for 10 minutes to blend flavors. I prefer my green pepper a little crunchy so I do not add it until the last minute of heating.

Yield: 1 cup

Garbanzo Beans and Broth*

2 cups	garbanzo beans
5 cups	water
5–6	bay leaves* (optional)
1/4 cup	chopped onion
1/2 teaspoon	minced garlic
1 teaspoon	sea salt

1. Rinse beans to remove dirt and dust. Soak beans 8–12 hours in refrigerator in 7 cups of water to allow beans to more than double in size.
2. Just before cooking, rinse beans thoroughly until rinsing water is clear. Drain.
3. Transfer beans to standard-size slow cooker. Add all ingredients except salt. Cook on low for 10–12 hours or on high for 4 1/2–5 hours until beans are tender but not mushy.
4. After cooking, remove the bay leaves. Just before serving, add salt and stir. Garbanzo beans freeze and reheat well for future meals.

Yield: 6 1/2 cups

Serving suggestions:

1. Serve as side dish with meal or use in Day 2 recipes, such as Garbanzo Bean Soup, Garbanzo Bean and Potato Soup, Minestrone Soup, and Stuffed Green Peppers.
2. Drain and serve on lettuce salad. You may use garbanzo bean broth in place of water in Zucchini Salad Dressing.
3. Temporarily transfer garbanzo beans to Day 4 and use in Beans and Beans (page 263).

*Special Note: Bay leaf belongs to the Laurel Family with avocado and cinnamon. Eating bay leaf on Day 2 breaks the rotation since cinnamon is used in many recipes on Day 3 and a few on Day 1. You can make your own decision about bay leaf. I personally use it without any concern regarding when I have or plan to consume cinnamon.

Garbanzo Bean and Potato Soup

1 cup	Garbanzo Beans and Broth (recipe above)
1 cup	potatoes, peeled, diced
2 tablespoons	green pepper, chopped
1/4 teaspoon	summer savory
to taste	sea salt

1. In saucepan, partially cook potatoes in a small amount of water and salt.
2. Add rest of the ingredients to the potatoes. Simmer for 10 minutes or until the potatoes are done. I prefer my green pepper a little crunchy so I do not add it until the last minute of simmering.

Yield: 2 cups

Recipe idea from The Yeast Connection Cookbook by Crook & Jones, p. 188.

Minestrone Soup

3 cloves	garlic, minced
2 teaspoons	olive oil
1 quart	tomato quarters or pieces (unsalted)
1 cup	onion, chopped
2 cups	eggplant, peeled, 1/2-inch cubed
2 cups	zucchini squash, peeled, 1/2-inch cubed OR 1 1/2 cups sliced okra
1 1/2 cups	Garbanzo Beans and Broth, drained, reserve broth (page 161)
2 cups	liquid (approximately 3/4 cup of bean broth and 1 1/4 cups water)
1/2 teaspoon	leaf oregano
1/2 teaspoon	basil
1/2 teaspoon	marjoram
1 3/4 teaspoons	sea salt

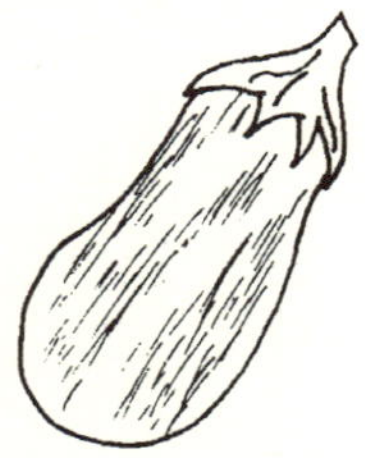

1. In 5-quart Dutch-oven kettle, sauté garlic in oil until soft. Add rest of the ingredients except salt. Heat to boiling, reduce heat, and cover. Simmer 3 hours. Stir occasionally. Just before serving, add salt (about 1/4 teaspoon per 1 cup) and stir.

2. To complement the meal, serve this delicious soup with Baked Cod and kiwi fruit. Freeze leftovers for an even quicker meal later.

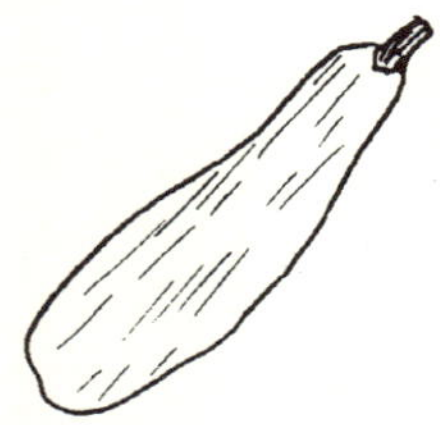

Yield: 6 1/2 cups

Special Note: I have prepared this recipe in a slow cooker but the flavor was not as delicious as with the method described above.

Vegetable Shrimp Soup

2 pints	tomato juice OR 1 pint of tomato juice and 2 cups of water
1 cup	zucchini squash, peeled, diced
1 cup	eggplant, peeled, diced
1 cup	potatoes, peeled, diced
1/2 teaspoon	summer savory
1/4 teaspoon	sea salt
1/2 pound	Fresh Shelled Shrimp (page 181)

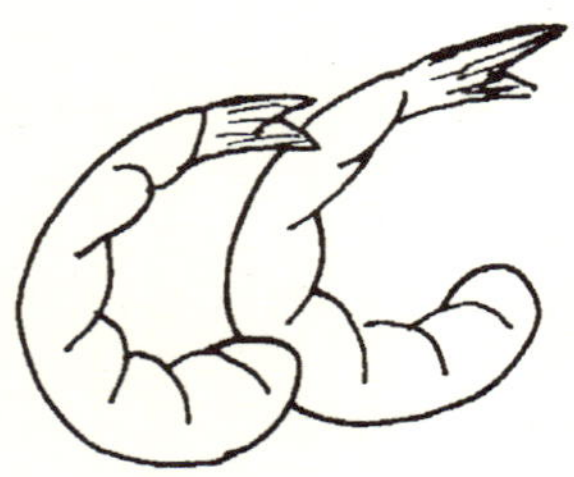

Combine all ingredients except shrimp in saucepan. Heat to boiling, reduce heat, cover. Simmer 20–25 minutes until potatoes are almost tender. Add prepared shrimp and simmer 5 minutes longer.

Yield: 6 cups

Vegetable Shrimp and Bean Soup

Prepare the same as Vegetable Shrimp Soup except substitute 1 cup of Garbanzo Beans and Broth (page 161) for the potatoes.

Vegetable Beef Soup

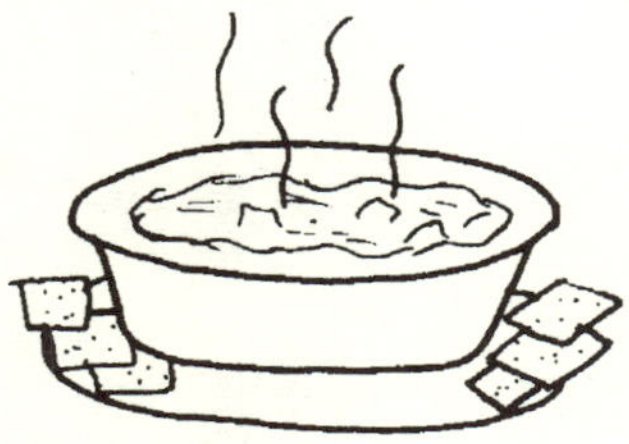

1 pint	tomato juice
2 cups	Beef Broth (page 166)
1 cup	zucchini squash, peeled, diced
1 cup	eggplant, peeled, diced
1 cup	cooked roast beef, diced
1 cup	potatoes, peeled, diced
1/2 teaspoon	summer savory
1/4 teaspoon	sea salt

Combine all ingredients in saucepan. Heat to boiling, reduce heat, cover, and simmer 25–30 minutes or until potatoes are tender.

Yield: 6 cups

Vegetable Beef and Bean Soup

Prepare the same as Vegetable Beef Soup except substitute 1 cup of Garbanzo Beans and Broth (page 161) for the potatoes.

Nightshade Beef Soup

1 pint	tomato juice
2 cups	Beef Broth (page 166)
2 cups	eggplant, peeled, diced
1 cup	cooked roast beef, diced
1 cup	potatoes, peeled, diced
1 cup	green peppers, diced
1/2 teaspoon	summer savory
1/4 teaspoon	sea salt

Combine all ingredients in saucepan. Heat to boiling, reduce heat, cover, and simmer 25–30 minutes or until potatoes are tender.

Yield: 6 cups

Nightshade Beef and Bean Soup

Prepare the same as Nightshade Beef Soup except substitute 1 cup of Garbanzo Beans and Broth (page 161) for the potatoes.

Chili*

1 pound	ground beef or ground buffalo
1/2 cup	onion, chopped
1 can	Muir Glen brand organic tomato puree (16 ounces)
4 cups	cooked kidney beans, drained (see below)*
2 cups	liquid (kidney bean broth and water)
2 cups	eggplant, peeled, diced
1/2 cup	green pepper, chopped
2 teaspoons	chili powder
1 teaspoon	Watkins Salsa Seasoning Blend or other Mexican blend spices
1 1/2 teaspoons	sea salt

1. In large kettle or skillet, cook ground meat and onions until done. Stir often to chop meat and brown evenly.
2. Add the rest of the ingredients except salt. Heat to boiling, reduce heat, cover, and simmer at least 30 minutes. Stir occasionally. Add more water if needed. Just before serving, add salt to taste and, if desired, add more seasonings.

Yield: 8 cups

Kidney Beans for Chili

1 1/2 cups	kidney beans
3 cups	water

1. Rinse beans to remove dirt and dust. Soak beans 8–12 hours in refrigerator in 7 cups of water to allow beans to more than double in size.
2. Just before cooking, rinse beans thoroughly until rinsing water is clear. Drain.
3. Transfer beans to standard-size slow cooker. Add water. Cook on low for 7–8 hours until tender but not mushy.

Yield: 4 cups cooked beans and 1 1/2 cups liquid to use in Chili recipe above

*Kidney beans are usually eaten on Day 4. Be sure to omit kidney beans on your Day 4 just before or after eating Chili on your Day 2.

Enthusiasm is a mental sunshine that keeps everything in us alive and growing.

Beef or Buffalo Fajita

4	Amaranth Tortillas (page 158)
8 ounces	beef or buffalo—round steak (pounded to tenderize) or minute steak cut meat into thin strips (approximately 1 cup)
1/2 cup	onion, thinly sliced
1 cup	green pepper strips
1 1/2 cups	zucchini squash, cut into strips
1–2 teaspoons	sunflower or olive oil
as needed	sea salt
as desired	summer savory
as desired	fresh tomato, diced, seasoned with a small amount of Watkins Salsa Seasoning Blend or other Mexican blend spices (optional)
as desired	Guacamole (page 196) (optional)
as desired	Picante Sauce (page 196) (optional)

1. Prepare or thaw tortillas.
2. Prepare tomato, Guacamole, and/or Picante Sauce if desired.
3. Preheat electric skillet to 300°F.
4. Prepare meat and vegetables as described above.
5. Add oil to preheated electric skillet. Stir fry meat, stirring often to brown evenly. You may cover with splatter screen (information on page 60) when not stirring.
6. Add vegetables and sprinkle with salt and savory. Stir often to cook meat and vegetables evenly. I prefer my vegetables crunchy.
7. Serve immediately. I have found the easiest way to serve fajitas is to begin with the tortilla on your plate. Spread approximately 3/4 cup of filling in the center of the tortilla lengthwise but about 1 inch from one side as Diagram A shows. Fold the 1-inch edge side over first, then fold the 1/3 side edges over the filling as Diagram B shows. Lift and hold with both hands. Eat and enjoy.

Yield: approximately 3 cups of filling, ample amount for 4 tortillas

Diagram A

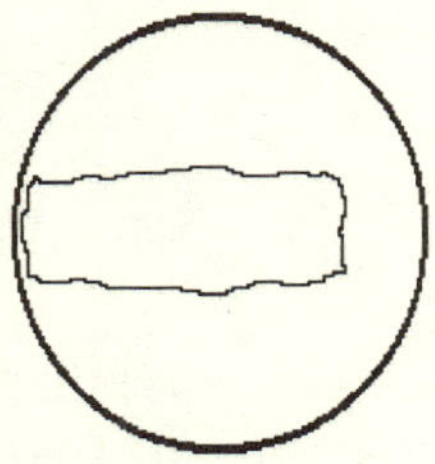

Diagram B

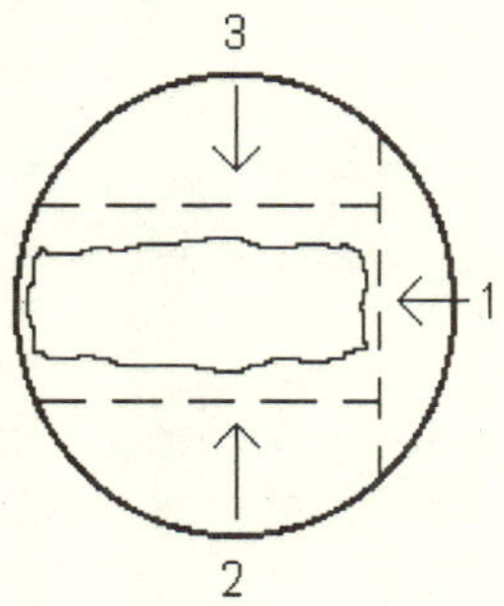

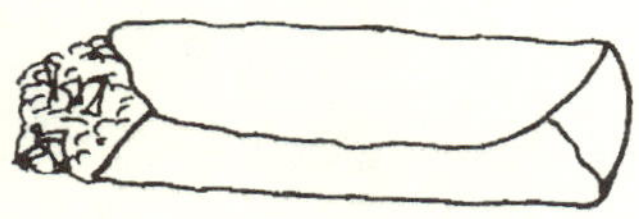

Roast Beef or Buffalo and Broth

2–3 pound	beef or buffalo roast (arm, blade, rump, chuck, etc.)
1 teaspoon	sea salt
1/2 teaspoon	summer savory
1	onion, chopped large (optional)

Method 1

1. Sprinkle salt and savory over meat on all sides. Place seasoned roast in standard-size slow cooker. If desired, add onion. Add water to cover roast or to within 1-inch of top of roast. Cook on low for 8-10 hours.

2. Serve with potatoes and salad. You may serve some of the broth over the meat and potatoes.

3. After the meal, strain leftover broth through fine-meshed strainer and chill. After chilling, remove the fat that is solid on the top. Freeze broth in ice cube trays. After frozen, transfer to a cellophane bag. Also, you may measure out specific amounts needed for recipes and freeze in glass jars. The broth is used in many recipes such as Beef Stew, wheat-free gravy, and beef soups. Also, freeze leftover meat in cellophane bags for future quick meals such as amaranth tortilla sandwiches, Hot Beef Sandwich, and beef soups.

Method 2

Another way to prepare roast is to use Reynolds cooking bags. Just follow the directions provided with the bags. They say that you can use these bags in the microwave, but I prefer to cook meat in the oven. Also, I do not shake flour in the bags, but I do add more liquid than called for in the directions. Strain and freeze the leftover broth as described above.

Hot Beef Sandwich

Garbanzo Bean Griddle Bread (page 155)
leftover cooked Roast Beef or Buffalo (recipe above)
Whipped Mashed Potatoes (recipe below)
Beef Gravy (recipe below)

Prepare ingredients and assemble open face on dinner place by placing heated meat over griddle bread. Then top with potatoes and gravy.

Beef Gravy

1 cup	Beef Broth, concentrated (recipe above)
1/4 cup	garbanzo bean flour

Use 2 cups of Beef Broth that was prepared when cooking a roast in a slow cooker and boil it in saucepan to yield 1 cup. Or use 1 cup of broth that was prepared when cooking a roast in roasting pan or Reynolds roasting bag. Add flour and stir with a whisk while cooking over medium heat to thicken. Taste and add salt as needed.

Whipped Potatoes

Scrub, peel, and dice potatoes. In saucepan, cook on low in a small amount of salted water until tender. Using a Braun hand blender, whip potatoes with a small amount of cooking water and Clarified Butter. If desired, add some Brazil Nut Milk (page 154).

Beef Stew*

1 pound	beef stew meat
2 teaspoons	olive or sunflower oil
1/2 teaspoon	sea salt
1/4 teaspoon	summer savory
2 cups	Beef Broth (page 166) OR water
1/2 cup	onion, chopped
1 pint	tomato quarters or pieces
1 1/2 cups	eggplant, peeled, 1/2-inch cubed
3/4 cup	zucchini squash, peeled, 1/2-inch cubed
2 cups	potatoes, peeled, 1/2 inch diced
1/2 cup	green peppers, diced (optional)
1/2 cup	peas*, frozen or fresh (optional)
1/2 cup	water
1 tablespoon	potato starch

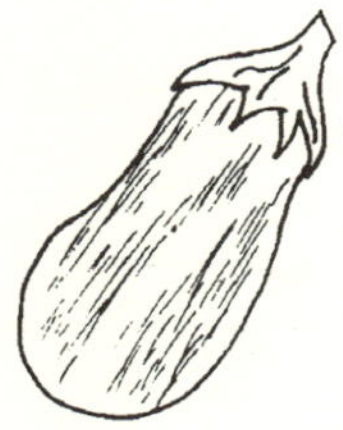

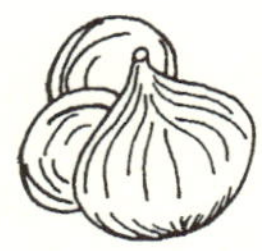

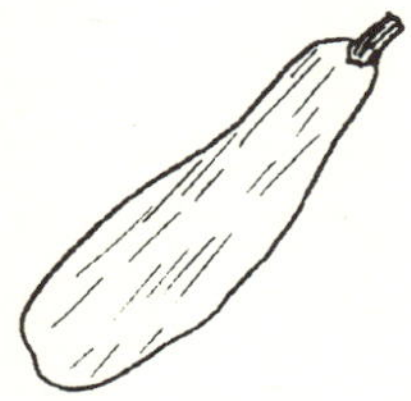

1. Trim any excess fat from meat. If needed, cut into approximately 1/2 inch cubes. In a 5-quart Dutch-oven kettle, brown meat in the oil. Season with salt and summer savory. Stir occasionally to brown cubes on all sides.
2. Add liquid and onion. Bring to boil. Reduce heat. Cover. Simmer for 20 minutes. Stir occasionally.
3. While meat is cooking, prepare vegetables as described above. Add tomatoes, eggplant, and zucchini to meat and simmer 10 minutes more. Now add potatoes to stew and simmer an additional 10 minutes or until potatoes are almost done. If needed, add more broth or water.
4. If you are using green peppers, add and stir. Continue to cook another 5 minutes.
5. Whisk water and potato starch together. Then add potato starch mixture slowly to stew while stirring. Continue to cook to thicken the broth, stirring continually. If you are using peas, add them now during the cooking time for the thickener.
6. Serve when potatoes are tender.

Yield: approximately 6 cups or 4 servings

Special Note: I have prepared this recipe several times with additional eggplant, zucchini, and water when I am extra hungry. The vegetables above may be exchanged for other vegetables as desired. Try to have some contrasting colors. If your family does not like the rust color appearance, remove the stew to be served to the person with CRC to another dish and add Kitchen Bouquet to the remainder to improve color for serving to family and guests.

*Special Note: If you add peas, you need to avoid eating peas on your Day 4 just before and after serving this recipe on Day 2.

Minute Steak with Garbanzo Bean Gravy

2 servings	minute steak beef or buffalo (approximately 1/3 pound each)
as needed	garbanzo bean flour
2 teaspoons	sunflower oil
to season	sea salt and summer savory

Ingredients for the gravy:

2 tablespoons	garbanzo bean flour
2 cups	water
1/4 teaspoon	sea salt

1. Preheat electric skillet to 350°F. Add oil. This recipe was developed using a stainless steel electric skillet; others may require more oil.
2. Roll meat in the flour. Place in hot skillet. Sprinkle with seasonings as desired to taste. Cover with a splatter screen (information on page 60). Brown the meat for 2 minutes—the browner the meat, the browner the gravy—but be careful not to dry the meat out or burn it. Turn meat, cover with splatter screen, and brown for another 2 minutes.
3. While the second side is browning, combine the gravy ingredients and blend with small whisk or fork. After browning meat, add the gravy mixture to skillet. Loosen any stuck meat pieces with a spatula. Cover and reduce heat to between simmer and 200°F. Simmer for 15–20 minutes, however do check on it from time to time.

Yield: 2 servings

Easy Steak Dinner

1 pound	beef round steak, cut into strips
1/3 cup	arrowroot starch
	OR 1/2 cup garbanzo bean flour
1 teaspoon	sea salt
1/4 teaspoon	summer savory (optional)
1 large	onion, sliced (approximately 2 cups sliced onion rings)
2 cups	green pepper strips, fresh or frozen
2 cups	zucchini squash, peeled and sliced, fresh or frozen
1 quart	tomato quarters or pieces

1. Prepare meat and vegetables as described above. Partially frozen meat will cut into thin strips easier. Layer beef strips in bottom of standard-size slow cooker. Add thickener and seasonings. Stir to coat meat with the flour.
2. Layer onions, green peppers, and zucchini on the top of the meat mixture. Do Not Stir. Pour tomato pieces and juice as evenly as possible over the layered meat and vegetables. Again, Do Not Stir.
3. Cover and cook on high for 4–5 hours or on low for 8–10 hours. Serve over boiled potatoes or cooked garbanzo beans. Leftovers may be frozen and reheated slowly. The appearance is not as pretty after freezing, but the taste is still wonderful.

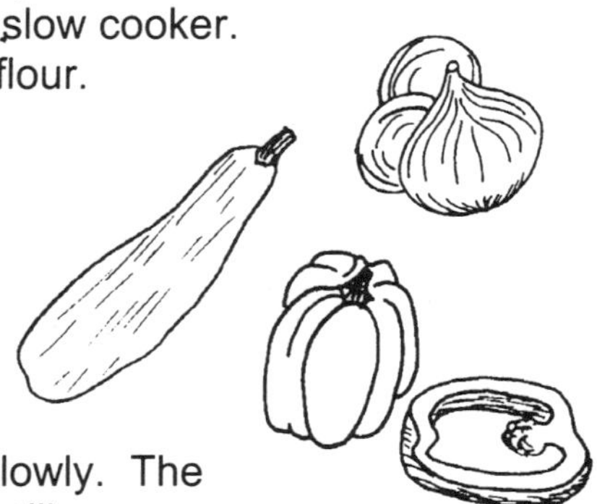

Yield: 4 servings

Easy Rabbit Dinner

Prepare the same as Easy Steak Dinner (except omit savory) substituting deboned rabbit for steak. I substitute 1 rabbit for 1 pound of steak. In addition, I soak rabbit several hours or overnight in salt water to remove most of the wild game taste.

Stuffed Green Peppers

1 pound	ground beef or buffalo
1 cup	Muir Glen brand organic tomato puree
1 cup	water
1/4 cup	onion, diced
2 cups	zucchini or eggplant, peeled, diced, fresh or frozen
1 1/2 cups	Garbanzo Beans and Broth, drained (page 161)
1 3/4 teaspoons	sea salt
1/4 teaspoon	minced garlic
1/2 teaspoon	Watkins Salsa Seasoning Blend or other Mexican blend spices
as needed	green peppers, choose peppers with somewhat flat bottoms so they will stand up in the casserole dish after being stuffed

1. In skillet, cook ground meat, until meat is done. Stir often to chop meat and brown evenly.

2. Add rest of the ingredients except green peppers. Bring to boil. Reduce heat, cover, and simmer 30 minutes. Stir occasionally. Taste and add more spices as desired.

3. While meat mixture is simmering, prepare green peppers. Wash peppers and cut off tops (stem end). Next, remove seeds and the center bitter membranes to which they are attached. I find it easy to remove this membrane by first cutting most of it free with a sharp knife and then using a teaspoon to scrape it out without cutting or damaging the green pepper. Rerinse to remove all seeds and loose pieces of membrane.

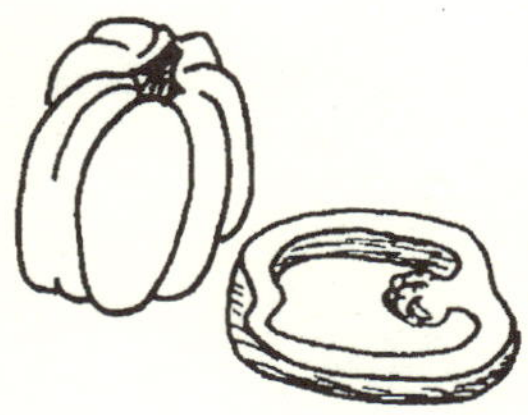

4. Steam prepared peppers in steamer pan for 8–10 minutes. Remove from pan and chill in ice water to stop the cooking process. Drain.

5. When the sauce is ready, fill the peppers. Place stuffed peppers in covered casserole dish(es) that is tall enough to allow for the height of the peppers. Bake covered in 350°F. oven approximately 30 minutes or until pepper is tender and stuffing is at serving temperature. Serve immediately. If needed, melt a little shredded taco cheese on top of the peppers not served to the person with CRC.

6. Stuffed peppers can be frozen before baking for future quick meals. Also, you can prepare green peppers and freeze them unstuffed when they are in season so you may enjoy this dish year round.

Yield: 6 cups of stuffing, usually enough for 12 small- to medium-size peppers

Tacos

1 pound	ground beef or buffalo
1 cup	Muir Glen brand organic tomato puree
1 cup	water
1/4 cup	onion, chopped
1 teaspoon	sea salt
1/4 teaspoon	garlic, minced
1/2 teaspoon	Watkins Salsa Seasoning Blend or other Mexican blend spices
as needed	Amaranth Tortillas (page 158)

<u>Toppings</u>

as needed	tomatoes, fresh, diced
as needed	lettuce, shredded
as desired	onions, diced
as desired	Guacamole (page 196)
as desired	Picante Sauce (page 196)

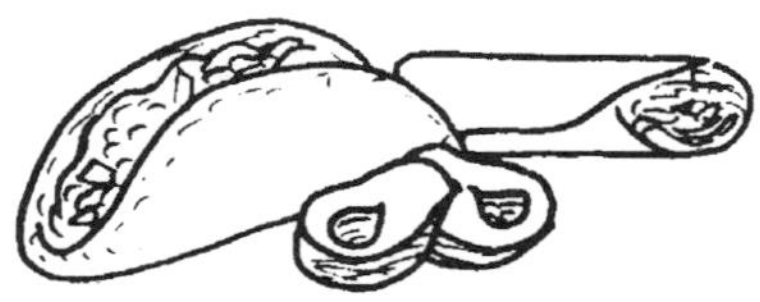

1. If desired, prepare onions, Guacamole, and/or Picante Sauce. Chill.
2. Prepare or thaw tortillas.
3. In a skillet, cook ground meat until done. Stir often to chop meat and brown evenly. Add remaining ingredients except for tortillas and toppings. Simmer 30 minutes. Stir occasionally. Taste and, if desired, add more spices.
4. While meat mixture is simmering, prepare tomatoes and lettuce. Refrigerate until needed. Often I stir 1/8 teaspoon of Watkins Salsa Seasoning Blend into the diced tomatoes.
5. To serve—layer meat mixture, lettuce, tomatoes, onions, Guacamole, and/or Picante Sauce in amount desired on 1/2 of tortilla. Fold, lift, and hold with both hands. Eat and enjoy.

Yield: 2 1/4 cups of taco meat

The ability to beat the odds lies within us all.

Destiny is not a matter of chance; it is a matter of choice.

Enchiladas

8	Amaranth Tortillas (page 158)

Filling Ingredients:

1 pound	ground beef or buffalo
1 cup	Muir Glen brand organic tomato puree
1 cup	water
1 cup	eggplant, peeled, cubed
1/4 cup	onion, diced
1/2 cup	green pepper, diced
1 teaspoon	sea salt
1/2 teaspoon	Watkins Salsa Seasoning Blend or other Mexican blend spices
1/4 teaspoon	minced garlic

Sauce Ingredients:

1 cup	Muir Glen brand organic tomato puree
1/4 cup	onion, diced
1/4 cup	green pepper, diced
1 teaspoon	sea salt
1/4 teaspoon	chili powder
1/8 teaspoon	Watkins Salsa Seasoning Blend or other Mexican blend spices
1/8 teaspoon	minced garlic

Topping Ingredients:

as desired	shredded lettuce
as desired	diced fresh tomatoes

1. Prepare or thaw tortillas.
2. In skillet, cook ground meat until done. Stir often to chop meat and brown evenly.
3. Add rest of the filling ingredients. Heat to boiling, reduce heat, cover, and simmer at least 30 minutes. Stir occasionally. Filling yields 4 cups.
4. While filling is simmering, combine all sauce ingredients in a 3 cup or larger measure and add enough water to yield 3 cups.
5. Spread 1/2 cup of filling mixture lengthwise on the center third of tortilla. Fold tortilla from each side on top of mixture. Carefully transfer enchilada to covered casserole dish and place folded side down. I prefer to use a 10-inch Corning shallow baking dish. If you crowd them you can get 4 enchiladas in the dish. Pour sauce evenly over enchiladas, 3/4 cup sauce per enchilada.
6. Bake in 350°F. oven for approximately 30 minutes or until sauce is bubbling and enchilada filling is at serving temperature.
7. While enchiladas are baking, prepare lettuce and tomatoes. Refrigerate until needed. Often I stir a small amount of Watkins Salsa Seasoning Blend into the diced tomatoes.
8. To Serve: Cut each enchilada in half crosswise. Then use 2 large metal spatulas to transfer enchiladas to dinner plates. Top with lettuce and tomatoes.

Special Note: If your family is not large enough to eat all 8 tortillas, simply freeze the filling and sauce separately for an future quick meal.

Yield: 8 enchiladas (4 cups of filling and 3 cups of sauce)

Amaranth Pizza Crust

Ingredients	5 inch	7 inch
amaranth flour	3 tablespoons	1/3 cup
arrowroot starch	1 tablespoon + 2 teaspoons	3 tablespoons
baking soda	1/8 teaspoon	1/4 teaspoon
vitamin C crystals	1/16 rounded teaspoon	1/8 rounded teaspoon
sea salt	2 pinches	scant 1/8 teaspoon
water	scant 2 tablespoons	scant 3 tablespoons
olive oil	1 1/2 teaspoons	1 tablespoon
pizza sauce	1/2 cup	3/4 cup

Ingredients	12 inch	10 X 14 inch
amaranth flour	1 cup	1 1/4 cups
arrowroot starch	1/2 cup	2/3 cup
baking soda	5/8 teaspoon	3/4 teaspoon
vitamin C crystals	3/8 teaspoon	1/2 teaspoon
sea salt	scant 1/4 teaspoon	1/4 teaspoon
water	1/2 cup	2/3 cup
olive oil	2 tablespoons	2 tablespoons + 1 1/2 teaspoons
pizza sauce	2 cups	2 1/2 cups

Combine the 5- and 7-inch pizza crust recipe to yield approximately a 10-inch pizza crust. 10 x 14-inch recipe can also be made into six 5-inch crusts.

1. Have your pizza sauce completely ready and warm.
2. Preheat oven to 350°F.
3. Measure oil according to chart below and place in center of stainless steel pizza pan or baking sheet. Set aside.

1/2 teaspoon for 5-inch
3/4 teaspoon for 7-inch
1 teaspoon for 10- and 12-inch
1 1/4 teaspoons for 10 X 14-inch

4. In mixing bowl, whisk together dry ingredients. Make a "well" in the center
5. Add water and oil. Stir with rubber spatula, making sure all dry ingredients are moistened.
6. Using fingers, spread oil on pizza pan to within one inch of edge. Make sure hands are lightly coated with oil before beginning next step.
7. With your lightly oil coated fingers, touch dough. If dough seems a little too soft and is sticky to your fingers, you have probably added too much liquid, which is easy to do. I suggest that you mix between 1 teaspoon and 1 tablespoon more flour into your dough before proceeding with the next step.
8. Transfer dough to pizza pan or baking sheet. Press dough out in a circular shape, maintaining even thickness and pressing out from the center in all directions. Push outer edge of dough circle up on outer edge of pizza pan to form crust edge, or create an edge if forming on a flat surface. Dough should be about 3/8 inch thick. If dough appears thin in spots, press surrounding dough toward thin area to remedy.

continued on next page

Amaranth Pizza Crust (continued)

9. Wash hands to remove oil.

10. Pour warm pizza sauce onto crust and spread out to cover crust surface. Add toppings according to sauce recipe.

11. Bake at 350°F. for 20-25 minutes (see chart):

20 minutes for 5-inch or 7-inch pizza
25 minutes for 10-inch, 12-inch, or 10 x 14-inch pizza

Special Note: Be aware when measuring tablespoons of water that it may tend to "round up" on the measuring spoon. Be sure to check that your tablespoon of water is a LEVEL tablespoon.

Recipe idea from Mastering Food Allergies newsletter, May 1991.

Meat and Vegetable Pizza Sauce

Sauce Ingredients

4 cloves	garlic, minced
1 1/2 teaspoons	olive oil
1 pound	ground beef or ground buffalo
1/2 cup	onion, chopped
1 cup	green pepper, chopped
3 1/2 cups	your choice of Day 2 vegetables: eggplant, zucchini, okra I prefer: 2 1/2 cups eggplant, peeled, 1/2-inch cubed 1 cup zucchini squash, peeled, 1/2-inch cubed
1 can	Muir Glen brand organic tomato puree (16 ounces)
2 cups	water
1 1/4 teaspoons	sea salt
1/4 teaspoon	summer savory
2 teaspoons	basil
1 1/2 tablespoons	leaf oregano
1/4 teaspoon	crushed cayenne (red) pepper

Topping Ingredients

as desired	green peppers, chopped or stripped
as desired	Spaghetti Squash (page 185)

1. In large skillet or kettle, sauté garlic in oil until soft. Add ground meat, and cook until meat is done. Stir often to chop meat and brown evenly.

2. Add rest of the ingredients. Heat to boiling, reduce heat, and cover. Simmer at least 1 hour. Stir occasionally. Taste and, if desired, add more seasonings.

3. Prepare Amaranth Pizza Crust (page 172). Pour warm sauce onto crust and spread out to cover crust surface. Sprinkle with desired amount of green peppers. Also, string spaghetti squash over the top to give the appearance of cheese. Bake according to pizza crust recipe.

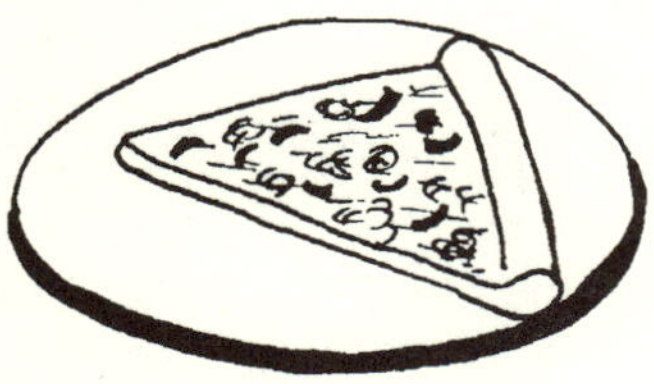

Yield: 6 cups of sauce, freeze leftover sauce for a quick pizza later

Special Note: Vegetables in this recipe may be prepared and frozen when they are in season.

Taco Pizza Sauce

Sauce Ingredients

1 pound	ground beef or buffalo
1 cup	Muir Glen brand organic tomato puree
1 cup	water
1/4 cup	onion, chopped
2 cups	eggplant, peeled, chopped
1/2 teaspoon	sea salt
1/4 teaspoon	garlic, minced
3/4 teaspoon	Watkins Salsa Seasoning Blend or other Mexican blend spices

Topping Ingredients

1/2 cup	onions, diced
4–5 cups	lettuce, shredded
2 cups	tomatoes, fresh, diced
as desired	Guacamole (page 196)
as desired	Picante Sauce (page 196)

1. Prepare Guacamole and Picante Sauce. Chill.
2. In skillet, cook ground meat until done, stir often to chop meat and brown evenly. Add remaining sauce ingredients. Bring to boil, reduce heat, cover, and simmer 30 minutes. Stir occasionally. Taste and, if desired, add more spices.
3. While sauce is simmering, prepare Amaranth Pizza Crust (page 172). Pour warm sauce onto crust and spread out to cover crust surface. Sprinkle with additional onions. Bake according to pizza crust recipe.
4. While pizza is baking, prepare tomatoes, lettuce and onions. Refrigerate until needed. Often, I stir 1/8 teaspoon of Watkins Salsa Seasoning Blend or other Mexican blend spices into the diced tomatoes.
5. Cut pizza into desired serving pieces. Top with desired amount of prepared topping.

Yield: 4 cups of sauce, enough for two 12-inch pizzas

Tofu Lasagna*

3 cloves	garlic, minced
3/4 cup	onion, chopped
1 teaspoon	olive oil
1 pound	ground beef or buffalo
1 1/2 teaspoons	sea salt
1 can	Muir Glen brand organic tomato puree (16 ounces)
2 cups	water
1 1/2 teaspoons	basil
1 tablespoon	oregano
1/2 teaspoon	summer savory
1 pound	soft tofu, drained, thinly sliced*
1 medium	eggplant, peeled, thinly sliced

To Prepare Sauce:

1. In large skillet or kettle, sauté garlic and onion in oil until soft. Add ground meat cook until meat is done. Stir often to chop meat and brown evenly.

continued on next page

Tofu Lasagna (continued)

2. Add all other ingredients except tofu and eggplant. Heat to boiling, reduce heat, cover, and simmer at least 30 minutes. Stir occasionally. Taste and, if desired, add more seasonings. Sauce yields approximately 4 1/2 cups.

To Prepare Lasagna:

3. Oven temperature—350°F. Preheating not necessary.
4. Layer lasagna in a Corning 10-inch covered casserole dish:
   - 1 cup of sauce, spread evenly over bottom of dish
   - thin slices of eggplant to cover sauce (can be straight from freezer)
   - thin slices of tofu to cover eggplant
   - 1 1/2 cups of sauce, spread evenly over tofu
   - thin slices of eggplant to cover sauce
   - thin slices of tofu to cover eggplant
   - approximately 2 cups of sauce to cover everything completely
5. Bake covered for approximately 50–60 minutes or until sauce is bubbling in center as well as on sides and all ingredients are fork tender. Remove lasagna from oven and allow it to set approximately 5 minutes before serving. Cut 4x4 and remove with spatula. Leftovers can be frozen. For best quality, thaw and reheat leftovers slowly in a covered dish. If you prepare this recipe in individual serving dishes, you may freeze unbaked. Thaw completely and bake as usual.

Yield: 4 servings

*Tofu is usually eaten on Day 4, so you need to avoid eating soy on your Day 4 just before and after eating this recipe on your Day 2.

Special Note: If desired, you may add Soy Lasagna Noodles (page 251) that I use in my Day 4 Shrimp Tofu Lasagna.

If your family would prefer Lasagna with noodles and a little cheese, you can prepare the recipe in individual serving dishes (such as Grab-It bowls). When using lasagna noodles, layer uncooked noodles in place of eggplant for the first layer and along with eggplant for the second layer. When using cheese, sprinkle a little mozzarella cheese after each layer of tofu.

Low Carbohydrate Lasagna

Use sauce ingredients from Tofu Lasagna recipe—except use only 1 1/2 cups of water

3 layers	summer squash, sliced approximately 1/4 inch thick
3–6 layers	amaranth greens, washed and drained (page 44)
	OR spinach leaves (see * explanation on Vegetarian Lasagna on page 176)

1. Prepare sauce as in steps 1 and 2 in Tofu Lasagna recipe above, except use only 1 1/2 cups of water. Sauce yields approximately 4 cups.
2. Oven temperature—350°F. Preheating not necessary.
3. Layer lasagna in a Corning 10-inch covered casserole dish.
   - 3/4 cup of sauce, spread evenly over bottom of dish
   - 1 layer of squash slices to cover sauce (can be straight from freezer)
   - 1–2 layers of amaranth greens
   - 1 cup of sauce, spread evenly
   - repeat squash, greens, and 1 cup sauce layers 2 more times using remaining sauce on top of final layer
4. Bake and serve as described in step 5 in Tofu Lasagna (recipe above).

Vegetarian Lasagna*

5 cloves	garlic, minced
1 cup	onion, chopped
1 tablespoon	olive oil
1 can	Muir Glen brand organic tomato puree (16 ounces)
2 cups	water
3 cups	eggplant, chopped
1 cup	green pepper, chopped
4 teaspoons	leaf oregano
2 teaspoons	basil
1 1/2 teaspoons	sea salt
as desired	amaranth greens, washed and drained (page 44) OR spinach leaves*
1 recipe	Soy Lasagna Noodles (page 251)**
1 pound	soft tofu, drained, thinly sliced lengthwise (12 slices)**

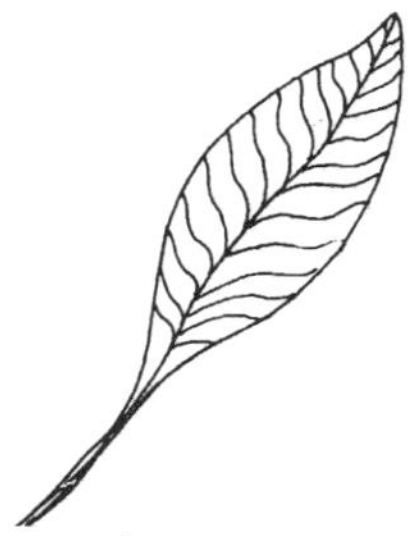

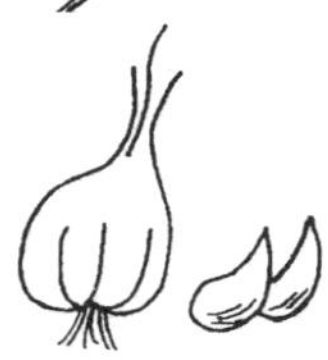

To prepare sauce:

1. In a large kettle sauté garlic and onion in oil until soft.
2. Add tomato puree, water, eggplant, green peppers and seasonings. Heat to boiling, reduce heat, cover and simmer at least 1 hour. Stir occasionally. Taste and add more seasonings, if desired. Measure sauce and add more water if sauce does not yield 4 1/2–5 cups.

To prepare lasagna:

3. Oven temperature—350°F. Preheating not necessary.
4. Layer ingredients in following order in a Corning 10-inch square covered casserole dish. (This recipe can also be prepared in 6 covered Corning Grab-It Bowls.)
   - 1 cup sauce, spread evenly
   - 2–3 layers of amaranth greens or spinach leaves
   - 1 layer of Soy Lasagna Noodles
   - 6 slices of tofu
   - 1 1/2 cups sauce, spread evenly
   - 1 layer of Soy Lasagna Noodles
   - 2–3 layers of amaranth greens or spinach leaves
   - 6 slices of tofu
   - 2 cups sauce, spread evenly
5. Cover and bake for 60–70 minutes until sauce is bubbling and all ingredients are fork tender. Remove from oven, cool covered for 5 minutes to set up. Cut into desired portions and serve with a spatula. Leftovers may be frozen. For best quality, thaw and reheat slowly in a covered dish. If you prepare recipe in the individual bowls, you may freeze them unbaked. Thaw bowls completely and bake as usual.

Special Notes:

If you wish, you may prepare this recipe in individual serving dishes for other family members and replace the soy noodles with uncooked whole-wheat or spelt lasagna noodles. You can also replace 1 layer of tofu with mozzarella cheese.

I prefer to use an 8-cup measure to mix sauce ingredients so I can check the yield and evenly distribute it between layers.

continued on next page

Vegetarian Lasagna (continued)

*If you use spinach you need to plan ahead to omit spinach on your Day 3 before and omit all foods from the Goosefoot Family (beet, chard, quinoa, spinach) from your Day 1 just before and Day 3 after enjoying spinach in this recipe on your Day 2 (see table below).

**Soy is usually eaten on Day 4 so you need to avoid eating soy on your Day 4 just before and after eating this recipe on your Day 2.

Yield: 4–6 servings

Vegetarian Pizza

1/2 recipe	sauce only from Vegetarian Lasagna (page 176)
as needed	amaranth greens, washed and drained Or spinach leaves*
12-inch	Amaranth Pizza Crust (page 172)
as desired	green peppers, chopped
as desired	Spaghetti Squash (page 185)

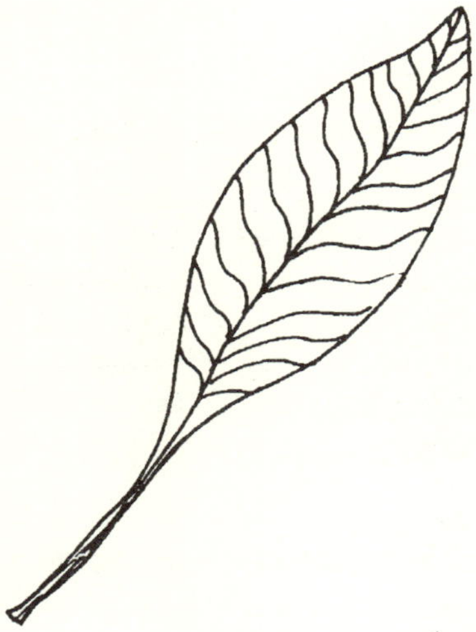

1. Prepare sauce according to Vegetarian Lasagna recipe. I also add 4 pinches of crushed red pepper. Keep warm.
2. Prepare Amaranth Pizza Crust according to recipe. Layer amaranth greens to cover crust (1 or more layers—your choice). Pour warm sauce onto crust and spread out to cover greens and crust surface.
3. Sprinkle with desired amount of peppers. String spaghetti squash over top to give appearance of cheese. Bake according to pizza crust recipe.

Yield: one 12-inch pizza

Special Note: It is easier to prepare a single recipe of sauce and freeze half of it for a quick pizza later.

*If you use spinach you need to plan ahead to omit spinach on your Day 3 before and omit all foods from the Goosefoot Family (beet, chard, quinoa, spinach) from your Day 1 just before and Day 3 just after enjoying spinach in this recipe on your Day 2 (see table below).

Day 1	Day 2	Day 3	Day 4
		omit spinach	

Day 1	Day 2	Day 3	Day 4
omit all Goosefoot Family	have Pizza or Lasagna with spinach leaves	omit all Goosefoot Family	

Spaghetti and Meat Sauce

(Two Variations)

4 cups	With Vegetables 6 cups	YIELD
2 cloves	3 cloves	garlic, minced
1 teaspoon	1 teaspoon	olive oil
1 pound	1 pound	ground beef or buffalo
1/2 cup	1/2 cup	onion, chopped
3/4 cup	3/4 cup	green pepper, chopped
none	3 1/2 cups	your choice of Day 2 vegetables—eggplant, zucchini, okra I prefer: 2 1/2 cups eggplant, peeled, 1/2-inch cubed 1 cup zucchini squash, peeled, 1/2-inch cubed
1 can	1 can	Muir Glen brand organic tomato puree (16 ounces)
2 cups	2 cups	water
1 1/4 teaspoons	1 1/2 teaspoons	sea salt
1/4 teaspoon	1/4 teaspoon	summer savory
1 1/2 teaspoons	2 teaspoons	basil
1 tablespoon	4 teaspoons	leaf oregano
scan 1/4 teaspoon	1/4 teaspoon	crushed cayenne (red) pepper
1–2 tablespoons	1–2 tablespoons	thickener—arrowroot starch, garbanzo bean flour, or potato starch (optional)

1. In large skillet or kettle, sauté garlic in oil until soft. Add ground meat and cook until meat is done. Stir often to chop meat and brown evenly.
2. Add rest of ingredients except thickener. Heat to boiling, reduce heat, and cover. Simmer at least 1 hour. Stir occasionally. Taste and, if desired, add more seasonings.
3. (Optional) Just before serving, dissolve your choice of thickener in a small amount of water. Add gradually, stirring continually to thicken the sauce. Add more thickener if desired. This is basically to add body to the sauce and to help remove the watery texture.
4. Serve with Spaghetti Squash (page 185) or temporarily transfer buckwheat to Day 2 and serve with purchased 100% buckwheat soba noodles. Leftover sauce can be frozen for future quick meals. After freezing and reheating you need to add more thickener.

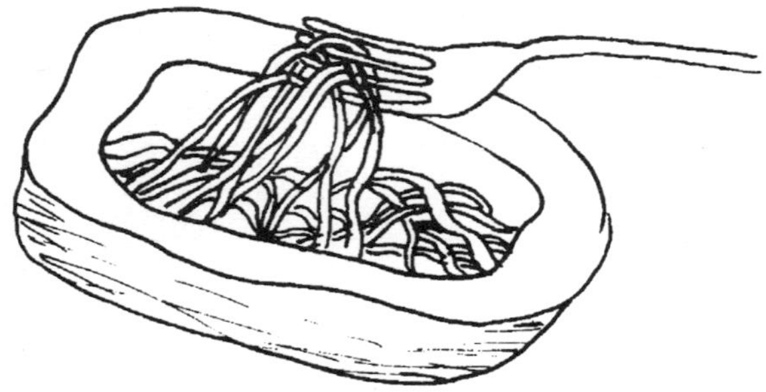

The darkest hour is only 60 minutes long.

Baked Fish for Day 2

Your choice of Day 2 fish fillets	cod (scrod), pollack, red snapper
Your choice of Day 2 seasonings	basil, garlic, oregano, savory, rosemary, and/or thyme
Your choice of Day 2 foods	sliced onion, green pepper strips, sliced zucchini squash, and/or, sunflower seeds
Your choice of Day 2 oil	olive oil, butter, or Clarified Butter (page 195)

Place fish fillets in covered casserole dish. Sprinkle with salt and seasonings. Garnish with your choice of other foods. Drizzle with approximately 1/2 teaspoon of oil per serving or dot with butter. Also, I usually add 1–2 tablespoons of water to casserole dish. Cover and bake for approximately 30 minutes at 350°F. until fish is flaky. Time will depend on thickness of fillet, whether fillet is frozen or thawed, and amount of other foods used. Garnish with a squeeze of fresh lemon and serve.

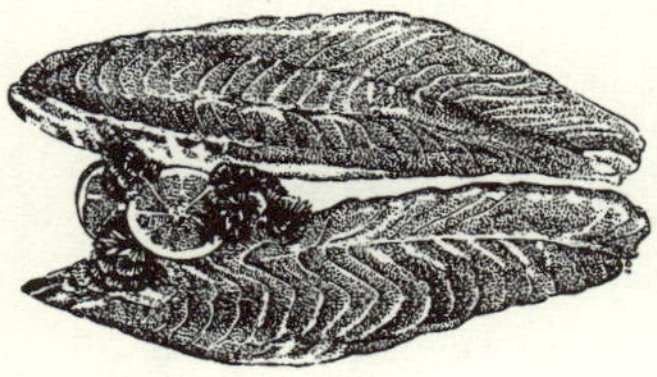

Grilled Shrimp

Prepare jumbo shrimp by following steps 1 and 2 of Fresh Shelled Shrimp recipe (page 181). Heat and brown shrimp on small electric grill to serving temperature. Turn often to prevent burning. I use a grill which has a thermostat for better temperature control which is especially needed for fish. Serve with a squeeze of fresh lemon, melted and seasoned Clarified Butter (page 195), and/or Picante Sauce (page 196).

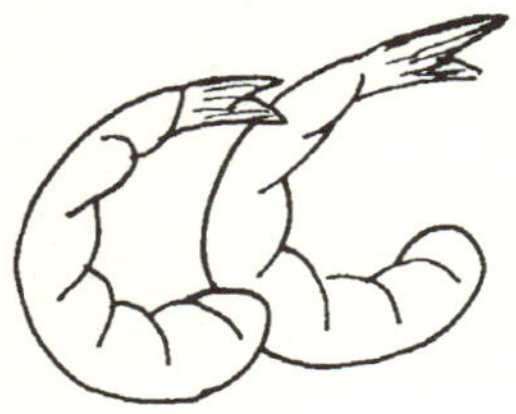

Spicy Baked Fish

1/2 pound	cod (scrod) or pollack fillet (2 servings)
2 cups	canned tomato quarters or pieces, drained OR 1 cup of fresh peeled tomatoes quarters
1/4 teaspoon	sea salt
1/2 teaspoon	leaf oregano
1/4 teaspoon	basil
1/4 teaspoon	minced garlic
2 cups	zucchini squash, peeled, sliced or diced OR 1 cup sliced okra
1/2 cup	onion, sliced or chopped (optional)

Place fish fillets in a shallow covered casserole dish. (I use a 10-inch square Corning casserole dish.) Combine tomatoes and seasonings. Add rest of vegetables and stir. Pour vegetable mixture evenly over fish. Cover and bake approximately 45 minutes until fish is flaky and vegetables are tender.

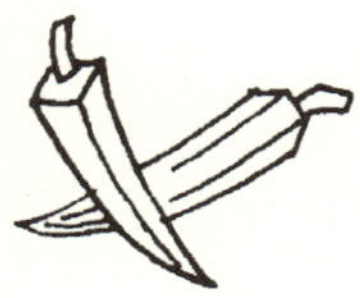

Suggestion: Save tomato juice to drink or freeze to add to soup.

Yield: 1 pound of fish equals 3–4 servings

Sunflower "Mayo"

1/2 cup	raw, hulled sunflower seeds
1 cup	water
1 teaspoon	unbuffered, corn-free vitamin C crystals
1 tablespoon	arrowroot starch
1/4 teaspoon	sea salt
1/4 teaspoon	garlic powder (optional)

1. Blend sunflower seeds in blender on highest speed until they become a fine powder, approximately 1–2 minutes. Stop once or twice to scrape sides and bottom of blender jar.
2. Add rest of the ingredients. Blend on highest speed for a minute longer, stopping once or twice to scrape sides and bottom of blender jar.
3. Pour mixture into small saucepan. Cook over medium heat, stirring constantly, until mixture thickens. I prefer to stir with a whisk to keep mixture smooth.
4. Chill. If necessary, you may store in a glass jar in the refrigerator for a week. If too thick, you may add additional water. Taste and add more garlic powder if you desire.

Yield: 1 1/3 cups

Recipe idea from The Yeast Connection Cookbook by Crook & Jones, p. 208.

Creamy Italian Salad Dressing

1 1/3 cups	Sunflower "Mayo" (recipe above)
2 teaspoons	leaf oregano
1 teaspoon	basil
1/4 teaspoon	garlic powder
1/4 teaspoon	sea salt

Prepare "Mayo." Add seasonings. Stir. Chill. Add small amount of water if too thick.

Yield: 1 1/3 cups

Lemon/Oil Dressing

The person with CRC usually cannot use commercial salad dressing. I have found mixing 1 teaspoon of sunflower oil with 1/2 teaspoon of freshly squeezed lemon juice to be rather tasty.

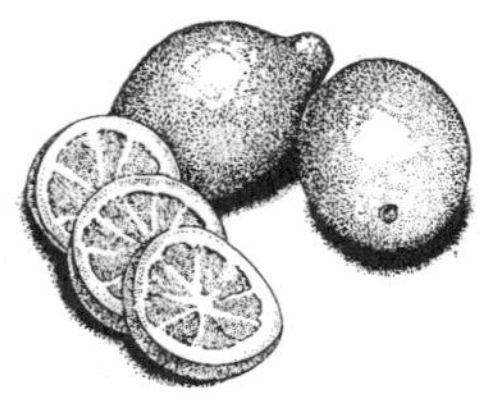

I have also found it difficult to always have fresh lemon juice on hand, so I developed the following recipe method.

Lemon Juice—Tips on Preparing and Storing

Wash lemons, cut in half crosswise, and squeeze juice using a hand juicer. Remove large pulp pieces and seeds. Pour into any dish with sides that will allow the juice to be only about 1/4–1/2 inch thick. Freeze, then cut into 1-inch squares and keep frozen in a bag for later use. Each square thaws very quickly to mix with oil for use in salad dressing. Save time and prepare several lemons at a time. Also, you can peel the lemons as you would an orange and run them through a juicer.

Zucchini Salad Dressing

1 cup	zucchini squash, peeled, diced
1/2 cup	water
1/2 teaspoon	unbuffered, corn-free vitamin C crystals
1 1/2 teaspoons	sunflower oil
2 pinches	sea salt
as desired	garlic or onion powder (optional)

1. Combine all ingredients, except garlic or onion powder, in blender. Blend on highest speed for 1–2 minutes until smooth. Stop once or twice to scrape sides and bottom of blender jar.

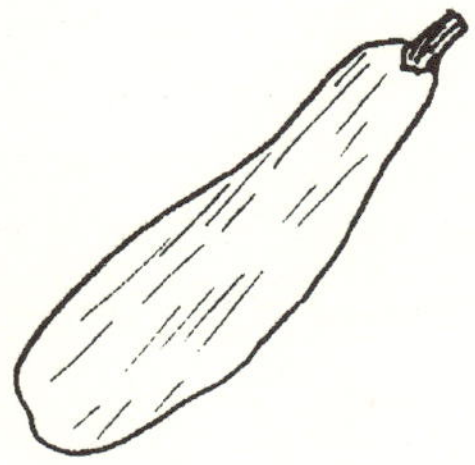

2. Chill. If necessary, you may store in a glass jar in the refrigerator for a week. Just before pouring desired amount on my salad, I add a sprinkle of garlic or onion powder to just the amount I plan to use.

Yield: I cup

Special Note: You may prepare this salad dressing with frozen zucchini also. Just measure out your 1 cup of frozen zucchini, place in blender, add the rest of the ingredients. Blend a few seconds, stir, and allow it to thaw for a minute or so. Repeat this process until zucchini is completely thawed and dressing has a nice consistency. Also, interestingly enough, you may freeze leftover dressing for later use. I freeze in ice cube trays, 1 tablespoon per cube. After freezing, I remove the cubes from the tray and keep them frozen in a cellophane bag. Then thaw just the amount desired.

Recipe idea from The Yeast Connection Cookbook by Crook & Jones, p. 207.

Fresh Shelled Shrimp
(Cooking Directions)

1. In large saucepan or kettle, bring salted water to boil. Reduce heat to medium-high. Rinse shrimp and add to boiling water. Cook for 2–3 minutes until shrimp turns a gentle pink color.

2. Drain and chill in ice water until shrimp is cold throughout. Peel and devein. To peel, pinch tail and break shell to remove it. To devein, make a shallow cut lengthwise down the back of each shrimp. Remove sand vein with point of knife and rinse shrimp.

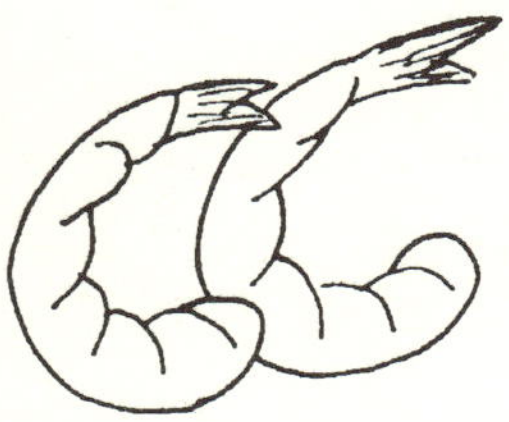

3. Dice shrimp for most recipes. I often cook 1–2 pounds and freeze in 1/4 pound amounts so I can prepare many shrimp recipes with ease. These recipes include: Shrimp Cocktail, Shrimp Vegetable Salad, Tossed Shrimp Salad, Shrimp Salad Sandwich, Chef Salad, and Vegetable Shrimp Soup. Also, I sometimes temporarily move shrimp to Day 4 to make Shrimp Tofu Lasagna.

Shrimp Cocktail

1/4 pound	Fresh Shelled Shrimp (page 181) per serving
as desired	Picante Sauce (page 196)

Prepare shrimp and Picante Sauce. Chill. Serve in stem cocktail glass for that romantic dinner at home. Or take chilled Picante Sauce with you and order a Shrimp Cocktail for an appetizer at that romantic outing.

Chef Salad

lettuce, assorted variety, torn
cucumbers, sliced
zucchini squash, sliced
green peppers, rings, stripped, or diced
red onions, rings or diced
sunflower seeds
peas, fresh or frozen, thawed and drained*
Garbanzo Beans and Broth, drained (page 161)
Fresh Shelled Shrimp, diced, chilled (page 181)
leftover cooked roast beef, diced or stripped
Zucchini Salad Dressing (page 181)
Creamy Italian Dressing (page 180)

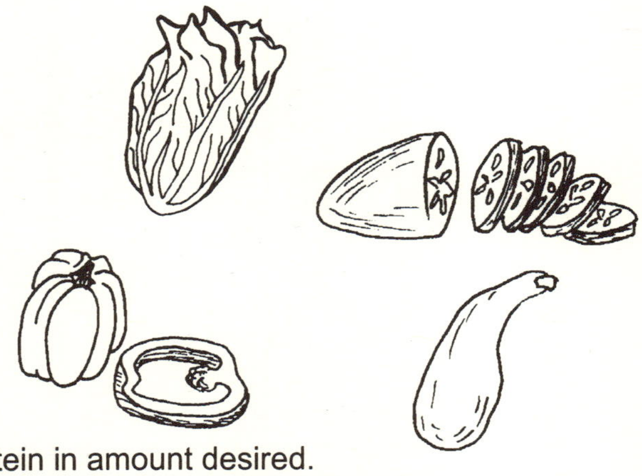

Clean and prepare your choice of vegetables and protein in amount desired. Assemble as desired. Serve with dressing of your choice and crackers for a complete light meal on a hot summer day.

*If you choose peas with your Chef Salad, you need to avoid eating peas on your Day 4 just before and after having peas with this salad.

Shrimp Vegetable Salad*

1/4 pound	Fresh Shelled Shrimp (page 181)
1/2 cup	peas, fresh or thawed and drained frozen*
1 cup	zucchini squash or cucumber, peeled, diced (or 1/2 cup of each)
1/4 cup	green pepper, diced
1/4–1/2 cup	Sunflower "Mayo" (page 180)
as desired	lettuce leaves
	OR
2 cups	lettuce, washed, drained, torn, loosely measured

1. In bowl, combine shrimp, peas, zucchini, cucumber, and green peppers. Toss gently. Add 1/4 cup of "Mayo" and mix to coat vegetables and shrimp. Chill.
2. Serve on bed of lettuce leaves.

   OR

   Just before serving, add 2 cups of lettuce and another 1/4 cup of "Mayo." Serve immediately.

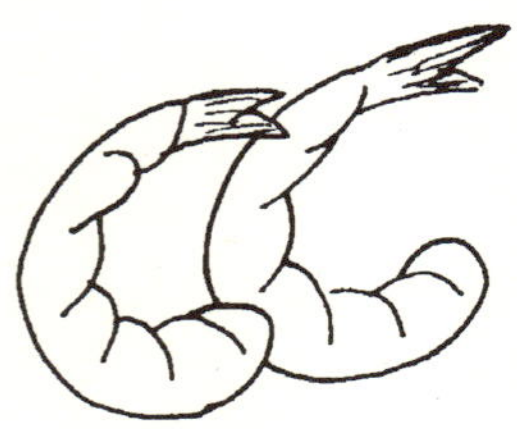

Serve with Amaranth Crackers for a complete light and easy meal.

Yield: 1 serving—2 cups without lettuce or 3 cups with lettuce

*To eat peas in this salad on Day 2, you need to avoid eating peas on your Day 4 just before and after serving this recipe.

Shrimp Salad

1 cup	Fresh Shelled Shrimp (page 181)
3/4 cup	cucumber, peeled or unpeeled, diced
1/2 cup	green pepper, diced
1/4 cup	Sunflower "Mayo" (page 180)
1/4 teaspoon	sea salt

Combine all ingredients and chill. Serve on bed of lettuce as a salad or as my favorite, a sandwich on an Amaranth Tortilla (page 158) with lettuce. Makes enough for 4 tortillas.

Yield: 2 cups

Tossed Shrimp Salad

1/4 pound	Fresh Shelled Shrimp (page 181) per serving
as desired	lettuce, washed, drained, torn
as desired	sliced cucumber
as desired	sliced zucchini
as desired	green pepper strips
as desired	red onion rings
as desired	sunflower seeds
as desired	Zucchini Salad Dressing (page 181) OR Creamy Italian Dressing (page 180)

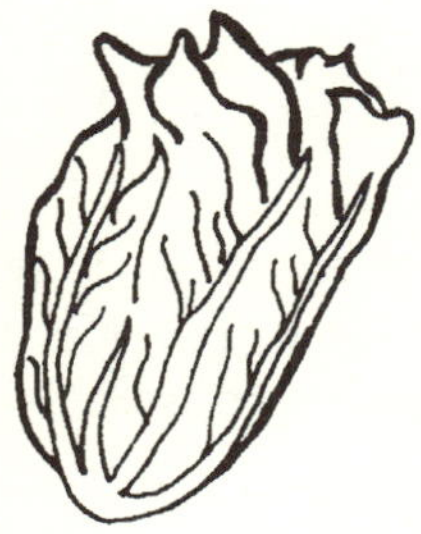

Prepare all ingredients as described above in amounts desired.
Toss salad and add dressing. Serve with Amaranth Crackers for a complete light meal.

Kidney Bean Salad*

Bean Preparation

1 cup	kidney beans
2 cups	water

Follow steps 1–3 on Kidney Beans for Chili (page 164). This will yield 3 1/4 cups cooked beans and broth or 2 1/2 cups drained kidney beans—enough for a double batch of Kidney Bean Salad. Extra cooked kidney beans can be frozen for a future quick salad. I do suggest that the liquid be frozen with the beans. When ready to use, thaw and drain to prepare the salad recipe below.

Salad Preparation

1 1/4 cups	cooked, drained kidney beans*
1 cup	cucumber, peeled or unpeeled, diced
1/2 cup	green peppers, diced
1/4 cup	Sunflower "Mayo" (page 180)
1/4 teaspoon	onion powder
1/4 teaspoon	sea salt

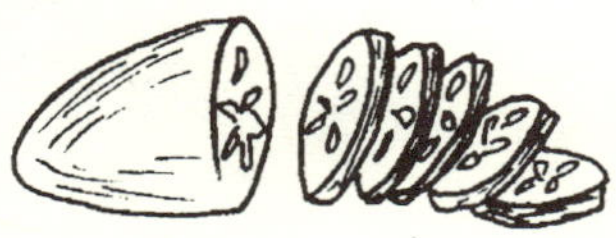

Combine all ingredients and chill.

Yield: 2 1/2 cups

*Realize that kidney beans are usually eaten on Day 4 so you need to avoid kidney beans on your Day 4 just before and after eating this salad on your Day 2.

Mixed Vegetable Salad

2 cups	your choice of diced vegetables: zucchini, cucumber, green pepper
1/2 teaspoon	onion powder
	OR 2 tablespoons finely diced onion
1/3 cup	Sunflower "Mayo" or Creamy Italian Dressing (page 180)

Combine ingredients, chill, and serve.

Yield: 2 cups

Potato Salad

2 cups	potatoes, peeled, diced
1/2 teaspoon	sea salt
2/3 cup	green or red pepper, diced
2/3 cup	cucumber
1/2 teaspoon	onion powder
	OR 2 tablespoons finely diced onion
1/3 cup	Sunflower "Mayo" (page 180)

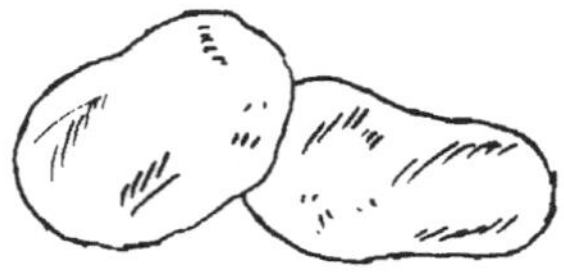

In saucepan, cook diced potatoes in small amount of water with salt on medium until tender. Drain and chill. Add rest of ingredients. Stir and chill. Sprinkle with paprika if desired.

Yield: 2 1/2 cups

Stir-Fry Vegetables for Day 2

zucchini squash, slant cut
onion, sliced into rings
green peppers, strips
sunflower or pumpkin seeds
cherry tomato
amaranth greens, torn into small pieces
olive or sunflower oil
sea salt
garlic powder, savory, basil, marjoram, and/or cayenne (red) pepper

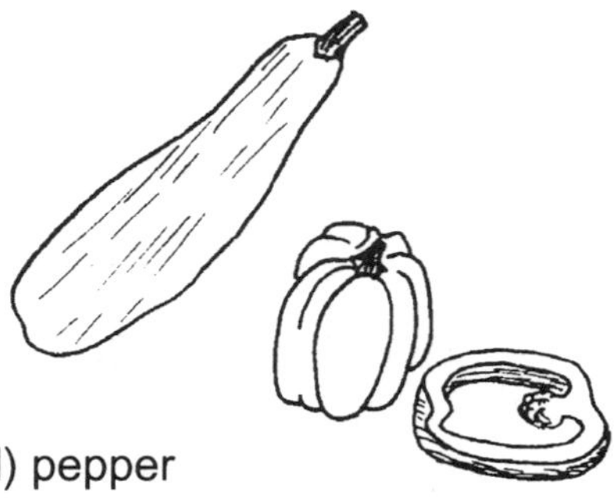

1. Preheat well-seasoned cast-iron skillet on medium (see on How to Season Cast Iron on page 63) or electric skillet to 300°F.
2. Prepare vegetables in amounts desired.
3. Add oil to preheated skillet (cast-iron skillet will require less oil). Add vegetables (except cherry tomato and amaranth greens) and nuts. Sprinkle with seasonings. Stir often to cook vegetables evenly. Add tomato and amaranth near end of cooking time just prior to serving. I prefer my vegetables crunchy and the tomatoes and amaranth greens just barely warm. Serve immediately.

Spaghetti Squash—How to Cook and Serve

1. Wash spaghetti squash, remove stem, and place in 9 X 13-inch baking dish. Add approximately 1/2-inch of water to baking dish.
2. Bake at 350ºF. for approximately 1 1/2–2 hours until the shell yields to gentle pressure. During the cooking time turn the squash by a one-quarter or one-half turn every 30 minutes. Also, do not allow the pan to become dry. Add more water if needed.
3. Remove from oven and allow to cool approximately 10 minutes.
4. Cut in half lengthwise. The knife will cause the cooked squash to fold over the seeds in the center so use a fork or spoon to gently push this back to expose the seeds. With scissors, cut the strands that attach to the seeds then remove seeds from the center with a large spoon.
5. With 2 table forks, start picking at the cooked squash. It will separate from the shell into strands that resemble spaghetti pasta, thus the name. Place desired amount on plate and top with sauce. Spaghetti squash has a somewhat sweet flavor.

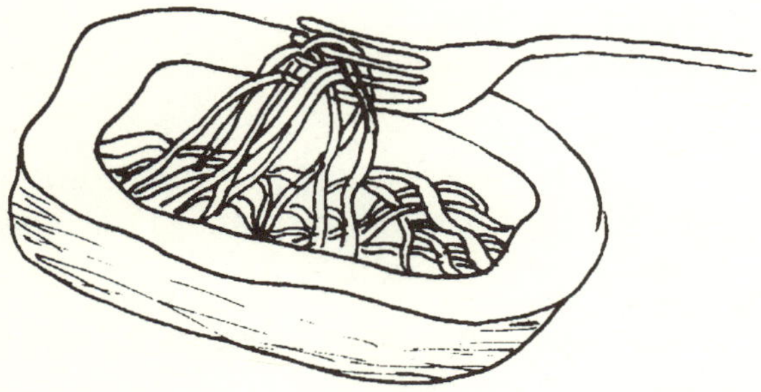

Special Notes:

I usually bake as many squash as my oven will hold at one time. Then I freeze the squash for many meals throughout the year (see Tips on Freezing and Reheating Spaghetti Squash).

If you desire, you may dry roast the spaghetti squash. Bake as above without water. It will usually cook in less time, but you need to turn the squash more often to prevent burning. I do not prefer this method because I feel that I can taste a slight burnt flavor in the cooked squash and the kitchen has a slight burnt odor.

Also, you can bake the squash in the microwave on full power for approximately 30 minutes. Turn the squash one quarter of a turn every 5 minutes. I do not prefer this method because microwaves bake somewhat unevenly.

Spaghetti Squash—Tips on Freezing and Reheating

To Freeze: Transfer long stands of cooked spaghetti squash with forks on to stainless steel baking sheets. I usually pile strands together in piles approximately 6 inches long and 1 inch high. Place sheets in freezer until the squash is frozen at least enough to hold together. Use a metal spatula to loosen squash from baking sheet and transfer to cellophane bags. Return to freezer.

To Reheat: Thaw squash at room temperature for a couple of hours or in the refrigerator for several hours or overnight. Drain. Heat in a covered casserole dish in microwave on half power until warm. Or heat in a 300ºF. oven in a covered casserole dish until warm. Serve with hot sauce.

For Pizza: Thaw and drain squash as described above under Reheat. Spread a thin layer on completed pizza to resemble cheese-like appearance. Do not place too much squash on your pizza or it will seem too sweet and not spicy enough. I love the appearance and flavor.

Cream of Potato Soup*

2 cups	potatoes, peeled, diced
1/4 cup	onions, chopped
1/2 teaspoon	sea salt
2 tablespoons	potato starch or flour
3/8 cup	chopped Brazil or macadamia nuts* (3/8 cup = 1/4 cup + 2 tablespoons)
1 tablespoon	butter or Clarified Butter (see page 195)
3 cups	liquid (potato broth and water)

1. In medium-size saucepan, cook potato, onion, and salt in a small amount of water until potatoes are almost done. Drain. Reserve liquid.
2. Combine potato starch, nuts, butter, and approximately 1/4 cup of liquid in blender. Blend on highest speed for 1–2 minutes until well blended. Stop once or twice to scrape sides and bottom of blender jar. Add rest of the liquid and blend a few seconds longer.

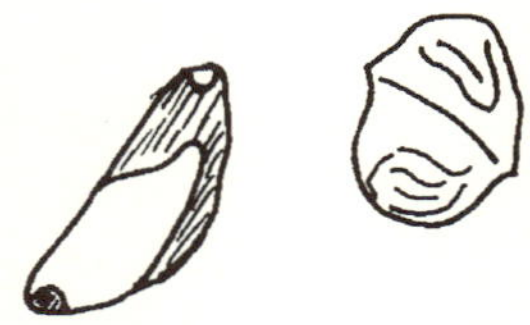

3. Transfer nut milk mixture to the saucepan you used to cook the potatoes. Cook over medium heat, stirring constantly until mixture thickens. I prefer to stir with a whisk to keep mixture smooth.
4. Add partially cooked potatoes and continue cooking until they are tender. Taste and add more salt if desired.

Yield: approximately 5 cups

Creamed Potatoes*

3 cups	potatoes, diced
3 tablespoons	onion, finely diced
3 tablespoons	green peppers, finely diced
3/4 teaspoon	sea salt
2 tablespoons	potato starch or flour
3 tablespoons	chopped Brazil or chopped macadamia nuts*
1 tablespoon	butter or Clarified Butter (see page 195)
1 1/4 cups	liquid (potato broth and water)

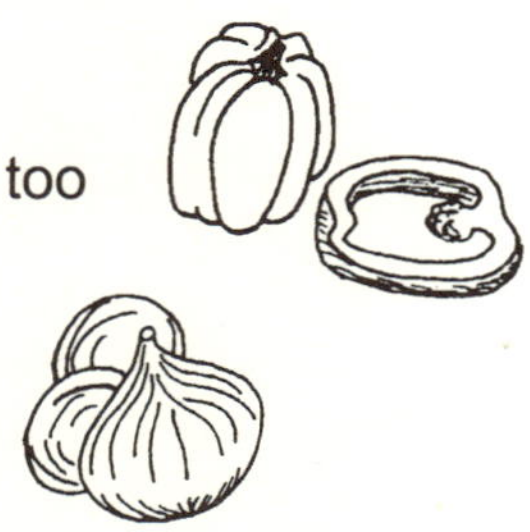

Prepare same as Cream of Potato Soup (recipe above). If mixture is too thick, add a small amount of water.

Yield: approximately 3 3/4 cups

*Brazil and macadamia nuts are unassigned "Fun Foods" on this rotational diet, see explanation on pages 30–31.

Scalloped Potatoes*

2 cups	potatoes, peeled, thinly sliced, and rinsed
2 tablespoons	onions, diced or thinly sliced
1/2 teaspoon	summer savory
1 tablespoon	potato starch
2 tablespoons	chopped Brazil or macadamia nuts*
1 tablespoon	butter or Clarified Butter (page 195)
1/2 teaspoon	sea salt
1 cup	water

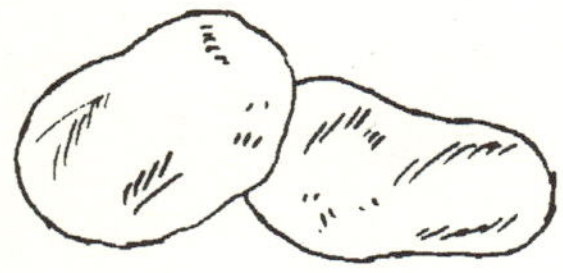

1. Oven temperature—350°F. Preheating not necessary.
2. Oil 1 1/2-quart covered casserole dish with sunflower oil.
3. Wash, peel, and thinly slice potatoes. I use my Black & Decker® Handy Shortcut™ Micro-Processor with the slicer disk. The bowl which catches the potatoes holds 2-cups so measuring is easy. Rinse and drain potatoes.
4. Layer potatoes, onions, and summer savory in oiled casserole dish.
5. Combine potato starch, nuts, butter, salt, and approximately 1/4 cup water in blender. Blend on high for approximately 1–2 minutes until well blended. Stop at least once to scrape sides and bottom of blender jar. Add rest of the water to the blender and blend for a couple seconds. Pour blended mixture into casserole dish and stir gently.
6. Bake covered for 1 1/2 hours or until potatoes are tender.

Yield: approximately 3 cups

*Brazil and macadamia nuts are unassigned "Fun Foods" on this rotational diet, see explanation on pages 30–31.

Fried Potatoes

3 medium-size	potatoes OR *plan*over, peeled, baked potatoes
1/4 cup	onions, finely diced
1/2 cup	green peppers
2 teaspoons	sunflower oil
sprinkle	ground cayenne (red) pepper
as needed	butter or Clarified Butter (page 195)

1. Wash and peel potatoes. Cut potatoes lengthwise twice (like quartered apples). Then slice each quarter 1/4-inch thick. Should yield approximately 2 cups. Steam potatoes in steamer pan for only 1–2 minutes.
2. Preheat electric skillet to 350°F. Add oil, potatoes, onions, green peppers, and cayenne pepper. Cover with splatter screen. Cook for approximately 10 minutes, stirring potatoes every 2 minutes. Use a metal spatula to loosen browned potato from skillet. Add butter or Clarified Butter about half way through the cooking process. Be careful not to burn the potatoes or vegetables but only brown them and make the potatoes crispy.

Yield: 3–4 servings

Fried Eggplant

1 medium	eggplant, peeled, sliced 3/8-inch thick
1/4 cup	arrowroot starch
1/4 cup	water
3/4 cup	Amaranth Cracker crumbs (page 156)

1. Preheat griddle. I use a well-seasoned cast-iron griddle (see How to Season Cast Iron on page 63). Griddle is hot enough when water dances when sprinkled on the griddle. Lightly oil griddle after preheating.
2. Prepare cracker crumbs. Peel and slice eggplant.
3. Stir together starch and water in small shallow bowl that is large enough for one slice of eggplant.
4. Dip each slice of eggplant into starch mixture and then place on a plate of cracker crumbs. Press to help crumbs stick to eggplant. Coat both sides of eggplant. Place on lightly oiled, preheated griddle. Cook 7–10 minutes on each side. Be careful not to burn the cracker breading. Keep warm in oven but do serve soon. Remove any loose crumbs that are left on the griddle. Lightly oil griddle again and repeat until all slices of eggplant are cooked.
5. Leftovers may be frozen. I prefer to freeze a single layer on a baking sheet. After frozen, transfer to cellophane bag. Keep frozen until ready to use (do not thaw). I enjoy the *plan*overs as Italian Fried Eggplant (page 189) or reheated on the griddle and serve for a interesting breakfast or vegetable side dish. When I reheat, I place the frozen fried eggplant on a cold griddle. While the griddle is heating the eggplant begins to thaw and heat. Turn often to prevent burning, especially after griddle is hot.

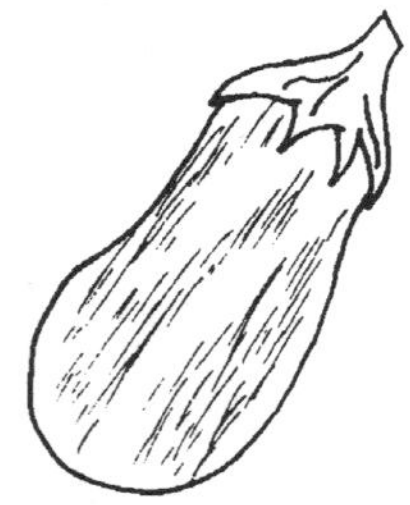

Yield: 4 or more servings as vegetable side dish

Special Note: I usually use 2 griddles and prepare 6–7 eggplant using 3 recipes of cracker crumbs during the summer to freeze for winter use.

Steamed Amaranth Greens

1. Wash leaves. Trim any bad spots from leaves. If leaves are very large, you may desire to remove the thick center stem.
2. In a saucepan that will hold the leaves with minimal folding required, bring a small amount of water to a boil. Add leaves. Sprinkle with salt and/or garlic powder. Cover and cook on medium for 10–15 minutes. Serve immediately.
3. If desired, you may drizzle a teaspoon of flaxseed or olive oil per serving over the leaves just before serving.

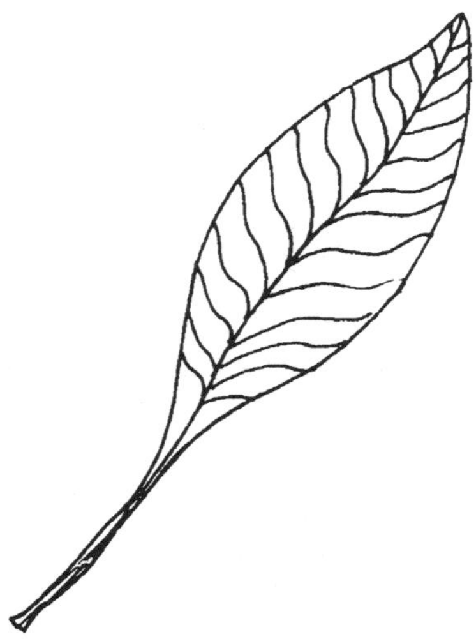

Italian Eggplant
(Two Variations)

	With Amaranth Cracker Crumbs	
3/4 cup	3/4 cup	Muir Glen brand organic tomato puree
1 1/4 cups	1 1/4 cups	water
1/4 cup	1/2 cup	green pepper, finely chopped
1/4 cup	2 tablespoons	onion, finely chopped
1/2 teaspoon	1/2 teaspoon	sea salt
1/4 teaspoon	1/4 teaspoon	minced garlic
1/2 teaspoon	3/4 teaspoon	basil
3/4 teaspoon	1 teaspoon	leaf oregano
2 1/2 cups	2 cups	eggplant, peeled, diced OR 8 3-inch peeled, and sliced eggplant (1/2 inch thick)
none	1/2 cup	Amaranth Cracker crumbs , separated (page 156)

1. Oven temperature—350°F. Preheating not necessary.

2. Combine tomato puree, water, green pepper, onion, and seasoning in a small bowl or 2 cup measurer.

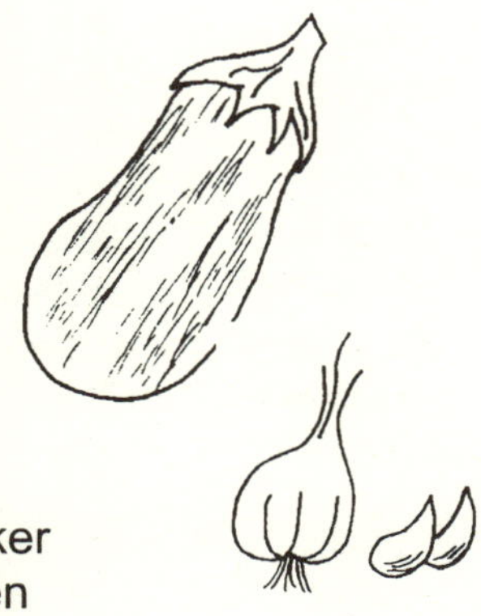

3. Layer eggplant into a covered, shallow baking dish. I use my 10-inch square Corning casserole dish. Note: If using slices, some may need to be cut in half to fit into the dish. If you have leftover eggplant you may freeze it in slices or cubes for later use.

   OR

   For Amaranth Cracker Crumb Version: Sprinkle 1/4 cup of cracker crumbs in the bottom of the baking dish. Layer eggplant and then sprinkle rest of crumbs evenly over the eggplant.

4. Pour tomato mixture evenly over the eggplant. Bake covered for 40–50 minutes or until sauce bubbles and eggplant is tender. Time will depend upon if the eggplant is fresh or frozen. I freeze eggplant diced and in slices when the vegetable is in season so I can enjoy this dish year round. Leftovers may be frozen, but I prefer to freeze the tomato mixture and eggplant separately and prepare as desired for a quick vegetable.

Yield: 4–6 vegetable servings or 2 vegetarian casserole servings

Serving suggestion: If needed, during the last 5 minutes of baking time, remove the eggplant to be served to the person with CRC to another dish and then sprinkle mozzarella and/or Parmesan cheese on the remainder for the family or guests.

Special Note: This can be can be prepared in the microwave, but I believe that the flavor blends better when baked in the oven.

Italian Fried Eggplant

Prepare the same as Italian Eggplant with Amaranth Cracker Crumbs substituting approximately 8 3-inch slices of Fried Eggplant (page 188) for the cracker crumbs and diced or sliced eggplant (since eggplant varies in size, I fill the bottom of my Corning 10-inch casserole dish).

Italian Tomato Vegetable Casserole

1 cup	Muir Glen brand organic tomato puree
1 cup	water
1 1/2 cups	eggplant, peeled, 1/2 inch diced
1 1/2 cups	zucchini squash, peeled, 1/2 inch diced
1/4 cup	onion, chopped
1/2 teaspoon	sea salt
1/4 teaspoon	minced garlic
1/2 teaspoon	basil
1 teaspoon	leaf oregano

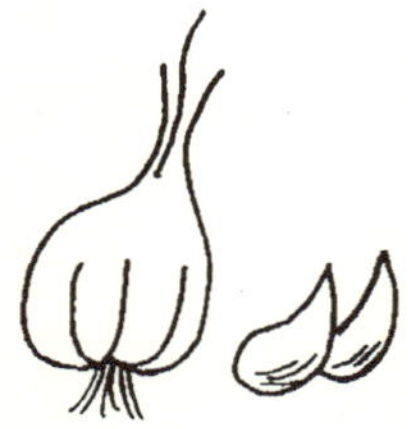

In saucepan, combine all ingredients. Bring to boil, reduce heat, and cover. Simmer 20 minutes or until the vegetables are tender and flavors are well blended. Leftovers may be frozen.

Yield: 3 1/2 cups

Italian Nightshade Casserole

1 cup	Muir Glen brand organic tomato puree
1 cup	water
2 cups	eggplant, peeled, 1/2 inch diced
1/2 cup	green pepper
1/2 teaspoon	sea salt
1/4 teaspoon	minced garlic
1/2 teaspoon	basil
1 teaspoon	leaf oregano

In saucepan, combine all ingredients. Bring to boil, reduce heat, and cover. Simmer 20 minutes or until the vegetables are tender and flavors are well blended. Leftovers may be frozen.

Yield: 2 1/2 cups

Zucchini or Okra with Tomato

2 cups	canned tomato quarters or pieces
2 cups	zucchini squash, peeled, sliced
	OR 1 cup sliced okra
1/2 cup	onions, chopped (optional)
1/8 teaspoon	sea salt
1/4 teaspoon	summer savory
1/4 teaspoon	leaf oregano (optional)
1/8 teaspoon	basil (optional)
1/8 teaspoon	minced garlic (optional)

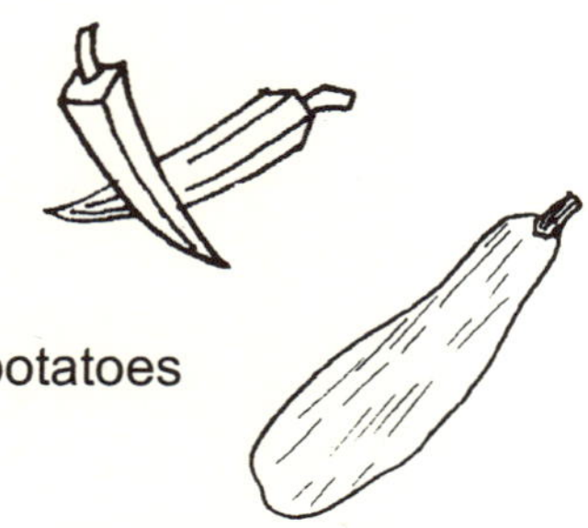

In saucepan, combine all ingredients. Heat to boiling, reduce heat, and cover. Simmer for 15 minutes to blend flavors and cook the squash or okra. I enjoy serving this dish over baked or boiled potatoes as a substitute for gravy or butter. Leftovers may be frozen.

Yield: 2 cups

Kiwi Sauce Method 1

Wash and peel. I prefer to use a serrated knife. Blend on low speed in blender adding 1 kiwi at a time. Or place in bowl and blend with a Braun hand blender.

Kiwi Sauce Method 2

Wash and peel as in method 1. Run fruit through Champion Juicer assembled for homogenizing.

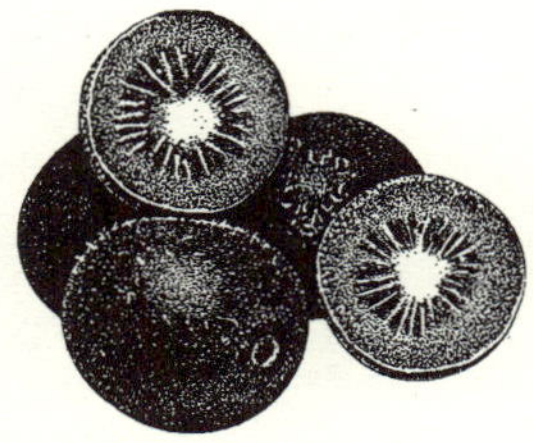

Special Note: 3 kiwi yield approximately 1/2 cup.

Tips on Freezing Kiwi Sauce

An easy way to freeze the kiwi sauce for later use is to freeze in ice cube trays, approximately 1 tablespoon per cube. After the sauce is frozen, remove from the trays and keep frozen in a cellophane bag until ready to use.

Zucchini Amaranth Cookies

1/2 cup	amaranth flour
1/4 cup	arrowroot starch
1/2 teaspoon	baking soda
1/4 teaspoon	sea salt
1/4 teaspoon	unbuffered, corn-free vitamin C crystals
1/8 teaspoon	allspice
1/4 cup	Kiwi Sauce (recipe above) OR pineapple sauce
1 tablespoon	olive oil
3/4 cup	zucchini squash, peeled, shredded*

1. Preheat oven to 375°F.
2. In mixing bowl, whisk together dry ingredients.
3. Add Kiwi Sauce and oil to dry ingredients. Stir thoroughly but do not beat. At this point, mixture will be a little stiff.
4. Add prepared squash. Mix.
5. Drop by teaspoon onto an oiled cookie sheet. Flatten each cookie a little with a fork. Do not make cookies more than 1 inch in diameter. Bake 18–20 minutes. Remove cookies from oven but allow them to cool on the cookie sheet to continue baking. Cookies freeze well. Thaw at room temperature for 15 minutes or so before serving. Do not thaw in microwave or they will become soggy and taste undone.

Yield: 15 cookies

Special Note: Prepare only this small batch at one time because you do not want the batter to set before baking. The idea is to bake them crispy on the outside yet soft but not doughy on the inside. The trick is to make them small, flatten just enough, and bake as long as possible, but do not burn them on the bottom. Also, I bake them on the upper rack in the oven to help prevent burning.

*Special Note: If you desire, you may freeze squash when in season. Premeasure shredded squash (3/4 cup) and package. Then thaw and drain thoroughly before preparing these cookies.

Amaranth Carob Cookies*

1 cup	amaranth flour
1/2 cup	arrowroot starch
1/4 cup	carob powder, sift after measuring*
3/4 teaspoon	baking soda
1/2 teaspoon	unbuffered, corn-free vitamin C crystals
1/4 teaspoon	sea salt
1/2 teaspoon	stevia, white powder concentrate*
1/2 cup	water
2 tablespoons	olive oil or sunflower oil

1. Preheat oven to 350°F.
2. Oil cookies sheets.
3. In mixing bowl, whisk together dry ingredients. Make "well" in the center.
4. Add water and oil to dry ingredients. Stir with rubber spatula, making sure all dry ingredients are moistened.
5. Lightly oil fingers. Form dough into 1-inch balls. Place on cookie sheet approximately 2 inches apart. Flatten with fork or bottom of glass.
6. Bake 10 minutes. Immediately remove cookies to cooling rack to cool.

Yield: 18 cookies

*Realize that stevia and carob are usually eaten Day 4, so you need to avoid eating them on your Day 4 just before and after these cookies on your Day 2.

Sunflower Seed Butter

3 cups	raw, hulled sunflower seeds
2 tablespoons	sunflower oil

1. Chill sunflower seeds in freezer at least overnight. Leave seeds in the freezer until ready to process.
2. Assemble Champion Juicer for homogenizing. Use the funnel for easier insertion of the seeds.
3. In bowl, stir sunflower seeds and oil to evenly coat the seeds. Run approximately 1/4 cup of seeds through at a time. The Champion Juicer manufacturer recommends to discontinue making seed butter if the juicer body becomes excessively warm. I prefer to process only 3 cups of seeds, quit, and clean up the juicer.
4. Store in wide-mouth, glass pint jar. Spread on crackers or tortillas and use in Carob Sunflower Candy (page 193).

Yield: almost 2 cups of sunflower butter

Carob Sunflower Candy*

1 1/3 cups	Sunflower Seed Butter (page 192)
1/3 cup	carob powder,* after measuring, sift to remove lumps
1/4 teaspoon	stevia,* white powder concentrate
1/3 cup	water
1/2 cup	ground sunflower seeds

1. In a bowl, whisk together carob powder and stevia. Add water and mix until smooth. Add sunflower seed butter and mix thoroughly. Mixture will be sticky at first but will become firmer as you mix.

2. Divide batter in half and form into 2 large balls. Cut each portion into eight wedges. Shape each wedge into a ball and cut each into thirds. Shape each third into a ball. Roll each ball in the ground sunflower seeds. Chill and serve. Candy may be frozen, but do not store past approximately 1 month.

Yield: 48 pieces, great to serve in place of fudge at holiday times

*Realize that carob powder and stevia are usually eaten on Day 4 so you need to avoid them on your Day 4 just before and after eating this recipe on Day 2.

Special Note: My way of sifting carob powder is to place the measurement of carob powder into a mesh strainer with a bowl under it. Then stir the powder to work it through the mesh and into the bowl.

Amaranth Pie Crust

3/4 cup	amaranth flour
1/4 cup	arrowroot starch
1/4 cup	cold water
3 tablespoons	olive oil (cold but best if not solid)
1/4 teaspoon	sea salt

1. Chill medium-size bowl and whisk.

2. Combine flour and starch in a small, unchilled bowl. Set aside.

3. Whisk together water, oil, and salt in chilled bowl until opaque and slightly thick.

4. Add flour mixture to liquids and stir with rubber spatula or fork until dough clumps together into a ball and is well mixed.

5. Transfer dough to an 8-inch pie pan. Press dough with oil-coated fingers to form pie shell, making sides and bottom as evenly thin as possible. Chill until filling is prepared and ready to bake.

Special Note: This crust recipe may also be pressed into the bottom of an 8-inch square baking dish to use with Tofu "Cheesecake" recipes. See Day 4 recipes.

Recipe idea from Mastering Food Allergies newsletter, September 1990.

Lemon Pudding*

1 quart	Mountain Sun brand organic Lemonade*
3 tablespoons	freshly squeezed lemon juice (approximate amount of juice from 1 lemon)
1/2 cup	arrowroot
1 teaspoon	alcohol-free lemon flavor (optional)
as desired	grated lemon rind

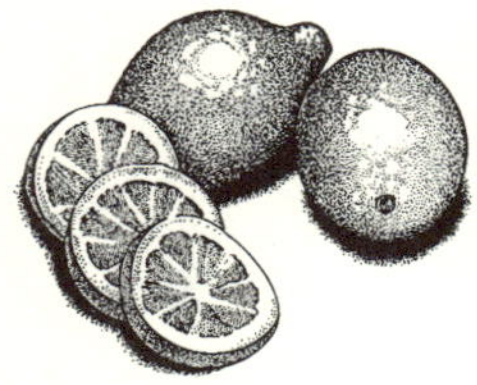

Combine all ingredients in large saucepan. Stir with whisk to dissolve arrowroot. Cook over medium heat until thickened. Stir with a whisk almost constantly (especially toward end). Portion into individual bowls. Chill.

Yield: 4 1/4 cups

*Realize that this brand of lemonade contains wild honey so you need to omit eating honey on your Day 4 just before and after enjoying this recipe on your Day 2. According to Mountain Sun, they add approximately 12% (by weight) honey to their juices. Using this information, I calculated that would equal about 1 tablespoon of honey per 1 cup of juice.

Thanks to Elva Waters for her assistance in developing this recipe.

Grapefruit Spritzer

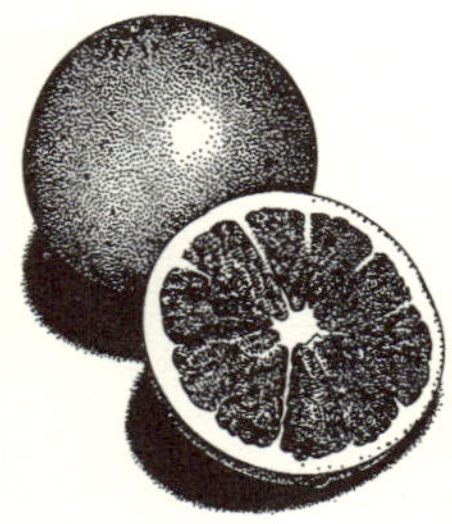

1 bottle	carbonated, unflavored mineral water, chilled (12 ounces)
1/4 cup	unsweetened grapefruit juice concentrate

Combine and serve immediately.

Yield: 1 3/4 cups

Quick Catsup*

1 can	Muir Glen brand organic tomato paste (8 ounces)
2/3 cup	water
1/4 teaspoon	sea salt
3/4 teaspoon	onion powder
3/4 teaspoon	leaf oregano
1/2 teaspoon	unbuffered, corn-free vitamin C crystals
1/8 teaspoon	garlic powder
1/8 teaspoon	ground cloves
1/8 teaspoon	ground cumin*
1/8 teaspoon	dry mustard*

Combine ingredients and chill. This is thick catsup. Dilute with more water if desired. Freeze leftovers in ice cube trays. After frozen, remove and keep frozen in cellophane bag. Thaw as needed.

Yield: 1 2/3 cups

*These seasonings are assigned to Days 1 and 3. However since they are in such small amounts, I personally do not concern myself with this minor break in rotation.

Garlic

Many of my recipes use fresh garlic. Fresh garlic is my preference over dehydrated minced garlic or garlic powder in these recipes. However, if time is a premium, you may choose to substitute dehydrated minced garlic or garlic powder for fresh minced garlic. (I do not recommend using garlic salt.) See the garlic product bottle for the suggested amount to substitute for each clove of garlic.

Mincing Fresh Garlic:

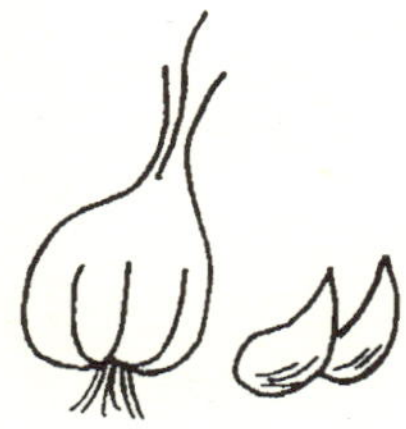

1. Separate clove of garlic from bud (head).
2. Peel and rinse clove.
3. Hold clove between index finger and thumb on cutting board. Using a sharp paring knife, slice garlic as thin as possible.
4. Cut each thin slice into very narrow strips.
5. Using a French knife, rock blade back and forth to finely mince the garlic strips. To rock the French knife, use the fingers of your left hand to hold the tip of the blade firmly on cutting board. With your right hand lift the blade from board to rock up and down several times across the garlic. Stop several times to remove garlic from blade. Gather garlic into pile on cutting board and repeat rocking procedure. (Rocking procedure described is for a right-handed person. Reverse if you are left handed.)
6. Gather minced garlic into a thin layer in the central area of the cutting board. Place the flat side of the French knife over garlic and gently smash pieces. This will help to release the garlic flavor.

Clarified Butter

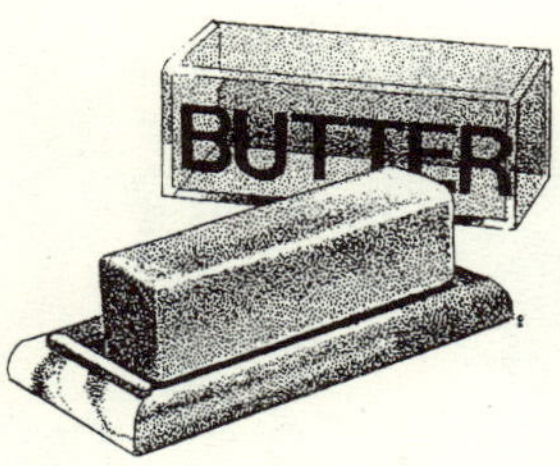

To make clarified butter, heat 1/4 to 1 pound of unsalted butter to a slow boiling point until it foams well. Remove from heat and allow it to cool until the milk solids fall to the bottom of the pan or float to the top. Carefully skim off the floating white milk solid residue and discard. Gently pour the clear yellow liquid into a storage container and discard the residue on the bottom of the pan or skillet. Generally, 1/4 pound of unsalted butter will yield around 2/3 cup of clarified butter.

Using a pan or skillet that will allow the melting butter to have a little depth works best to facilitate the separation process. In addition, you may process more than 1 pound of unsalted butter at one time, but don't start with so much that it begins to burn on the bottom of the pan before it can completely melt and uniformly reach a boiling stage.

Allow the clarified butter to cool thoroughly before storing it in a container with a tight-fitting lid. To maintain freshness and prevent possible mold formation, keep the container tightly closed when it is not being used, always use a clean utensil to dip into it, and store it in the refrigerator. Since clarified butter is partially saturated, it is firm when cold and you may wish to let the amount to be used set at room temperature to soften (it thaws very quickly).

While this recipe is relatively simple to make, clarified butter is also available commercially at health-food stores and through mail-order sources under product name Ghee.

Picante Sauce

1 can	Muir Glen brand organic tomato puree (16 ounces)
1 cup	water
1/4 cup	green pepper, finely chopped
2 tablespoons	onion, finely chopped
1 teaspoon	chili powder
1 teaspoon	leaf oregano
1 teaspoon	sea salt
1/2 teaspoon	minced garlic
1/2 teaspoon	Watkins Salsa Seasoning Blend or other Mexican blend spices

1. In saucepan, combine all ingredients. Heat to boiling then reduce heat some. Cover with splatter screen (information on page 60) and boil gently for 10 minutes or longer to blend flavors and reduce sauce to 1 cup. Stir often, especially at the end.
2. Chill and serve with Enchiladas, Tacos, Taco Pizza, Breakfast Burrito, or Beef Fajita.
3. Freeze leftovers for future use. I freeze in ice cube trays, 1 tablespoon per cube. After frozen, I remove the cubes from the tray and keep frozen in a cellophane bag. Thaw just the amount desired.

Yield: 2 cups

Guacamole*

1	ripe avocado*
2 tablespoons	onion, chopped
2 tablespoons	green pepper, chopped
1/4 teaspoon	chili powder
1/8 teaspoon	minced garlic
2 pinches	sea salt
2 pinches	unbuffered, corn-free vitamin C crystals
1	tomato, diced

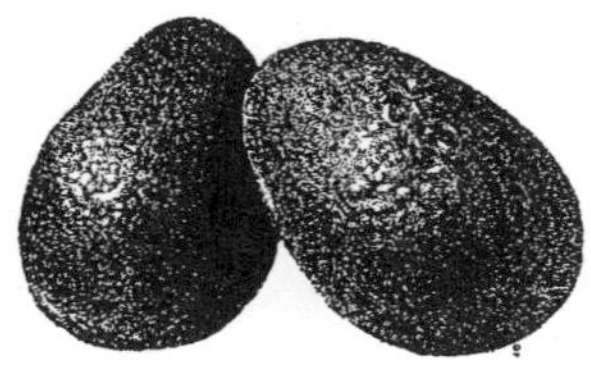

1. Cut avocado in half, remove the pit, and scoop the flesh into a blender.
2. Add rest of the ingredients except tomato. Blend until smooth. Place into a small bowl, and stir in diced tomatoes. Cover and chill. Serve as a dip with crackers.

   OR

   Do not stir in the tomatoes and serve with Enchiladas, Tacos, Taco Pizza, or Beef Fajita.

Yield: approximately 2/3 cup without tomato

<u>Special Notes</u>:
For a chunky guacamole, I place all the ingredients except tomatoes in my Black & Decker® Handy Shortcut™ Micro-Processor using the knife blade.

I have successfully frozen Guacamole without tomato to use later. After freezing, it turns a darker color. Stir in a pinch or so more of unbuffered, corn-free vitamin C crystals to lighten.

*Avocado belongs to the Laurel Family with bay leaf and cinnamon. Eating avocado on Day 2 breaks the rotation since cinnamon is used in many recipes on Day 3 and a few on Day 1. You can make your own decision about eating avocado on Day 2. I personally eat this only occasionally because I prefer Picante Sauce (recipe above) with my Mexican food.

10. FOODS, MEAL PLANNING, AND RECIPES FOR DAY 3

Foods for Day 3

Animal Protein

103 flounder, turbot
106 salmon, trout
121 duck, goose
126 turkey, turkey egg

Vegetables

28 spinach
36 cauliflower, Brussels sprouts, rutabaga, kale
65 carrots, parsnips

Grains, Flours, and Baking Foods

6 barley, corn, millet, oat, rye, wild rice
28 quinoa
47 tapioca starch
52 cream of tartar

Fruit

34 avocado
40a apple
40b plum, prune, cherry
52 raisin, grape

Sweeteners

40a apple
28 FOS—NutriFlora™

Oils

22 walnut oil
36 canola oil

Herbs and Spices

34 bay leaf
65 caraway, fennel

Seeds and Nuts

22 walnut
23 filbert (hazelnut)

Foods That Float Between Days 1 & 3

65 parsley
34 cinnamon

Recipe Table of Contents for Day 3

Biscuits, Crackers, & Etc. Bread

Cereals, Grains, & Nongrains

Muffins and Pancakes

Protein Dishes

Protein Dishes (continued)

Vegetables, Salads, & Dressing

Desserts

Miscellaneous

Meal Planning for Day 3

Quick & Easy Meals

- Egg Drop Soup with Vegetables
  Barley or Quinoa Biscuit

- Salmon Patties
  Basic Millet with Caraway
  raw carrot slices

- ground turkey patty
  Basic Quinoa
  steamed Brussels sprouts

- Grilled Fish for Day 3
  Steamed Parsnips
  steamed spinach with flaxseed oil

- Salmon Millet Dinner

Quick and Easy Meals with Advanced Planning

- Millet or Quinoa Turkey Vegetable Stew
  Barley or Quinoa Biscuit

- Turkey Vegetable Salad
  Quinoa Muffin

- Turkey Parsnip Soup
  crackers or muffin

- Turkey Salad with spinach on
  Quinoa Tortilla
  beets (floated from Day 1)

- Salmon Salad with spinach
  on Rudolph's Rye Bread
  Vegetable/Apple Salad

- Quinoa Tortilla with *plan*over
  Roast Turkey
  Day 3 Pasta Salad

- Creamed Turkey on Rye Toast

Easy Meals

Turkey Oatmeal Loaf
Day 3 Pasta Salad
spinach salad

Turkey Barley Soup
Barley Biscuits

Baked Fish for Day 3
Stir-Fry Vegetables for Day 3
rye pasta with flaxseed oil
or Whipped Parsnips

Spinach Chef Salad with
Carrot-Caraway Salad Dressing
muffin or crackers

Turkey Quinoa Pasta Salad or Stew
Apple Quinoa Crisp

Rainbow Trout
Basic Millet
fresh spinach with
Carrot-Caraway Salad Dressing

Lower Carbohydrate Meals

Salmon Cauliflower Chowder

Salmon or Turkey Vegetable Salad
with or without Pasta

Egg Drop Soup with Vegetables

Spinach Chef Salad with
Carrot-Caraway Salad Dressing

Grilled or Baked Fish for Day 3
steamed spinach with flaxseed oil

Breakfast Ideas

your choice of muffins, pancakes, biscuits, or cooked cereal
(see Recipe Table of Contents for Day 3)

Rolled Oat Waffles with Applesauce

Puffed Millet cold cereal with Macadamia or Brazil Nut Milk (These nuts are unassigned "Fun Foods," see explanation on pages 30–31.)

Arrowhead Mills Bits of Barley cereal

fresh fruit

any *plan*over Day 3 vegetable, fish, casserole, or soup

turkey eggs cooked you favorite way or float chicken eggs from Day 1

Millet or Quinoa Pudding

Snack Ideas

- carrot sticks
- cauliflower buds
- Oat Bran or Quinoa Muffins
- Quinoa Crackers
- filberts or walnuts
- Barley, Oat, or Quinoa Biscuits
- Apple Salad
- Oat or Quinoa Apple Crisp
- Millet or Quinoa Pudding
- fresh fruit

Meals Away from Home

Turkey Parsnip Soup with fresh spinach and crackers

Turkey Vegetable Salad
Quinoa Muffin

Salmon Vegetable Salad
Oat Bran Muffin

Quinoa Tortilla sandwich with *plan*over Roast Turkey and fresh spinach
Vegetable/Apple Salad

Quinoa Salad (best to add the apple in the morning before you leave instead of the night before)
*plan*over Roast Turkey

Salmon Cauliflower Chowder
carrot sticks

Special Occasion Meals

Brunch–
Egg (Cheese-free) Soufflé
carrot sticks
Oat Scones
Pau D'Arco tea

Easy Thanksgiving Feast–
Cranberry Spritzer (moved from Day 4)
Roasted Turkey
Dill "Stove-Top" Stuffing (floated from Day 1)
steamed broccoli, cauliflower, and/or carrots (broccoli floated from Day 1)
Apple Salad
Kamut® Dinner Rolls (floated from Day 1)
Butternut Squash Pie (squash moved from Day 4)
Dacopa beverage
—I have prepared this menu with the addition of canned cranberries and Libby's Pumpkin Pie for family and company and they were all delighted and "stuffed."

Luncheon with Grandparent–
Salmon Cauliflower Chowder
raw carrot slices
Granola Bar
iced Pau D'Arco tea

Recipes for Day 3

Creamy Millet Cereal I

1/3 cup	hulled whole millet grain
1/4 teaspoon	sea salt
2 cups	water (room temperature)

1. Wash millet (page 36). Combine ingredients in a 1-quart size slow cooker.* Cook overnight and awake to enjoy this ready-to-eat, mouth-watering cereal.

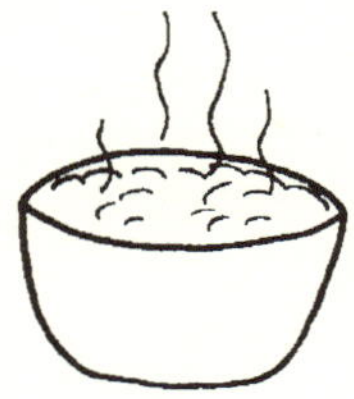

2. Stir before serving. This cereal resembles cooked quick oatmeal, but a little yellow in color. If desired, add fruit of the day to sweeten. I prefer this cereal with 2–3 tablespoons of peeled, diced apple.
3. Leftovers may be frozen and reheated for another quick breakfast or used as my favorite Millet Pudding (page 229).

*This recipe is too small to cook in a standard-size slow cooker, but it can be easily doubled or tripled if desired. Cook on low if slow cooker has two settings. Also, see page 61 for more information on slow cooker.

Recipe idea from Mastering Food Allergies newsletter, December-January, 1988.

Yield: 2 cups

Creamy Millet Cereal II

1/4 cup	hulled whole millet grain
1/8 teaspoon	sea salt
1 1/2 cups	water

1. Bring water and salt to boil in a small saucepan.
2. Wash millet (page 36), add to saucepan and stir. Reduce heat. Cover and simmer for 20 minutes. The cereal resembles yellow hominy, but is smaller and has a grainy texture. Also, this cereal is not as creamy as Creamy Millet Cereal I.

Yield: 1 cup

Sometimes I've believed as many as six impossible things before breakfast.
Lewis Carroll

Quinoa Cereal I

1/3 cup	whole quinoa
2 tablespoons	quinoa flour
1/4 teaspoon	sea salt
1/4 teaspoon	FOS (optional)
2 cups	water (room temperature)

Quinoa Cereal II

3/8 cup	whole quinoa (3/8 cup = 1/4 cup + 2 tablespoons)
1/4 teaspoon	sea salt
1/4 teaspoon	FOS (optional)
2 cups	water (room temperature)

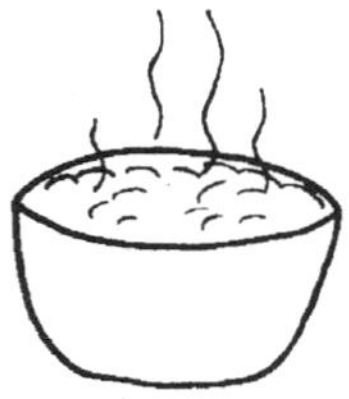

1. Rinse quinoa thoroughly (page 36). Combine your choice of the above ingredients in a 1-quart size slow cooker. Cook overnight and awake to enjoy this ready-to-eat, mouth-watering cereal.
2. Stir before serving. I enjoy these cereals best served with 2 tablespoons of unsweetened applesauce and a dash of cinnamon per serving.
3. Leftovers may be frozen and reheated for another quick breakfast or used in Quinoa Pudding II (page 231).

*This recipe is too small to cook in a standard-size slow cooker, but it can be easily doubled or tripled if desired. Cook on low if slow cooker has two settings. Also, see page 61 for more information on slow cooker.

Recipe idea for Quinoa Cereal I is from Mastering Food Allergies newsletter, December-January, 1988.

Yield: 2–2 1/4 cups (2 servings)

Quinoa Cereal III

1/2 cup	whole quinoa
2 1/2 cups	water
1/4 teaspoon	sea salt

1. Rinse quinoa thoroughly (page 36).
2. Bring water and salt to boil. Stir in rinsed quinoa. Cover. Reduce heat and simmer for 20–25 minutes. Stir occasionally. Add more water if needed. Serve as described in Quinoa Cereal I and II.

Yield: 2 1/2 cups

Oat Bran Cereal

1 cup	water
1/8 teaspoon	sea salt (or slightly less)
1/3 cup	oat bran

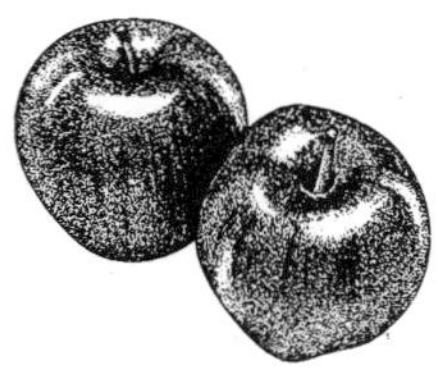

In saucepan, heat water and salt to boiling. Add oat bran, stir, reduce heat, and cook for 1–2 minutes. Stir constantly so it does not boil over or stick. Cover, remove from heat, and allow to set 3–5 minutes to thicken. Serve with cinnamon, maple granules, and/or peeled, diced apple.

Yield: 1 cup

Oatmeal Cereals*

Rolled Oats in Microwave

2 2/3 cups	water
1/2 teaspoon	sea salt
1 1/2 cups	old fashioned rolled oats

In large kettle, heat water and salt to boil. Add oats, stir, and cover. Cook in microwave for 4 minutes on cookmatic level 5 or medium power. Allow to set 3–5 minutes to thicken. Serve with cinnamon, maple granules, and/or peeled, diced apple.

Yield: 3 cups

Rolled Oats Cooked on Stove Top

3 cups	water
1/2 teaspoon	sea salt
1 1/2 cups	old fashioned rolled oats

In large kettle, heat water and salt to boil. Add oats, stir, and reduce heat to medium high. Cook at a gentle boil for 5 minutes, stirring constantly. Remove from heat, cover, and allow to set 3–5 minutes to thicken. Serve with cinnamon, maple granules, and/or peeled, diced apple.

Yield: 3 cups

Oat Granola

1 cup	rolled oats
1 cup	oat bran
1/4 cup	walnuts, chopped
2 tablespoons	maples granules (optional)*
1/4 cup	water or apple juice
1/2 teaspoon	alcohol-free cinnamon extract (optional)
2 tablespoons	canola or walnut oil

1. In a mixing bowl, combine both oat cereals, nuts, and maple granules. Add cinnamon to either water or apple juice. Add this mixture gradually to the dry ingredients while stirring to evenly coat cereal mixture. Repeat the same process while gradually adding oil.

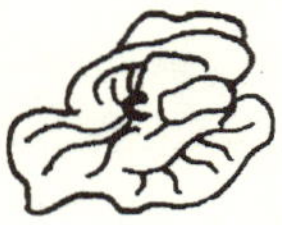

2. Scatter mixture lightly in 9x13-inch baking pan. Bake in oven at 250°F. for 45–60 minutes. Remove mixture from oven and stir every 10–15 minutes. Bake until cereal is dry and slightly crunchy, but be careful not to burn. Cool completely and store in glass jar in freezer.
3. Serving suggestions: Eat plain for a crunchy snack or as topping for Vanilla Rice Dream.** I also enjoy this as a topping on microwave-baked apple. Just peel and dice a fresh apple. Place apple in serving bowl, sprinkle with cinnamon, top with granola, and cook in microwave on high for 1–2 minutes or until apple is tender. Serve warm

Yield: 2 cups

*Maple is an unassigned "Fun Food" in this rotational diet, see explanation on pages 30–31.

**Realize that Vanilla Rice Dream breaks rotation since rice is a Day 1 food.

Rolled Oat Waffles

2 1/4 cups	water
1/4 teaspoon	sea salt
1/2 cup	old fashioned rolled oats (regular, uncooked)
1 tablespoon	walnut or canola oil
2 tablespoons	walnuts (optional)

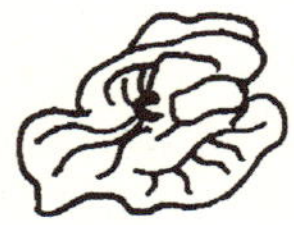

1. Combine ingredients in a bowl and allow to soak 30 minutes or overnight in refrigerator.
2. Preheat waffle iron. After preheating, I lightly oil my waffle iron* (your waffle iron may vary in the need for the oil).
3. Pour soaked mixture in blender and blend until light and foamy, then pour onto preheated, oiled waffle iron.
4. Bake for 12–15 minutes.
5. Serve with hot unsweetened applesauce, with or without cinnamon.

Yield: approximately three 8-inch Belgian waffles

Special Notes: Leftovers may be frozen and reheated. You may also use the waffles as bread for sandwiches.

*This recipe was developed using a nonstick Belgian waffle iron which due to my chemical sensitivities I can no longer use it. At publish date, I have not been able to try this recipe with a cast-iron or stainless steel waffle iron but I include this recipe for those who can use the nonstick finished pans.

Recipe idea from <u>*The Yeast Connection Cookbook*</u> *by Crook & Jones, page 140.*

Apples—How to Freeze

Sliced or diced apple is a wonderful sweetener for Day 3 cereals and puddings. However, often a whole apple is not needed, especially when sweetening only a single bowl of cereal. I follow this simple method to freeze apples so I can have them ready to sweeten cereals as well as make a quick dessert for Day 3.

<u>To Prepare</u>:

- Dissolve 1/4 teaspoon of vitamin C crystals in a medium-size bowl of water.
- Wash, peel, core, and rinse apples. Slice or dice. Soak in vitamin C water until ready to blanch. Drain just before blanching.

<u>To Blanch</u>:

- Fill bottom of a steamer pan with water to about 1/2 inch from the bottom of steamer insert. Add 1/4 teaspoon of vitamin C crystals. Heat water to boiling.
- Add 2 cups of prepared apples to insert of steamer pan. Cover and immediately begin timing. Steam over boiling vitamin C water for 2 minutes.
- Immediately drain and chill in ice water until cold.

<u>To Freeze</u>:

- Drain well.
- Place the amount desired for recipe in cellophane bag and freeze.

OR

Individually quick freeze on a baking sheet before placing in cellophane bag. See explanation on page 290 in the Canning and Freezing section of Chapter 12—Organics—The Only Way to Go!

Rice-Oat Pancakes

12 Dollar-size	24 Dollar-size	YIELD
1/2 cup	1 cup	brown rice flour*
3 tablespoons	1/4 cup + 2 tablespoons	oat flour
1/2 teaspoon	1 teaspoon	baking soda
1/4 teaspoon	1/2 teaspoon	sea salt
1/4 teaspoon	1/2 teaspoon	unbuffered, corn-free vitamin C crystals
1 tablespoon	2 tablespoons	ground flax seed
1/2 cup	1 cup	water
2 teaspoons	1/4 cup	canola oil

1. Preheat griddle. I use a well-seasoned cast-iron griddle (see How to Season Cast Iron on page 63). Griddle is hot enough when water dances when sprinkled on the griddle.
2. In mixing bowl, whisk together dry ingredients. Add water and oil to the dry ingredients. Stir with whisk for 15 seconds. Allow batter to set up to 30 seconds to thicken. Stir again
3. Dip batter onto the griddle using a tablespoon. Batter is thick, in fact so thick you need to shake it out of the spoon onto the griddle. Cook 2 minutes on first side until pancake bubbles and gets slightly dry around edges. Turn. Cook until dry on second side, approximately 1 minute.
4. Serve plain or with flaxseed oil and/or heated applesauce. You may freeze leftovers for future breakfasts and snacks.

*Rice is usually eaten on Day 1, so you need to avoid eating rice on your Day 1 just before and after eating this recipe on your Day 3.

Quinoa Pancakes

12 Dollar-size	24 Dollar-size	YIELD
1/2 cup	1 cup	quinoa flour
3 tablespoons	1/4 cup + 2 tablespoons	tapioca starch
1/2 teaspoon	1 teaspoon	baking soda
3 pinches	scant 1/4 teaspoon	sea salt
1/4 teaspoon	1/2 teaspoon	unbuffered, corn-free vitamin C crystals
1/2 teaspoon	1 teaspoon	FOS (optional)
1/2 teaspoon	1 teaspoon	ground cinnamon (optional)
1/2 cup	1 cup	water
2 teaspoons	4 teaspoons	canola oil

1. Follow steps 1 and 2 as above in Rice-Oat Pancake recipe.
2. Dip batter onto the griddle using tablespoon. Cook on first side until pancake is golden brown, approximately 1 1/2 minutes. Turn. Cook until golden brown on second side, approximately 1 minute. If your batter thickens, you may desire to stir in very small amounts of additional water. Also, you may need to add additional oil to griddle as you cook repeated batches.

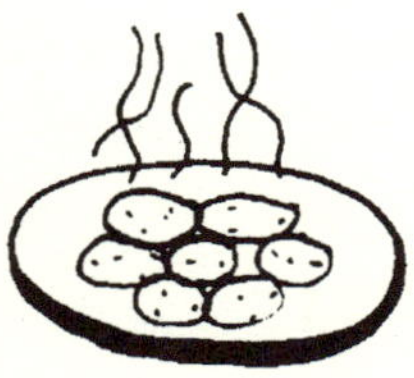

3. Serve plain or with flaxseed oil and/or heated applesauce.

Barley Biscuits

1 cups	barley flour
1/4 teaspoon	sea salt
1/2 teaspoon	baking soda
1/4 teaspoon	unbuffered, corn-free vitamin C crystals
1/3 cup	water
2 tablespoons	canola oil
1-2 tablespoons	barley flour to roll out biscuits

Quinoa Biscuits

3/4 cup	quinoa flour
1/4 cup	tapioca starch
1/4 teaspoon	sea salt
1 teaspoon	baking soda
1/4 teaspoon	unbuffered, corn-free vitamin C crystals
1 teaspoon	FOS
1/3 cup	water
2 tablespoons	canola oil
1-2 tablespoons	quinoa flour to roll out the biscuits

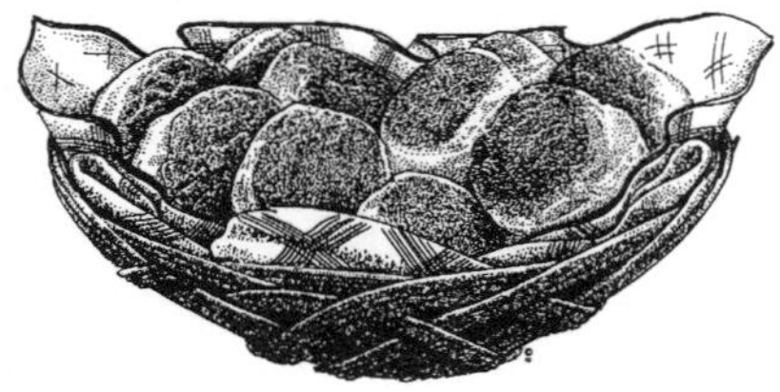

1. Preheat oven to 400°F.
2. In a mixing bowl, whisk together dry ingredients. Make "well" in center.
3. Add water and oil. Stir with rubber spatula or fork until dough clumps into a ball and flour is well mixed.
4. Knead dough lightly on a floured board using 1–2 tablespoons of flour. Pat out to 1/2 inch thick using more flour if needed.
5. Cut with biscuit cutter or drinking glass with a diameter of approximately 2 1/4 inches. Cut 3 biscuits. Form together the scraps of dough, pat out, and cut 2 more biscuits. If there is enough dough remaining, form it into another biscuit.
6. Bake on ungreased stainless steel baking sheet according to time chart below. These biscuits do not raise much but are very tasty.

15–18 minutes for Barley Biscuits
10–12 minutes for Quinoa Biscuits

Yield: 5–6 biscuits

Oat Biscuits

1 cup	oat flour
1/4 teaspoon	sea salt
1 teaspoon	baking soda
1/4 teaspoon	unbuffered, corn-free vitamin C crystals
1/4 cup	water
2 tablespoons	canola oil
1/4 cup	oat flour to roll out the biscuits

1. Preheat oven to 400°F.
2. In a mixing bowl, whisk together dry ingredients starting with only 1 cup of flour. Make "well" in center.
3. Add water and oil. Stir dough with rubber spatula or fork until dough clumps into a ball and flour is well mixed. This dough tends to take a lot of stirring to get mixed well.

<u>For Rolled Biscuits</u>:

4. Add 2 tablespoons more flour, mix. Then knead dough lightly on a floured board using at least 1–2 tablespoons more oat flour. Pat out to 1/2 inch thick using more flour if needed. Cut with biscuit cutter or drinking glass with a diameter of approximately 2 1/4 inches. Cut 3 biscuits. Form together the scraps of dough, pat out again, and cut 2 more biscuits. If there is enough dough remaining, form it into another biscuit.
5. Bake on ungreased stainless steel baking sheet for 15–18 minutes.
6. These biscuits do not raise much. I enjoy these biscuits served as shortbread topped with hot unsweetened applesauce and a dash of cinnamon.

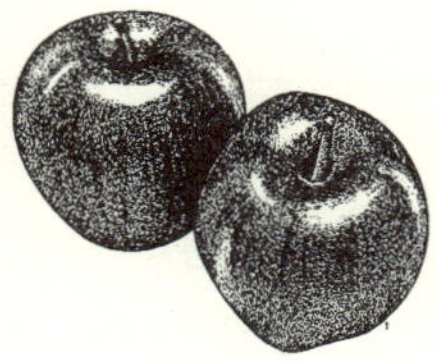

Yield: 5–6 biscuits

<u>For Drop Biscuits</u>:

4. Drop from teaspoon onto ungreased stainless steel baking sheet. Bake 10–12 minutes.

Yield: 12 small biscuits

Tears are the safety valve of the heart when pressure is laid on it.
Albert Smith

Oat Bran Muffins

6 Muffins	12 Muffins	YIELD
1 1/2 cups	3 cups	oat bran
1/4 cup	1/2 cup	raisins (optional)
1 1/2 teaspoons	1 tablespoon	baking powder (remember baking powder contains corn)
1/4 teaspoon	1/2 teaspoon	salt
3/4 cup	1 1/2 cups	unsweetened apple juice
2 tablespoons	1/4 cup	canola oil
1	2	eggs*
OR EGG SUBSTITUTE		
1 tablespoon	2 tablespoons	ground flax seed
3 tablespoons	3/8 cup	water (3/8 cup = 1/4 cup + 2 tablespoons)

(I prefer the flax seed substitute over the egg version.)

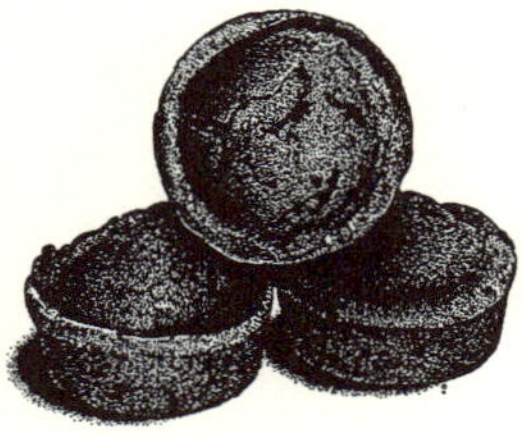

1. Preheat oven to 425°F.
2. Oil and flour (use oat flour) sides and bottom of stainless steel muffin cups.
3. In a mixing bowl, combine oat bran, baking powder, salt, and raisins. Mix well to coat raisins.
4. Whisk together apple juice, oil, and eggs (or substitute).
5. Add liquid mixture to dry ingredients and stir until just moistened. Allow to set approximately 5 minutes to absorb liquid.
6. Stir batter again and fill the prepared muffin cups. The muffin cups will be very full. These muffins do not raise and are rather heavy, but are delicious, moist, and filling. For the raisinless version, fill each muffin cup with 1/3 cup of batter. Bake 12–15 minutes.
7. Cool muffins in the pan(s) on wire rack for 5 minutes. Then turn muffins out of pan(s). Sometimes you need to take a sharp thin knife around the edges of the muffins to loosen them from the sides. Muffins are best served warm. They freeze and reheat well in the microwave.

Special Notes: As a person with CRC, I cannot tolerate dried fruits, so I prepare the recipe without raisins. After filling the muffin cups with the desired quantity of muffins without raisins, I stir some raisins into the remaining batter for others to enjoy. If these muffins are too sweet, especially for the person with CRC, replace 1/4–1/2 cup of the apple juice with water.

I have given Oat Bran Muffins as Christmas gifts to my neighbors and family.

*Realize that eggs are usually eaten on Day 1. If you choose to use eggs, remember to omit eggs on your Day 1 just before and after eating this version on your Day 3.

Quinoa Applesauce Muffins

6 Muffins	12 Muffins	YIELD
7/8 cup	1 3/4 cups	quinoa flour (7/8 cup = 3/4 cup + 2 tablespoons)
1/4 cup	1/2 cup	tapioca starch
1 teaspoon	2 teaspoons	baking soda
1/4 teaspoon	1/2 teaspoon	sea salt
1 teaspoon	2 teaspoons	ground cinnamon (optional)
1/4 teaspoon	1/2 teaspoon	unbuffered, corn-free vitamin C crystals
1/2 cup	1 cup	unsweetened applesauce
1/3 cup	2/3 cup	water
2 tablespoons	1/4 cup	canola oil

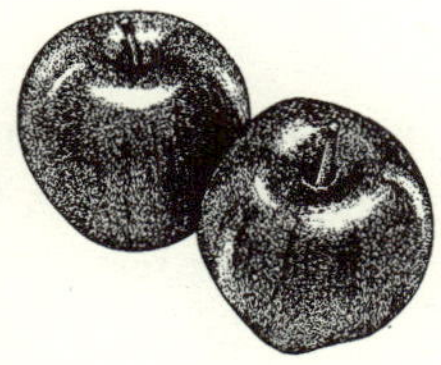

1. Preheat oven to 375°F.
2. Oil and flour bottom and sides of muffin cups.
3. In a mixing bowl, whisk together dry ingredients.
4. Add applesauce, water, and oil. Stir just to moisten. Batter will have some lumps, but they will bake out.
5. Equally portion batter into prepared muffin cups, slightly more than 1/4 cup of batter each. Bake 20–22 minutes.
6. Cool muffins in the pan(s) on wire rack for 5 minutes. Then turn muffins out of pan(s). Sometimes you need to take a sharp thin knife around the edges of the muffins to loosen them from the sides. Muffins are best served warm. They freeze and reheat well in the microwave.

Quinoa Muffins (No Fruit)

6 Muffins	12 Muffins	YIELD
1 cup	2 cup	quinoa flour
1/4 cup	1/2 cup	tapioca starch
1 teaspoon	2 teaspoons	baking soda
1/4 teaspoon	1/2 teaspoon	sea salt
1 teaspoon	2 teaspoons	ground cinnamon (optional)
1/4 teaspoon	1/2 teaspoon	unbuffered, corn-free vitamin C crystals
3/4 cup	1 1/2 cups	water
2 tablespoons	1/4 cup	canola oil

Prepare as you do Quinoa Applesauce Muffins, omitting the applesauce. Batter will yield slightly less than 1/4 cup per muffin cup.

Basic Quinoa

1 cup	whole quinoa
2 cups	water
1 teaspoon	FOS (optional)
1/4 teaspoon	sea salt

1. Rinse quinoa thoroughly (page 36). Combine all ingredients in 2 1/2-quart saucepan. Bring to boil on high. Cover. Reduce heat to between low and medium to allow the quinoa to simmer. Simmer 15 minutes.
2. Remove from heat. Stir to fluff. Serve immediately or cover and allow to set 5 minutes.

Yield: 4 cups

Special Note: For best results, quinoa should not be stirred or uncovered during the cooking process. If it is necessary to check the progress of the quinoa during the cooking time, do so quickly to minimize the loss of steam. Do not stir the quinoa as this will disrupt the even cooking of the grain. If tasting for doneness, use a fork to gently remove a small amount from the surface of the quinoa. Different stoves and different pans may require an adjustment in time, temperature, and/or amount of liquid used.

Quinoa Crackers

1 cup	quinoa flour
1/3 cup	tapioca starch flour
2 teaspoons	caraway seeds
1 teaspoon	baking soda
1/4 teaspoon	sea salt
1/4 teaspoon	unbuffered, corn-free vitamin C crystals
1/2 cup	water
3 tablespoons	canola oil

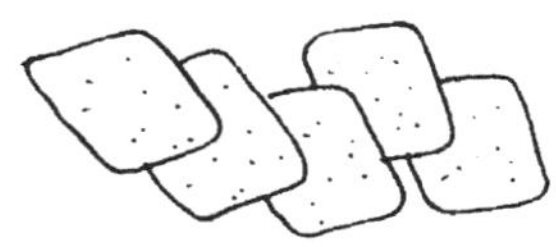

1. Preheat oven to 350°F.
2. Place 1 1/2 teaspoons of oil on a 14 x 10-inch stainless steel baking sheet and set aside. (This amount of oil is in addition to the amount listed above.)
3. In large mixing bowl, whisk together dry ingredients and caraway seeds. Make "well" in center.
4. Add water and oil. Stir dough with a rubber spatula or fork until dough clumps into a ball and flour is well mixed. If dough is sticky, add 1 more tablespoon of flour and mix.
5. Spread oil on baking sheet with fingers to within two inches of edge. As the dough is rolled out, it will push the oil to the edge of sheet. In addition, using your fingers to spread the oil will lightly coat them and aid in working with the dough.
6. Transfer dough to center of the baking sheet. Use your hands to form dough so it has no rough edges. Press dough out evenly in all four directions until it cannot be further spread with your hands, making sure to maintain rectangular shape.
7. If your baking sheet has sides on it, be sure the rolling pin will fit all the way down onto surface on both the width and length of the baking sheet and that its handles clear the edges.

continued on next page

Quinoa Crackers (continued)

8. Lightly dust rolling pin with flour and roll dough out from center to edges, being sure to press in all four directions and to keep dough at a uniform thickness. Occasionally run your hand across the top of the dough to feel if there are any thick areas that need to be evened out.

9. As the dough gets thinner, use the dull back side of a table knife to press edges of dough to maintain rectangular shape. Continue rolling and shaping until dough is about 1/8–1/4 inch thick and fills baking sheet. To help reduce possibility of extra-thin dough edge, use back side of a table knife to gently push all four edges of dough to make edge thickness uniform with remaining dough.

10. Using a pizza cutter, cut dough into squares as follows. Be sure to move pizza cutter slowly and with a back and forth motion to help avoid tearing dough if cutter goes directly across a caraway seed. Cut rectangle in half along dough length (see number 1 in diagram). Cut each half in half (see number 2), then cut each fourth in thirds (see number 3). This will create 12 strips.

11. Next cut rectangle in half along dough width (see number 4). Cut each half in half (see number 5) and each fourth in half (see number 6). This will create 8 sections and 96 individual crackers. Next use a sharp knife to be sure each cut on the outer edge of the rectangle is completely separated.

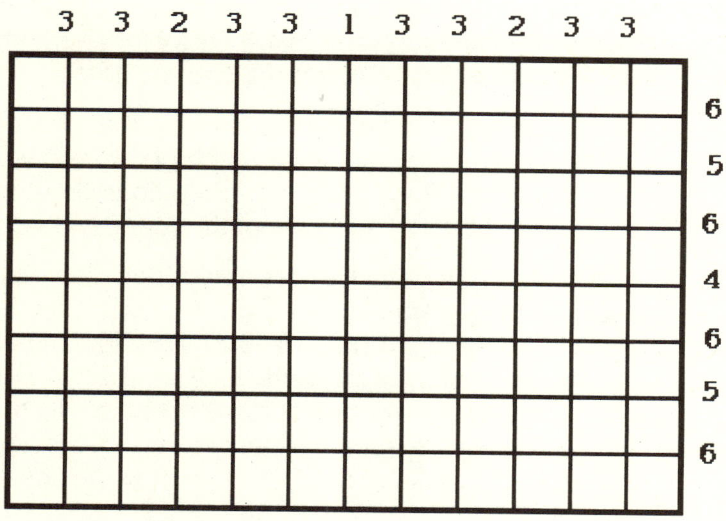

12. Prick holes in each square with fork. If you wish, you can salt the tops of the crackers with sea salt before baking.

13. Bake for 25 minutes. Remove baking sheet from oven and carefully remove outer circle of crackers if they are crispy. Return remaining crackers to oven for 5 minutes. To crisp crackers further, loosen crackers from baking sheet and return them to oven for at least 15 minutes with oven turned off.

14. Cool crackers on cooling rack by either leaving them on the baking sheet or removing and placing them directly on the cooling rack. After cool, store in the freezer. I prefer to use a wide-mouth quart jar. No need to thaw, eat straight from the freezer.

Yield: 96 crackers, almost a full quart

Quinoa Tortillas

5/8 cup	quinoa flour (amount needed to start) (5/8 cup = 1/2 cup + 2 tablespoons)
1/4 teaspoon	sea salt
1/4 cup	water
1/2 teaspoon	canola oil
1/2 cup	quinoa flour (amount needed for kneading and rolling)

Special Note: Before starting your tortilla preparation, I suggest you read Helpful Hints on Tortilla Preparation starting on page 79.

1. Preheat nonstick, unoiled griddle or skillet. I use a well-seasoned cast-iron griddle (see How to Season Cast Iron on page 63). Griddle is hot enough when water dances when sprinkled on the griddle.
2. In a curved-sided bowl, whisk together 5/8 cup (1/2 cup + 2 tablespoons) of flour and salt. Make a "well" in the center.
3. Add water and oil. Stir with rubber spatula or fork until dough clumps together into a moist ball. This dough ball is too sticky for kneading, so add 1 tablespoon more flour and mix in thoroughly with the rubber spatula or fork.
4. Scatter 1 tablespoon flour on rolling surface. Transfer dough to floured rolling surface and knead dough to work in as much of this additional flour as possible. Dough texture should resemble Play Doh. Add more flour if needed. Form dough into ball and cut into fourths. Flour the cut surfaces of the four dough portions with remaining flour.
5. Lightly flour rolling pin. Pat dough portion into circular shape, then roll out tortilla by pressing evenly from the center out in all directions and working to keep tortilla as round as possible. Keep dough well floured on both sides (you will need approximately 1/2 tablespoon of flour per tortilla). Turn dough over often by loosening with a spatula before flipping. Feel dough surface occasionally to be sure it is evenly thin. Finished tortilla will be very thin and approximately 7–8 inches in diameter. Using a pastry brush, gently brush both sides of tortilla to remove excess flour.
6. Cook each tortilla on preheated, unoiled griddle approximately 45 seconds on each side. You will note that the edge of the quinoa tortillas will curl up when cooking on the first side then flatten out when cooking on the second side. Cool each tortilla 1–2 minutes on cooling rack. Place the slightly cooled tortillas between two layers of a clean cotton towel.
7. Serve either whole or cut in half. Use your imagination to create a simple deli-like sandwich—for example: turkey, spinach, Filbert "Mayo," and/or shredded carrots are all good for Day 3. Also, use for salmon or turkey salad sandwich. Leftover tortillas may be frozen flat in a cellophane or plastic bag for future meals.

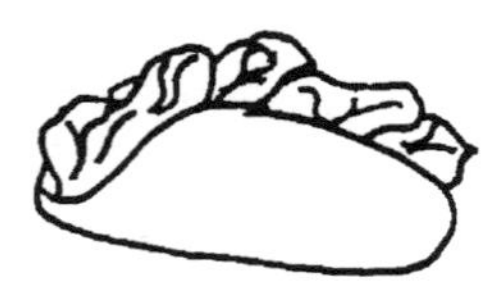

Yield: 4 tortillas, 7–8 inches in diameter

Recipe idea from The Yeast Connection Cookbook by Crook & Jones, p. 159.

Basic Millet

1 cup	hulled millet
2 cups	water
1/2 teaspoon	caraway seed (optional)
1/4 teaspoon	sea salt

1. Rinse millet (page 36). Combine all ingredients in 2 1/2-quart saucepan. Bring to boil on high. Cover. Reduce heat to between low and medium to allow the millet to simmer. Simmer 15 minutes.
2. Remove from heat. Stir to fluff. Serve immediately or cover and allow to set 5 minutes.

Yield: 4 cups

Special Note: For best results, millet should not be stirred or uncovered during the cooking process. If it is necessary to check the progress of the quinoa during the cooking time, do so quickly to minimize the loss of steam. <u>Do not stir</u> the millet as this will disrupt the even cooking of the grain. If tasting for doneness, use a fork to gently remove a small amount from the surface of the millet. Different stoves and different pans may require an adjustment in time, temperature, and/or amount of liquid used.

Roasted Basic Millet

Roasting intensifies the delicious taste of the millet and caraway seeds. Prepare as for Basic Millet except add a dry roasting step before cooking. To dry roast:

1. Transfer the rinsed and drained millet to a cold, heavy-bottomed pan. I prefer a well-seasoned cast-iron skillet (see How to Season Cast Iron on page 63). Stir in caraway seed. Place skillet on range. Turn burner to medium-high. Roast, stirring almost constantly, for approximately 4 minutes or until the millet has become rather dry.
2. Lower heat to medium low and continue to roast, stirring constantly for approximately an additional 4 minutes or until you can smell the intense aroma of the millet and caraway seed. Be careful not to burn the millet or allow it to become so hot that it pops.
3. Transfer the roasted millet to the boiling salted water and continue to cook as described in the above recipe.

Egg (Cheese-Free) Soufflé*

2	extra-large eggs, separated *
1 teaspoon	canola oil
1/4 cup	tapioca starch, packed
1/8 teaspoon	sea salt
1 tablespoon	water
3/4 teaspoon	homemade baking powder (see below)

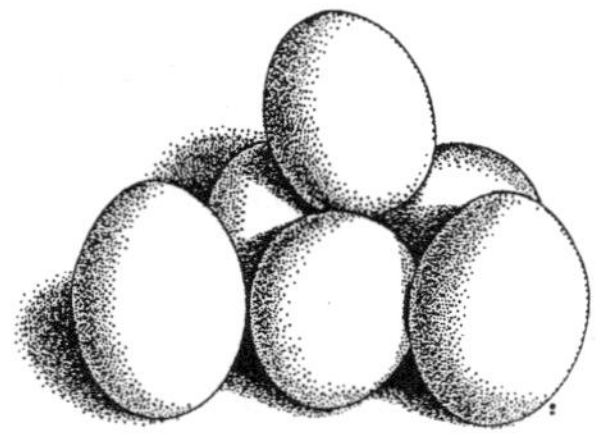

1. Preheat oven to 350°F.
2. Using 2 separate bowls, separate eggs. Place yolks in larger mixing bowl and whites in smaller bowl. Set bowl with egg whites in sink containing some warm water. Stir occasionally to bring the egg whites up to room temperature.
3. Oil bottom and sides of 9-inch square glass baking dish with the 1 teaspoon of oil.
4. Scoop tapioca starch into a 1/4 cup measure, rounding it. Tap edge of measure with knife a few times to aid in packing it. Then level off cup. Place into a small bowl, stir with whisk to unpack it. Set aside.
5. Beat egg whites until stiff. Set aside.
6. Beat yolks with whisk. Add salt, water, tapioca starch, and stir well. Add baking powder and stir. Fold in stiff egg whites.
7. Pour into prepared glass baking dish. Bake for 15 minutes or until a toothpick inserted in the center comes out clean. Serve immediately. This soufflé raises to be approximately 1 1/4 inches high and then falls to be about 3/4 to 1 inch high. Use a sharp knife to cut edges away from side of dish and to cut into 4 squares. Use a wide, sharp spatula to scrap the bottom of the dish when serving. This makes a delicious grain-free breakfast or serve with vegetables for a light lunch or brunch.

Yield: 2 Servings

*Realize that eggs are usually eaten on Day 1. Be sure to omit eggs on your Day 1 just before and after enjoying this recipe on your Day 3.

Recipe idea from Deb Buhr of Sumner, Iowa.

Homemade Baking Powder
(Used in Above Recipe)

1 teaspoon	baking soda
2 teaspoons	tapioca starch
2 teaspoons	cream of tartar

Mix all ingredients well and store in an airtight container until needed for above recipe.

Yield: 5 teaspoons

Turkey Parsnip Soup

3 1/2 cups	water
1 cup	Turkey Broth (page 221)
1 1/2 cups	cooked turkey, diced
1 1/2 cups	carrots, peeled, sliced thin or diced
3/4 cup	parsnips, peeled, sliced thin or diced
1/4 teaspoon	sea salt
as desired	fresh spinach leaves, torn (optional)

1. Combine all ingredients except spinach in a large saucepan. Bring to boil, reduce heat, cover, and simmer for 10–15 minutes or until vegetables are tender.

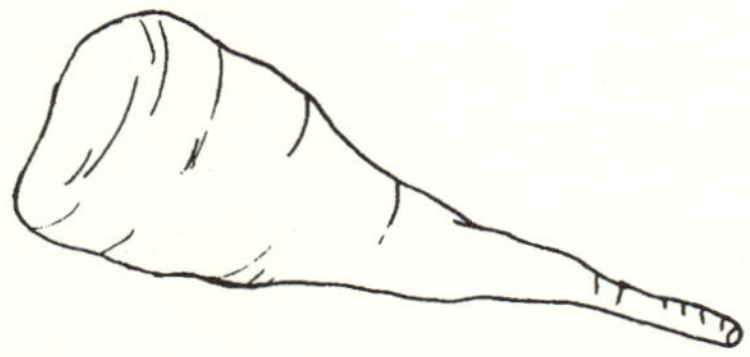

2. Garnish each bowl with fresh spinach.

Yield: approximately 4 1/2 cups without the spinach

Egg Drop Soup with Vegetables*

1 cup	Turkey Broth (page 221)
1 cup	water
2	eggs, beaten*
1/2 cup	carrots, peeled, diced small or thinly sliced
1/8 teaspoon	sea salt
1/2 cup	spinach, fresh leaves, torn small

1. In saucepan, heat turkey broth and water to simmering temperature.

2 Gradually pour in beaten egg in a thin stream while stirring the simmering broth. Add salt and carrots. Simmer a few minutes until carrots are just warm or tender. I prefer them crisp.

3. Garnish in each serving bowl with 1/4 cup fresh spinach. Serve with muffin, biscuit, or crackers for a complete light meal.

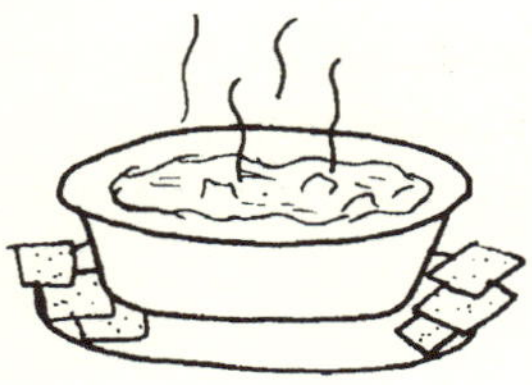

Yield: 2 cups

*Realize that eggs are usually eaten on Day 1. Be sure to omit eggs on your Day 1 just before and after eating eggs in this salad on your Day 3.

Turkey Quinoa Soup

4 cups	water
1 cup	Turkey Broth (page 221)
1/4 cup	whole quinoa, rinse and drain 2–3 times (page 36)
1 1/2 cups	cooked turkey, diced
1 1/2 cups	carrots, peeled, sliced thin or diced
1/4 teaspoon	sea salt
as desired	fresh spinach leaves, torn (optional)

1. Bring all ingredients, except spinach, to boil in a large saucepan. Reduce heat, cover, and simmer for 15 minutes or until the carrots and quinoa are tender. Taste and add more salt if desired.

2. Garnish each bowl with fresh spinach.

Yield: approximately 5 cups without the spinach

Turkey Barley Soup

5 cups	water
1 cup	Turkey Broth (page 221)
1/4 cup	pearled barley
1 1/2 cups	cooked turkey, diced
1 1/2 cups	carrots, peeled, sliced thin or diced
1/2 teaspoon	sea salt
as desired	fresh spinach leaves, torn (optional)

1. Bring water, broth, and barley to boil in a large saucepan. Reduce heat, cover, and simmer for 50 minutes.
2. Add the rest of the ingredients except spinach. Simmer for 10–15 minutes longer or until the carrots and barley are tender. Taste and add more salt if desired.
3. Garnish each bowl with fresh spinach.

Yield: approximately 5 1/2 cups without the spinach

Turkey Soup

3 cups	water
1 cup	Turkey Broth (page 221)
1 1/2 cups	cooked turkey, diced
2 cups	carrots, sliced thin or diced
1/4 teaspoon	sea salt
as desired	fresh spinach leaves, torn (optional)

1. Combine all ingredients except spinach in a large saucepan. Bring to boil, reduce heat, cover and simmer for 10–15 minutes or until carrots are tender. Taste and add more salt, if desired
2. Garnish each bowl with fresh spinach.

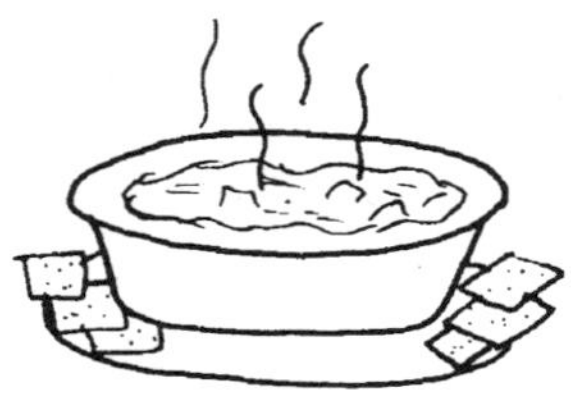

Yield: approximately 4 cups without the spinach

Turkey Quinoa Pasta Soup

1 cup	Turkey Broth (page 221)
1 cup	water
1 cup	carrots, fresh or frozen, peeled and sliced
1/2 cup	cauliflower, fresh or frozen, sliced or small florets
1/2 cup	cooked turkey meat, diced
as needed	sea salt
1/2 cup	wheat-free quinoa pasta

1. In saucepan, combine all ingredients except pasta. Simmer until vegetables are almost tender.
2. Cook pasta according to recipe Quinoa Pasta—How to Cook (page 227) and add to the simmering soup. Continue cooking and stir gently until pasta is just hot enough to serve. Do not overcook pasta.

Yield: 3 cups

Special Note: Prepare only amount to be served because quinoa pasta turns to mush when reheated.

Cream of Cauliflower Soup*

1 cup	water
3/8 teaspoon	sea salt
2 cups	cauliflower florets
1/4 cup	chopped macadamia or Brazil nuts*
2 tablespoons	tapioca starch
1 cup	water

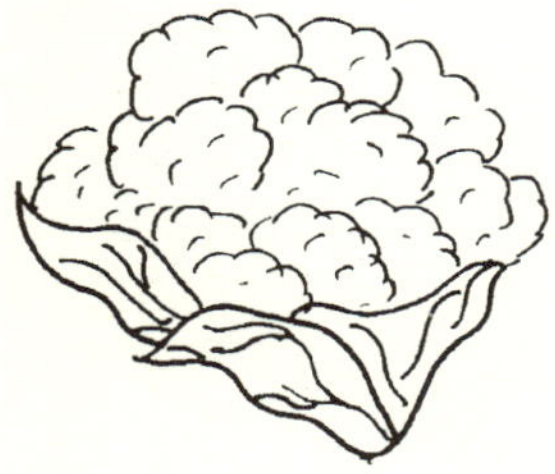

1. In saucepan, bring water and salt to boil. Reduce heat. Add cauliflower, cover, and simmer 5 minutes.
2. While cauliflower is cooking, combine nuts, starch, and approximately 1/3 cup of water in blender. Blend on highest speed for 1–2 minutes until well blended. Stop at least once to scrape sides and bottom of blender jar. Add the rest of the water and approximately 1/2 of the cooked cauliflower mixture to blender. Blend about 20 seconds on lowest speed.
3. Pour blended mixture into saucepan. Heat to serving temperature and to thicken. Stir almost constantly. Serve with crackers, biscuit, or muffin for a quick light lunch or as side dish with meal.

Yield: 2 3/4 cups

Salmon Cauliflower Chowder*

Prepare same as Cream of Cauliflower Soup except add 1–7 1/2 ounce jar of Chuck's Seafood salmon at step 3. Also, you may desire to increase salt to at least 1/2 teaspoon.

Yield: 3 2/3 cups

*Brazil and macadamia nuts are unassigned "Fun Foods" in this rotational diet, see explanation on pages 30–31.

Turkey Oatmeal Loaf

1 pound	ground turkey
1/2 cup	old fashioned rolled oats (regular, uncooked)
1/2 cup	water
1/2 cup	carrots, shredded
1/2 teaspoon	sea salt

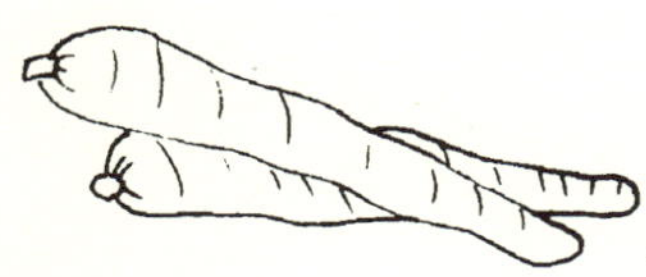

1. In large mixing bowl, combine all ingredients thoroughly. I prefer to mix with my hands while wearing disposable plastic gloves.
2. Shape meat mixture in 9 x 5-inch loaf pan, 9 muffin cups (1/3 cup of meat mixture per muffin cup), or 6 custard cups (1/2 cup of meat mixture per custard cup).
3. Bake at 350°F. for 50–60 minutes in loaf pan, 20–25 minutes in muffin pan, or 35–45 minutes in custard cups.

If you wish, ingredients may be mixed early in the day and stored in refrigerator to be cooked for evening meal.

Yields: 4 servings

Millet or Quinoa Turkey Vegetable Stew

1 pound	ground turkey
1 teaspoon	sea salt
1 cup	Turkey Broth (page 221)
1 1/2 cups	water
1/4 cup	hulled millet grain OR whole quinoa, rinsed (see page 36)
1 1/2 cups	parsnips, peeled and sliced or diced
2 cups	cauliflower, small florets or sliced
2 1/2 cups	carrots, peeled, sliced or diced
1/2 cup	water (optional)
2 tablespoons	tapioca starch (optional)

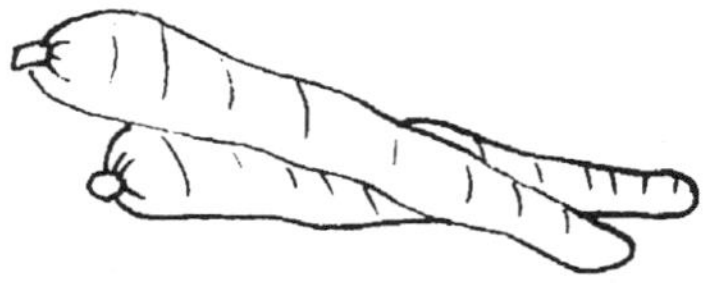

1. Combine ground turkey and salt in 5-quart Dutch-oven kettle. Cook until meat is done. Stir often to chop meat and brown evenly.
2. Add turkey broth, 1 1/2 cups of water, rinsed millet or quinoa, and prepared vegetable. Heat to boiling, reduce heat, cover, and simmer for 15–20 minutes or until millet or quinoa is done and vegetables are tender. Stir occasionally. Add more water if needed. Taste. Add more salt if needed.
3. If desired, in a small bowl, whisk together 1/2 cup of water and tapioca starch to blend. Add to stew and cook to thicken. Serve with or without biscuits. Freeze leftovers for future quick meals.

Yield: 6 1/2 cups

Special Note: I usually prepare this quick meal in the winter and use frozen vegetables. If fresh vegetables are used, you may need to add more water.

Turkey Quinoa Pasta Stew

1 cup	Turkey Broth (page 221)
1 cup	water
2 cups	carrots, fresh or frozen, peeled and sliced
1 cup	cauliflower, fresh or frozen, sliced or small florets
1 cup	cooked turkey meat, diced
as needed	sea salt
1 cup	wheat-free quinoa pasta

<u>Ingredients to thicken</u>:

2 tablespoons	tapioca starch
1/2 cup	water

1. In saucepan, combine all ingredients except pasta and thickening ingredients. Simmer until vegetables are almost tender.
2. Cook pasta according to recipe Quinoa Pasta—How to Cook (page 227).
3. Whisk together water and tapioca starch and add to the simmering stew. Continue cooking, stirring continuously, until thickened. Then add cooked pasta and stir gently until pasta is just hot enough to serve. Serve with Quinoa Biscuits (page 208).

Yield: 4 1/2 cups

Special Note: Prepare only amount to be served because quinoa pasta turns to mush when reheated.

Roast Turkey and Broth

1	12–15 pound turkey hen
1–2 tablespoons	sea salt
2–3 cups	water

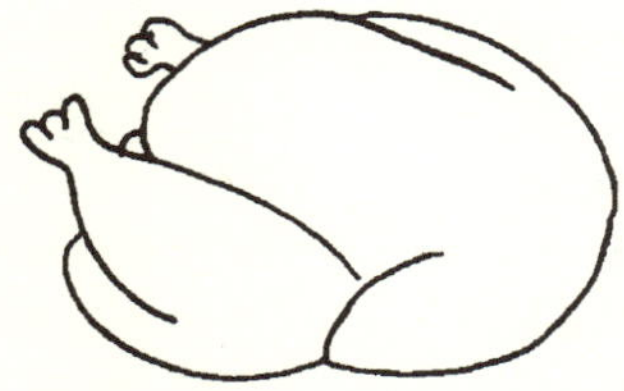

There are many ways to roast a turkey. I prefer to use a covered stainless-steel roasting pan or Reynolds Oven Cooking Bag.

1. Wash your bird inside and out. Remove any pin feathers from the skin. Rub the inside and outside of bird with salt. Tuck wings under back of bird or sew wing tips to breast. Tie legs together with heavy cotton string.
2. Place bird on roasting rack in roasting pan. Add water. Cover and roast at 325–350°F. Allow approximately 3 1/2–4 hours. Use a meat thermometer and roast until the internal temperature reaches 180°F. Be sure the thermometer is inserted into the thickest part of the meat and is not touching a bone. If turkey is not browning to your liking, roast uncovered for the last 15–30 minutes.

   OR

   Insert bird into Turkey-size Reynolds Oven Roasting Bag. I follow the directions that come with the bags except I do not shake flour in the empty bag but I do add 2–3 cups of water. Do not forget to make six 1/2-inch slits in top of bag.
3. After the meal, strain leftover broth through fine-meshed strainer and chill. After chilling, remove the fat that is solid on the top. Also, after the meal, remove remaining cooked meat from the bones. Break the carcass to fit into large kettle. Add approximately 2–3 cups of water. Simmer 1–2 hours until excess turkey is so tender that it falls off the bones. Add this broth to the broth that you got from roasting. Measure broth and add more water if needed to yield 9–11 cups of broth. Finally, measure out and freeze broth in 1 cup servings. This way the turkey broth is all ready for most recipes in this cookbook.

Easy Thanksgiving Feast

Menu	Preparation Schedule
Cranberry Spritzer	Day before–Chill ingredients. Combine ingredients just before serving.
Roast Turkey	Day before—Clean bird, sew wings, and tie legs. Place in oven 4 hours before serving.
Dill "Stove-Top" Stuffing	Day before—Prepare your choice of vegetables, and boil turkey neck for broth. If desired you may remove meat from neck and add. Prepare 20 minutes before serving.
steamed broccoli, cauliflower, and/or carrots	Day before—Prepare your choice of fresh vegetables. Cook 10 minutes before serving.
Apple Salad	Day before—Prepare "Mayo" and vegetables. In the AM—Dice apples, combine, and chill.
Kamut® Dinner Rolls	Day before—Measure ingredients. Begin mixing 1 hour before serving. Bake while turkey is being carved.
Cranberry Sauce	Day before—Chill.
Butternut Squash Pie /Libby's Pumpkin Pie	Day before—Prepare both.
Dacopa beverage	Prepare as needed before serving.

Creamed Turkey on Rye Toast

1 pound	ground turkey
1/2 teaspoon	sea salt
1 cup	Turkey Broth (page 221)
1/2 cup	water
2 cups	carrots, diced or sliced thin
1/2 teaspoon	cilantro
1/4 cup	water
3 tablespoons	tapioca starch

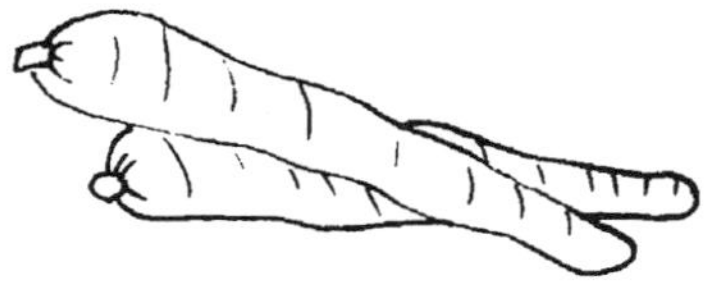

1. In large skillet, cook ground turkey and salt. Stir often to chop meat and brown evenly.
2. Add broth, first measurement of water, carrots, and cilantro. Heat to boiling, reduce heat, cover, and simmer for 10–15 minutes or until carrots are tender. Taste and add more seasonings if desired.
3. In small bowl, whisk together 1/4 cup water (second measurement of water) and tapioca starch to blend. Add to turkey and vegetable mixture and cook to thicken. Serve over toasted Rudolph's 100% Sour dough Rye Bread or with any Day 3 biscuits. Freeze leftovers for future quick meals.

Yield: 4 cups

Baked Fish for Day 3

Your choice of Day 3 fish fillets	flounder, fresh salmon
Your choice of Day 3 seasonings	funnel, ginger, caraway seeds and/or canola seed
Your choice of Day 3 foods	sliced apples, thinly sliced carrots, and/or thinly sliced parsnips

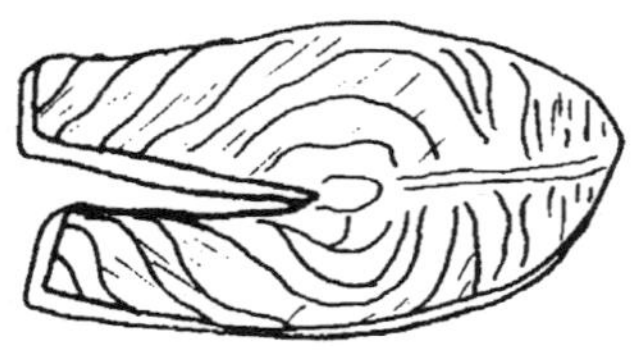

Place fish fillets in covered casserole dish. Sprinkle with salt and seasonings. Garnish with your choice of other foods. Add 1–2 tablespoons of water to casserole dish. Cover and bake for approximately 30 minutes at 350ºF. until fish is flaky. Time will depend on thickness of fillet, whether fillet is frozen or thawed, and amount of other foods used. Just before serving drizzle with flaxseed oil. Garnish with fresh spinach or parsley and serve.

Grilled Fish for Day 3

Day 3 fish fillet for grilling	fresh salmon steak
Day 3 oil	canola oil

Baste both sides of fish fillet with small amount of oil. Sprinkle both sides of fish fillet with salt. Cook on small electric grill. Turn often to prevent burning. I use a grill which has a thermostat for better temperature control which is especially needed for fish. Garnish with fresh spinach or parsley and serve.

Yield: 1 pound of fish equals 3 servings

Rainbow Trout
(Baked or Grilled)

To bake:
- Rainbow Trout is one fish that is cooked with the head and tail intact.
- Rinse trout thoroughly.
- Sprinkle inside with small amount of sea salt.
- Place trout in shallow covered casserole dish that is large enough to keep fish flat.
- Cover and bake at 350°F. for approximately 20 minutes or until trout is flaky and skin will remove easily.

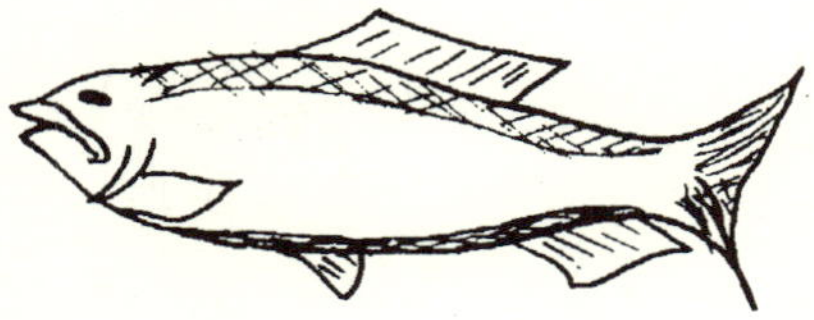

To Grill:
- Prepare trout same as for baking except place trout in aluminum foil.
- Fold ends and edges of foil around trout to make a folded seal.
- Place on a preheated counter-top electric grill on highest setting.
- Grill 10 minutes on first side, turn, and grill 7 minutes on second side.

To remove skin and bones:
- Using the edge of a fork, break through the skin along the back bone.
- Use two (2) table forks like tongs to pull the skin off the top of the trout.
- Slide the fork under the meat to remove the top fillet without the bone. Sometimes the fillet will come off in more than one piece.
- Carefully use fingers to pull the bone up from the tail. Look closely and remove any remaining small bones from the bottom fillet.
- Turn fish over and remove the skin from the bottom fillet.
- Serve immediately with a small amount of flaxseed oil. On occasion, I break rotation and sprinkle with garlic powder and use Clarified Butter (page 195) instead of oil.

Salmon Millet Dinner

1/2 cup	hulled millet
1 1/4 cups	water
1/2 teaspoon	sea salt
4 cups	Day 3 vegetables, fresh or frozen I prefer: 2 cups cauliflower, fresh or frozen, small florets 2 cups carrots, sliced
1 jar	Chuck's Seafood Salmon, flaked (7 1/2 ounces)

1. Rinse millet (page 36). Add all ingredients in order given to a 2 1/2 quart saucepan. Bring to boil. Cover. Reduce heat to between low and medium to allow food to simmer for 15 minutes. Do not peek during cooking time.
2. Stir and serve. Leftovers may be frozen. Thaw and reheat slowly or in microwave.

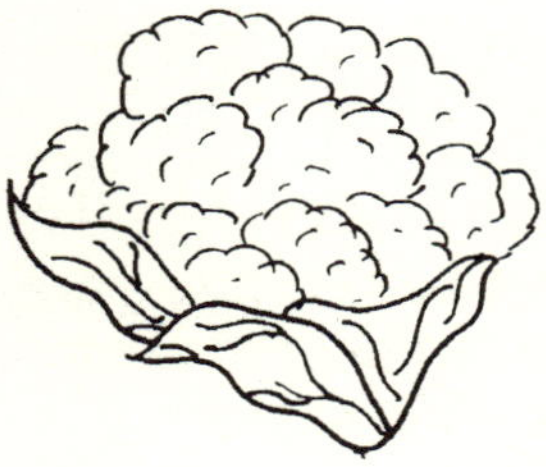

Yield: 5 cups

Salmon Patties

1 jar	Chuck's Seafood Salmon, flaked (7 1/2 ounces)
1/2 cup	shredded carrots
1/4 cup	tapioca starch
1/4 teaspoon	sea salt
1 teaspoon	canola oil

1. Preheat electric skillet to 350ºF. Add oil to preheated skillet.
2. Combine all ingredients except oil in bowl. Mix thoroughly. Divide into 6 portions. Patty each portion by forming into a ball and then flattening.
3. Cook for 3–5 minutes on each side until golden brown. Serve immediately.

Yield: 2 servings, 6 patties

Filbert "Mayo"

1/2 cup	filberts
1 cup	water
1 teaspoon	unbuffered, corn-free vitamin C crystals
1 tablespoon	tapioca starch
1/4 teaspoon	sea salt
as desired	caraway seed, fennel—depending on use (optional)

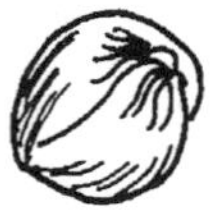

1. Blend filberts in blender on highest speed until they become a fine powder, approximately 1–2 minutes. Stop once or twice to scrape sides and bottom of blender jar.
2. Add rest of ingredients except caraway and/or fennel. Blend on highest speed for a minute longer, stopping once or twice to scrape sides and bottom of blender jar.
3. Pour mixture into small saucepan. Cook over medium heat. Stir constantly until mixture thickens. I prefer to stir with a whisk to keep mixture smooth.
4. Add caraway and/or fennel if desired. Chill. You may store in glass jar in refrigerator for a week, if necessary. Add a tablespoon of additional water if too thick.

Yield: 1 1/3 cups

Recipe idea from The Yeast Connection Cookbook by Crook & Jones, p. 208.

Carrot-Caraway Salad Dressing

1 cup	carrot, peeled, shredded
1/2 cup	water
1 1/2 teaspoons	canola oil
1/2 teaspoon	unbuffered, corn-free vitamin C crystals
2 pinches	sea salt
1/2 teaspoon	caraway seed

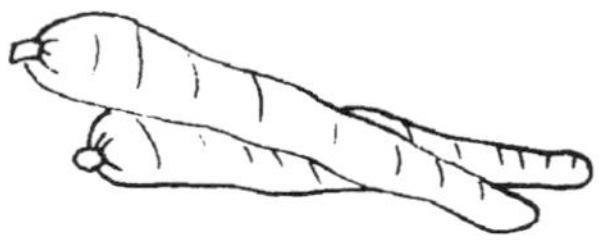

1. Combine all ingredients, except caraway seed, in blender. Blend on highest speed for 1–2 minutes until smooth, stopping once or twice to scrape sides and bottom of blender jar.
2. Pour dressing in glass jar or bottle. Add caraway and stir or shake. Chill. You may store in glass jar in refrigerator for a week, if necessary.

Yield: 1 cup

Salmon Salad

1/2 jar	Chuck's Seafood salmon, flaked (3 3/4 ounces)
1/3 cup	shredded carrots
few sprigs	fresh parsley, torn or cut into small pieces (optional)
2 tablespoons	Filbert "Mayo" (page 224)
to taste	sea salt

Combine and chill. Serve on bed of fresh spinach leaves as a salad or as my favorite, a sandwich on Rudolph's 100% Sourdough Rye Bread with spinach leaves. Makes enough for 2–3 sandwiches..

Yield: 3/4 cup

Salmon/Egg Salad

Add to the above recipe:

1 diced hard boiled egg* and an extra tablespoon of dressing. Serve as above as salad or sandwich.

Yield: 1 cup

Turkey Salad*

1/2 cup	cooked turkey, diced
1	egg, hard boiled, diced*
1/3 cup	shredded carrots
few sprigs	fresh parsley, torn or cut into small pieces (optional)
3 tablespoons	Filbert "Mayo" (page 224)
to taste	sea salt

Combine and chill. Serve on bed of fresh spinach leaves as a salad or as my favorite, a sandwich on a quinoa tortilla or Rudolph's 100% Sourdough Rye Bread with spinach leaves. Makes enough for 2–3 sandwiches.

Yield: 1 cup

*Realize that eggs are usually eaten on Day 1. Be sure to omit eggs on your Day 1 just before and after enjoying this recipe on your Day 3.

Nothing in life is to be feared.
It is only to be understood.
Marie Curie

Salmon or Turkey Vegetable Salad

1 cup	carrots, peeled, sliced or diced
1 cup	cauliflower, sliced or small florets
1/2 jar	Chuck's Seafood salmon, flaked (3 3/4 ounces)
	OR 1/2 cup of cooked diced turkey
1/4 teaspoon	sea salt
few sprigs	fresh parsley, torn or cut into small pieces (optional)
1/2 cup	Filbert "Mayo" (page 224)
	OR 1/3 cup of Carrot-Caraway Salad Dressing (page 224)
as desired	fresh spinach leaves

1. Prepare vegetables and dressing as described above.
2. In bowl, gently toss all ingredients except dressing and spinach. Add dressing and mix to coat all vegetables. Chill.
3. Serve on bed of spinach leaves or just before serving tear spinach leaves and toss into salad along with additional dressing. Makes a complete meal, but I also enjoy the salad with crackers or a muffin.

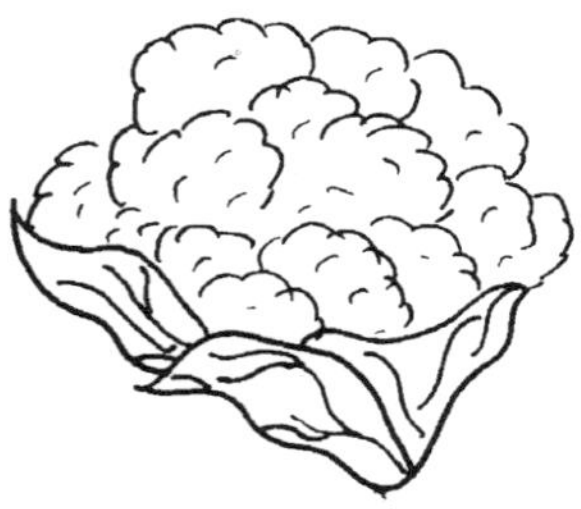

Yield: 2 1/2 cups

Variation: You may add some cooked pasta (100% rye or wild rice) with additional dressing.

Turkey Quinoa Pasta Salad

1/2 cup	wheat-free quinoa pasta
1 cup	carrots, peeled and sliced
1/2 cup	cauliflower, sliced or small florets
2	eggs, hard cooked, diced (optional)
1/2 cup	cooked turkey meat, diced
1/4 teaspoon	sea salt
1/4–1/3 cup	Filbert "Mayo" (page 224)
as desired	fresh spinach leaves

1. Cook quinoa pasta according to recipe Quinoa Pasta—How to Cook (page 227). Chill.
2. In bowl, combine and gently toss carrots, cauliflower, eggs, turkey, and salt. Chill.
3. Add chilled pasta to the other chilled ingredients and toss lightly. Add "Mayo" and mix carefully. Taste and add more salt if needed. Chill until ready to serve.
4. Wash and drain fresh spinach leaves. Serve salad on a bed of the leaves.

Yield: 2 1/4 cups

*Realize that eggs are usually eaten on Day 1. Be sure to omit eggs on your Day 1 just before and after eating eggs in this salad on your Day 3.

Day 3 Pasta Salad

2 cups Old Creek brand 100% Wheat-free pasta
I prefer: 1 cup Rye pasta
1 cup Wild Rice pasta.
1/2 cup shredded carrots
3/4 cup Filbert "Mayo" (page 224)

1. Cook pasta according to package directions. Chill
2. Add carrots and "Mayo." Stir and chill. Taste and add salt and/or more "Mayo" if desired.

Yield: 4 cups

Quinoa Pasta*—How to Cook

Preparing Quinoa Pasta for Cold Salads

1. Bring 1 1/2 cups of salted water to boil. Add 1/2 cup quinoa pasta. Reduce heat a little, to about medium high. Cook pasta for 3–4 minutes until tender. Stir almost continually.
2. Remove from heat, drain immediately. Then quickly put the cooked pasta into ice water to chill and to stop any further cooking. Drain. Refrigerate until ready to mix in salad.

Preparing Quinoa Pasta for Hot Dishes

1. Bring 1 1/2 cups of salted water to boil. Add 1/2 cup quinoa pasta. Reduce heat a little, to about medium high. Cook pasta for only 2–3 minutes, stirring almost continually. Pasta will not be tender yet.
2. Remove from heat, drain and rinse immediately. Add to simmering soup or stew. Heat only until pasta is tender.

Special Note: Over cooking this gluten-free pasta makes it mushy.

*Special Note: Wheat-free quinoa pasta ingredients are yellow corn flour, quinoa flour, and sesame flour. It comes in elbows and rotille. Because of the sesame, eating this quinoa pasta on Day 3 breaks rotation. I eat it occasionally without concern. You can make your own decision.

Spinach Chef Salad

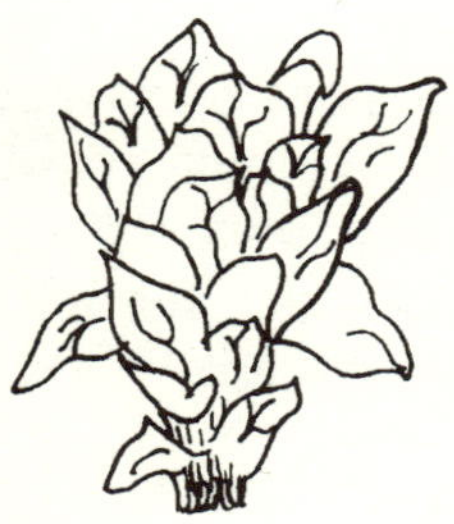

spinach, torn
carrots, shredded
cauliflower, sliced or florets
walnuts or filberts, chopped
eggs, hard-cooked, diced
salmon, flaked
cooked turkey, diced or strips
Carrot-Caraway Salad Dressing (page 224)
Filbert "Mayo" (page 224)

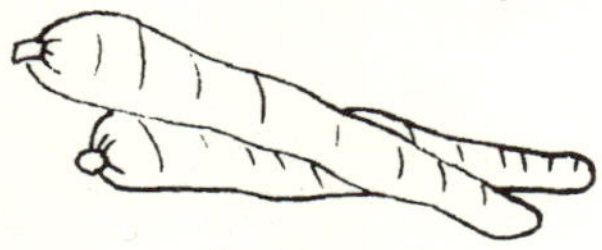

1. Clean and prepare your choice of vegetables in amount desired
2. Add eggs, salmon, and/or turkey and dressing in desired amounts.
3. Serve with Day 4 biscuits, crackers, or muffins for a complete light meal.

Quinoa Salad

1 cup	chilled Basic Quinoa (page 212)
1/2 cup	apple, finely diced
1/3 cup	carrot, shredded
few springs	fresh parsley (optional)

Combine all ingredients. Chill and serve. This is one of my favorite recipes for using leftover Basic Quinoa.

Yield: approximately 1 1/3 cups firmly packed

Apple Salad

1	small apple, peeled and diced (approximately 2/3 cup)
1–2 tablespoons	walnuts, chopped
2 tablespoons	Filbert "Mayo" (page 224)

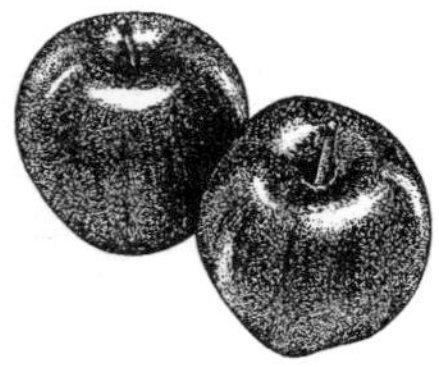

Combine, chill, and serve.

Yield: approximately 2/3 cup

Vegetable/Apple Salad

1	medium apple, peeled and diced (approximately 1 cup)
1/2 cup	shredded carrot
2 tablespoons	walnuts, chopped
3 tablespoons	Filbert "Mayo" (page 224)

Combine, chill, and serve.

Yield: approximately 1 1/2 cups

Variation 1: Add 1–2 tablespoons small flaked coconut.

Variation 2: Add 1 cup of fresh torn spinach leaves and more "Mayo."

Variation 3: Substitute 1/4 cup of diced celery for half of the carrots. However, do remember to avoid eating celery on your Day 1 just before and after eating this variation on your Day 3.

Parsnips

Parsnips are an old-fashioned vegetable being rediscovered now that complex carbohydrates are growing in popularity. Add parsnips to winter stews and soups (such as Millet or Quinoa Turkey Vegetable Stew and Turkey Parsnip Soup). Also try the following delicious recipe.

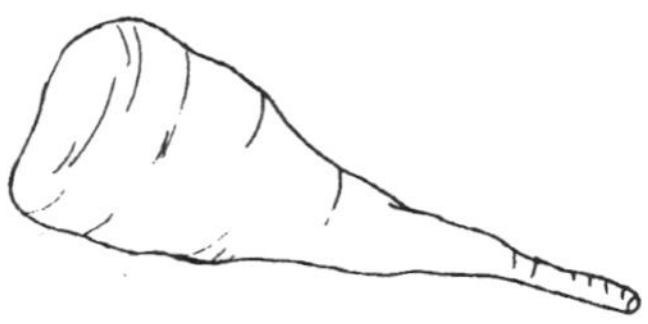

Steamed or Whipped Parsnips

Choose young, tender parsnips. Scrub, peel, and slice. In saucepan, steam with small amount of water and salt approximately 15 minutes until tender. (If you only have the choice of large parsnips, you may desire to remove the pithy center at the top before cooking.) If desired, whip as you would mashed potatoes. I prefer to use a Braun hand blender. Serve plain or season with flaxseed oil and/or caraway seeds.

Stir-Fry Vegetables for Day 3

cauliflower florets
Brussels sprouts, sliced, blanched or frozen
carrot, slant cut
filberts or walnuts, chopped coarse
canola and/or walnut oil
sea salt
caraway seed or fennel
spinach, torn small pieces

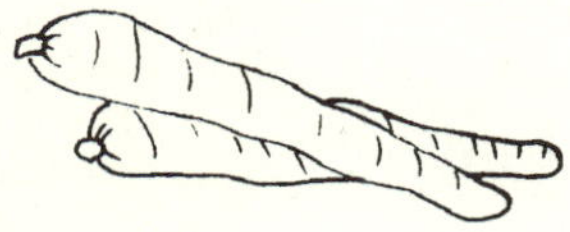

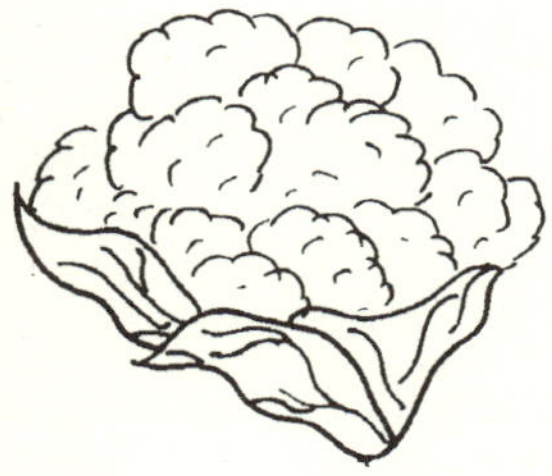

1. Preheat well-seasoned cast-iron skillet on medium (see How to Season Cast Iron on page 63) or electric skillet to 300ºF.
2. Prepare vegetables in amounts desired.
3. Add oil to preheated skillet (cast-iron skillet will require less oil). Add vegetables (except spinach) and nuts. Sprinkle with seasonings. Stir often to cook vegetables evenly. Add spinach near end of cooking time just prior to serving. I prefer my vegetables crunchy and the spinach just barely warm. Serve immediately.

Millet Pudding

1 cup	sliced or diced apple, peeled
1/4 cup	water
1/2 teaspoon	cinnamon
1–2 tablespoons	walnuts, chopped
1 cup	Creamy Millet Cereal (page 203)*
2 teaspoons	tapioca starch
1 tablespoon	water
1 teaspoon	alcohol-free vanilla flavoring

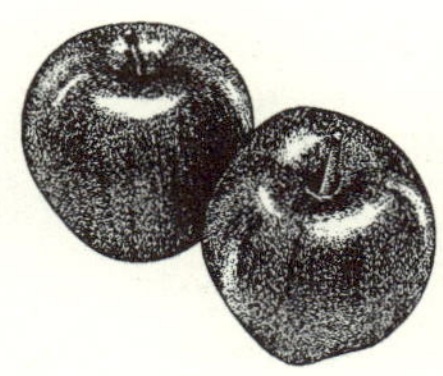

1. Layer apples, 1/4 cup of water, cinnamon, walnuts, and cooked millet in a 1-quart Vision saucepan. Do not stir. Cover.
2. Bring water to boil over medium heat. I prefer to use the glass Vision cookware so I can see when the water begins to boil.
3. Turn heat down to low and simmer for 15 minutes or until apples are tender.
4. Dissolve tapioca starch in 1 tablespoon of water and vanilla. Add to cooked mixture. Stir and cook until pudding thickens. Serve for breakfast or for dessert, either warm or cold. However, it is best warm. You may freeze leftover Millet Pudding for future quick desserts.

Yield: approximately 1 2/3 cups.

Special Note: Since I enjoy this pudding warm for breakfast, I will cook and freeze extra millet on Day 3. Then, I will pull the cooked millet from the freezer the day before I wish to eat it 4 or 8 days later and allow it to begin thawing in the refrigerator. The millet does not need to be completely thawed—just enough to chunk up with a fork. Also, most of the time I use frozen sliced apples (page 206). Once you have prepared this recipe a couple of times, you will not even need to measure the apples, cinnamon, and walnuts. You will just know what it looks like in the pan.

*If desired, you may use 1 cup cooked Basic Millet (page 215) however increase water to 3/4 cup and omit tapioca starch and second measurement of water as well as step 4.

Simply Delicious Oat Granola Bars

1/3 cup	undiluted apple juice concentrate
2 tablespoons	walnut or canola oil
2 cups	old fashioned rolled oats
2 tablespoons	walnuts
1/2 cup	oat bran
1/4 cup	small flaked unsweetened coconut (optional)
1/2 teaspoon	sea salt
2 teaspoons	cinnamon

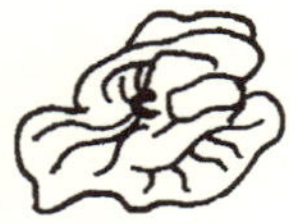

1. Oil an 8-inch square baking pan with approximately 1/4 teaspoon oil.
2. Preheat oven to 350ºF.
3. Measure apple juice concentrate in a 1-cup glass measure. Add water slowly until the liquid totals 1/2 cup. Add oil. Set aside.
4. Pour rolled oats into chopper cup of Black & Decker® Handy Shortcut™ food processor (the cup holds 2 cups so no need to measure). Chop for 10 seconds. Stop and stir with knife or handle of spoon. Chop for 5 seconds more. The oats should now be coarsely chopped. Pour into mixing bowl.
5. Add nuts to chopper and chop for approximately 15 seconds or longer until desired size.
6. Add chopped nuts, oat bran, coconut, salt, and cinnamon to mixing bowl. Toss to distribute ingredients evenly.
7. Pour liquid mixture evenly over oat mixture. With hands, toss ingredients to evenly coat oat mixture with liquids.
8. Transfer to prepared pan and spread evenly. Press mixture firmly in pan. I prefer to use both my hands, one on top of the other.
9. Bake 25 minutes. Cool completely. Cut 4x2. Enjoy for breakfast, dessert, or snack. Leftovers can be frozen. I individually bag the bars in cellophane bags. No need to thaw, you can just unwrap and enjoy. These granola bars do crumble a little, but for the most part they hold together.

Yield: 8 servings

Quinoa Pudding I

1 cup	Basic Quinoa (page 212)
1/2 cup	unsweetened applesauce
1/2 cup	water
2 tablespoons	chopped walnuts
3/4 teaspoon	ground cinnamon
1 teaspoon	alcohol-free vanilla flavoring

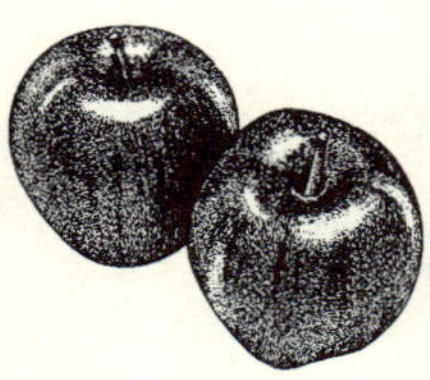

Combine all ingredients in small saucepan. Simmer on low heat for 5–10 minutes to combine flavors. If desired, add more water. Serve warm or cold.

Yield: 1 1/2 cups

Quinoa Pudding II

1 cup	Quinoa Cereal I or II (page 204)
1/4 cup	unsweetened applesauce
1–2 tablespoons	walnuts, chopped
1/2 teaspoon	ground cinnamon
1 teaspoon	alcohol-free vanilla flavoring

Combine all ingredients in small saucepan. Simmer on low heat for 5–10 minutes to combine flavors. Serve warm or cold.

Yield: 1 1/4 cups

Traditionally, scones were the backbone of Scottish and English tea parties. I like to serve them at informal brunches. These scones are flaky and taste great. They are even better the next day.

Oat Scones

2 1/4 cups	oat flour
1/2 teaspoon	baking soda
1/4 teaspoon	unbuffered, corn-free vitamin C crystals
3 tablespoons + 1 teaspoon	water
1/3 cup	canola oil
1/4 cup	raisins, boiled, drained, and cooled*
1/2 cup	rolled oats

1. Preheat oven to 325ºF.
2. In mixing bowl, whisk together 1 cup oat flour, baking soda, and vitamin C.
3. Add water and oil. Beat hard with a wooden spoon for 50 strokes.
4. Stir in raisins.
5. Add and stir in 1–2 tablespoons of additional oat flour. Repeat this step until dough forms a ball and is not sticky. Divide dough into 2 balls.
6. Scatter half of rolled oats on an ungreased cookie sheet. Place 1 ball on the top of them, and roll it to cover with the oats. Then flatten into a 6–7 inch circle about 3/8 inch thick. Turn a few times to coat well with oats. Cut dough into 8 wedges. Do not separate wedges.
7. Repeat with remaining dough and oats.
8. Bake for 25 minutes, or until light golden brown. Cool for 30 minutes on the baking sheet. Serve at room temperature.

*Variation I: Omit the raisins and add 1/8 teaspoon of stevia to dry ingredients. Realize that this variation breaks rotation. Stevia is a Day 4 food. However, I usually do not concern myself with the break in rotation.

Variation II: You can add 1/4 cup of rice flour** and reduce the oat flour to 3/4 cup in step 2.

Yield: 16 scones

** Rice is usually eaten on Day 1 so you need to avoid rice on your Day 1 just before and after enjoying this variation on your Day 3.

Recipe idea from The Allergy Self-Help Cookbook by Jones.

Apple Oat or Quinoa Crisp

Amount for:

Grab-It Bowl: 1 serving	Pie Pan: 4 servings	YIELD
1/2 cup	2 cups	apples, fresh or frozen, peeled, sliced
1/4 teaspoon	1 teaspoon	ground cinnamon
sprinkle	sprinkle	nutmeg
1 teaspoon	4 teaspoons	maple granules, optional

Ingredients for **OAT** crisp topping:

1/4 cup	1 cup	old fashioned rolled oats (regular, uncooked)
1 tablespoon	1/4 cup	oat bran
2 pinches	1/8 teaspoon	sea salt
1/8 teaspoon	1/2 teaspoon	ground cinnamon
sprinkle	sprinkle	nutmeg*
1 teaspoon	4 teaspoons	maple granules, optional*
1 1/4 teaspoons	5 teaspoons	canola oil

Ingredients for **QUINOA** crisp topping:

2 tablespoons	1/2 cup	quinoa flour
1 pinch	4 pinches	sea salt
1/8 teaspoon	1/2 teaspoon	ground cinnamon
sprinkle	sprinkle	nutmeg*
1 teaspoon	4 teaspoons	maple granules (optional)*
scant 1 teaspoon	1 tablespoon	canola oil
scant 1 teaspoon	1 tablespoon	water

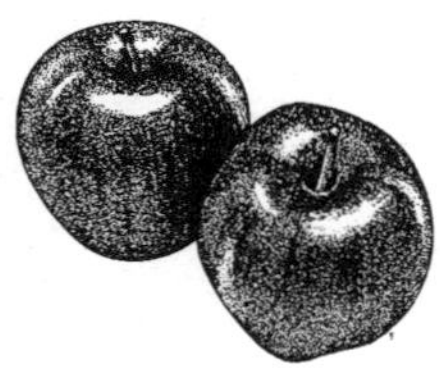

1. Preheat oven to 425°F.
2. Prepare apple slices; toss lightly with spices and maple granules. Layer in an oiled Corning Grab-It bowl or 8-inch pie pan.
3. In mixing bowl, whisk together dry topping ingredients.
4. FOR OAT: Gradually add oil while stirring mixture. Sometimes I use my hands to completely blend in the oil so that all the oatmeal is evenly moistened.

   FOR QUINOA: Add oil and water. Stir with fork or rubber spatula to coat flour mixture evenly with liquids. You may desire to use a pastry blender.
5. Sprinkle crisp mixture evenly over apples. Bake for 18–20 minutes or until apples are tender. Cooking time will depend on whether you use fresh or frozen apple slices.

Special Notes: I prefer to use eating apples rather than baking apples because an eating apple like red delicious will be more naturally sweet. This dessert will teach you that cinnamon, rather than sugar, is the key to apple crisp. Freeze leftovers for future cravings for a sweet treat.

To make this a real treat, serve with a small scoop of Vanilla Rice Dream non-dairy dessert. However do realize that rice is normally eaten on Day 1.

*Maple and nutmeg are unassigned "Fun Foods" on this rotational diet, see explanation on pages 30–31.

Butternut Squash, Sweet Potatoes, or Yams*
How to Prepare for Delicious Pie

To Prepare Sweet Potatoes or Yams:

1. Select nice firm potatoes with no sign of mold. Wash and scrub potatoes thoroughly. Peel and cut into small pieces. Steam or cook in microwave in small amount of water until very tender. Drain, but reserve the water. Using a hand blender (Braun), blend until you get a creamy mixture. Add some of the drained liquid if needed to blend or to get the texture of pumpkin. Measure into 1 cup portions and freeze in glass jars to be ready to prepare a pie in minutes.

To Prepare Butternut Squash:

1. Select ripe butternut squash. Ripe squash has a medium tan color whereas unripe squash is off white in color, sometimes with green lines.
2. Wash squash and cut in half lengthwise. Scoop out seeds and strings. I like to use a serrated grapefruit knife which has a curved end.
3. Place cut side down in shallow baking dish. Add a small amount of water (like 1/4 cup). Bake in oven at 350°F. for 30–60 minutes or until very tender. Baking time will depend on size of squash.

OR

3. Cook in microwave on full power for 5 minutes; turn one quarter turn; cook for 3–5 minutes longer until very tender. (Continue to turn one quarter turn every 5 minutes as needed.) Cooking time will vary depending on the size of the squash and difference in microwaves.
4. Allow squash to cool at least enough to handle. Scoop out the soft squash. Stir, no need to blend. Measure out into 1 cup portions and freeze extra in glass jars to prepare a pie in minutes.

Special Note: When I cooked 4 small butternut squash it yielded 3 cups. Since one cannot get butternut squash year round, you can purchase several butternut squash when in season, bake, and freeze filling in 1- or 2-cup portions all ready to make a quick pie.

*Sweet potato, yams, and butternut squash are usually eaten on Day 4. For sweet potatoes and yams, you just need to omit eating them on your Day 4 just before and after enjoying this pie on Day 3. For butternut squash, you need to omit butternut squash on your Day 4 before and all squash from your Day 2 before and Day 4 after enjoying this pie on Day 3.

Oatmeal Pie Crust

1 1/2 cups	old fashioned rolled oats (regular, uncooked)
1/2 teaspoon	sea salt
1/4 cup	canola oil
1 tablespoon	water

1. Preheat oven to 450°F.
2. Combine oats and salt. Stir to distribute the salt evenly.
3. Add oil gradually while stirring to evenly coat the oats.
4. Pour water as evenly as possible over the mixture and stir again.
5. Pour into an 8-inch pie pan. With your hands, press the oat mixture evenly onto the bottom and sides of the pie pan, making it as firm and compact as possible. Do not allow crust to go above 1/8 inch from the lip of the pie pan because oil from the crust will bubble out over the edge of the pie pan during baking.
6. Bake for 10 minutes, then cool for 10 minutes while allowing the oven temperature to cool down to 350°F. to bake the Butternut Squash, Sweet Potatoes, or Yam Pie.

Special Note: This recipe was developed for use with the squash and sweet potato pie. At publication date, I do not know what it would be like with any other filling. This crust does not form together like regular pie crusts. However, it will surprisingly do so after the filling is baked in the crust.

Recipe idea from Rotational Bon Appetité! by Hayes & Maynard, p. 38.

Quinoa Pie Crust

1/4 cup	ice water
3 tablespoons	canola oil, cold
1/4 teaspoon	sea salt
3/4 cup	quinoa flour
1/4 cup	tapioca starch
1/2 teaspoon	ground cinnamon

1. In small bowl, whisk together flour, starch, and cinnamon and set aside.
2. In curved-sided chilled mixing bowl, whisk together water, oil, and salt until mixture is slightly thick and opaque (whitish creamy color). Note: if water and oil are not cold, the mixture will not become thick and opaque.
3. Add flour mixture all at once to oil mixture and stir with a rubber spatula or fork until flour is evenly moist.
4. Oil the bottom and sides of a 9-inch pie pan. With oiled fingers, transfer dough to pan. Press dough firmly into bottom and sides as evenly thin as possible. If you get oil on the outside of the pie pan when spreading the dough, as I do, before baking wipe outside edges and bottom of pie pan with damp cloth. You may refrigerate until ready to bake.
5. Add a double recipe of Butternut Squash, Sweet Potato, or Yam pie filling (page 235) and bake according to that recipe.

Recipe idea from Mastering Food Allergies newsletter, September 1990.

Butternut Squash, Sweet Potato, or Yam Pie
A delicious substitute for Pumpkin Pie

1	egg, lightly beaten*
1 cup	Butternut Squash, Sweet Potato, or Yams for pie* (page 233)
1/4 teaspoon	sea salt
3/4 teaspoon	cinnamon
1/4 teaspoon	ginger*
1/8 teaspoon	cloves*
1/2 cup	unsweetened apple juice

1. Prepare Oatmeal Pie Crust (page 234).
2. Preheat oven to 350°F.
3. In a medium-size bowl, mix egg, prepared squash (or sweet potato or yam)(page 233), and spices to distribute the spices evenly as you would when preparing a normal pumpkin pie. (I prefer the butternut squash.)
4. Add apple juice and mix.
5. Mixture should yield 1 3/4 cups. Pour mixture into prebaked and cooled Oatmeal Pie Crust (page 234) and bake 45–50 minutes or until knife inserted into center of pie comes out clean. Cool. Serve with Vanilla Rice Dream, a non-diary dessert, if desired. (Realize Rice Dream also breaks rotation.)
6. These pies freeze well for future desserts. Before freezing, cut pie into serving pieces and loosen for ease in thawing just amount desired.

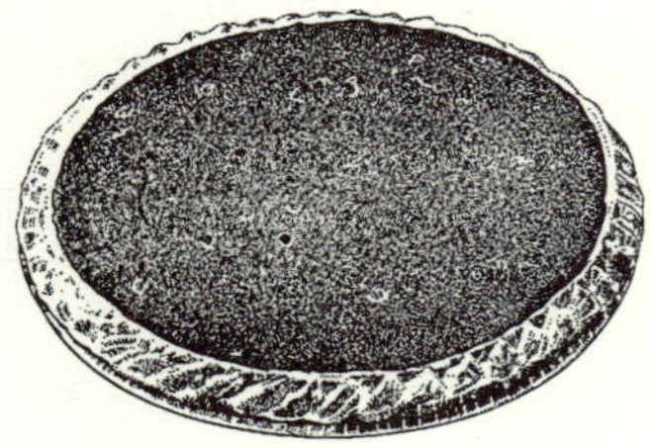

TO PREPARE THIS PIE IN OTHER CRUSTS such as Quinoa Pie Crust (page 234), double the recipe and bake 65–70 minutes.

*Realize these ingredients break rotation but careful planning can allow you to eat this recipe occasionally—especially for holidays.

- Eggs are usually eaten on Day 1 so you need to omit eating eggs on your Day 1 just before and after enjoying this pie on your Day 3.
- Sweet potato, yams, and butternut squash are usually eaten on Day 4. For sweet potatoes and yams, you just need to omit eating them on your Day 4 just before and after enjoying this pie on Day 3. For butternut squash, you need to omit butternut squash on your Day 4 before and all squash from your Day 2 before and Day 4 after enjoying this pie on Day 3.
- Ginger is an unassigned "Fun Food" on this rotational diet, see explanation on pages 30–31.
- Cloves are usually eaten on Day 2 so you need to omit eating cloves on your Day 2 just before and after enjoying this pie on your Day 3.

Applesauce Method 1

1. Wash fresh, ripe fruit. Peel, core, rinse, and drain.
2. Run fruit through Champion Juicer set up for homogenizing. This will make sauce very quickly. To prevent fruit from darkening, add approximately 1 teaspoon of unbuffered, corn-free vitamin C crystals to 8 cups of applesauce. It is best to add the vitamin C before the fruit begins to darken. I find it works best to add the vitamin C to about the first 2 cups of homogenized fruit. Then as I continue the process I add the additional applesauce, stirring after each addition.

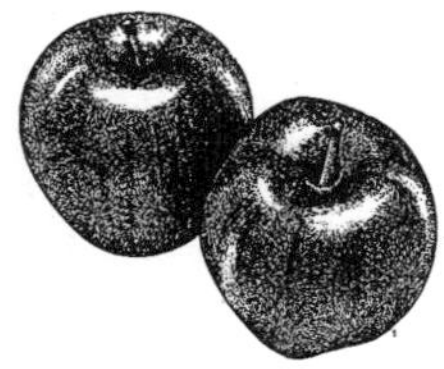

3. Transfer to saucepan. Cover with splatter screen and cook on medium to thicken to desired consistency.
4. Stir often to prevent sticking.

Applesauce Method 2

1. Wash fresh, ripe fruit. Peel, core, rinse, and drain.
2. Transfer to a saucepan. To prevent fruit from darkening, add unbuffered, corn-free vitamin C crystals, approximately 1 teaspoon for 8–10 cups of apple quarters. It is best to add the vitamin C before the fruit begins to darken so I suggest that you stir in the crystals when you have about 2 cups of quarters ready to cook. As you continue the process, stir the apple quarters after each addition. Cook on low until soft. Stir often to prevent sticking.
3. It is not necessary to add additional water to fruit before cooking since it will create its own juice as it cooks.
4. Blend in blender OR press through a canning sieve or food mill.
5. Return to saucepan, cover with splatter screen, and cook on medium to thicken to desired consistency.

Tips on Freezing Applesauce

An easy way to freeze the fruit sauce for later use is to freeze in ice cube trays, approximately 1 tablespoon per cube. After the sauce is frozen, remove from the trays and keep frozen in a bag until ready to use.

Pancake Fruit Sauce

For fruit sauce to serve with pancakes, I prefer to dilute the fruit sauce with water and heat before serving (about 2 tablespoons fruit sauce to 1 tablespoon water). This allows me to have more sauce on my pancakes with less sweetness.

11. FOODS, MEAL PLANNING, AND RECIPES FOR DAY 4

Foods for Day 4

Animal Protein

87	haddock
91	sea bass
95	mahi mahi
100	swordfish
102	ocean perch
130	squirrel
134	pork
135	venison
137	lamb, goat
	orange roughy

Vegetables

11	asparagus, leeks
27	sorrel
41	green beans, peas, lentils, soybeans & all beans not on Day 2
70	sweet potato
74	squash—acorn, butternut, & other squash not on Day 2
80	artichoke

Grains, Flours, and Baking Foods

1	agar agar, kombu
27	buckwheat
41	carob powder, kudzu (kuzu), and lentil, soy, navy, & pinto bean flours
80	Jerusalem artichoke flour

Fruit

27	rhubarb
45	orange, tangerine, tangelo
93	blueberry, cranberry

Sweeteners

27	buckwheat honey
41	clover honey
80	stevia

Oils

41	soy oil
80	safflower oil

Herbs and Spices

80	tarragon

Seeds and Nuts

41	roasted soy beans
48	cashew

Foods That Float Between Days 2 & 4

Herbs and Spices:

11	garlic
73	oregano
74	chili powder

Recipe Table of Contents for Day 4

Biscuits, Crackers, & Etc. Bread

Cereals, Grains, & Nongrains

Muffins and Pancakes

Protein Dishes

Vegetables, Salads, & Salad Dressings

Desserts

Miscellaneous

Meal Planning for Day 4

Quick & Easy Meals

Pork Cutlet and Bean Gravy
peas
green beans

Easy Meal Banquet

Pork Chop
sweet potato with flaxseed oil
green beans

Grilled Venison
Basic Buckwheat Groats
asparagus spears

Quick & Easy Meals with Advanced Planning

Stir-Fry Buckwheat and Vegetables
with or without Shrimp or Meat

Ham and Bean Stew

Pork and Buckwheat Pasta Casserole

Pork Fajita
asparagus spears

Venison and Buckwheat Pasta Casserole

Mexican Venison and Bean Stew

Pork and Bean Burritos

Buckwheat Tortilla with *plan*over
Roast Pork, sorrel, and Day 4 "Mayo"
asparagus spears

Easy Meals

Breaded Pork Chop
stir-fried Jerusalem artichoke
Baked Beans

Squash and Meatballs
green beans

Roast Pork or Venison
Basic Buckwheat Groats
green beans or asparagus spears

Tomato-Free Chili
green beans

Tofu and Asparagus in Black Bean Sauce

Scalloped Potatoes and Ham
green beans

Lower Carbohydrate Meals

Cream of Asparagus Soup
Orange Roughy

Stir-Fry Meal for Day 4

Baked or Grilled Fish for Day 4
asparagus spears

Easy Squirrel Dinner

Breakfast Ideas

Buckwheat Muffins, Pancakes, Bread, or Cereal (see Recipe Table of Contents for Day 4)

Lentils with fresh side (uncured, unsmoked bacon)

Split Pea Soup

Stir-Fry Buckwheat and Vegetables

fresh fruit

any *plan*over Day 4 vegetable, fish, casserole, or soup

Snack Ideas

- cucumber slices (floated from Day 2)
- Buckwheat Muffin
- Buckwheat Crackers
- roasted soybeans or cashews
- Carob Cake Brownies
- Buckwheat Yeast-Free Bread with Rhubarb Jelly
- Blueberry Tofu "Cheesecake"
- Orange Buckwheat Cake
- Carob Pudding
- Carob Shake
- Spritzer—3 varieties
- carob chunks

Meals Away from Home

Beans and Beans
cucumber slices (floated from Day 2)

Quick Bean Soup
raw Jerusalem artichoke with Macadamia Nut Dressing

Cucumber and Pea Salad with or without *plan*over Roast Pork or fresh side (uncured, unsmoked bacon)

Venison or Pork and Buckwheat Pasta Casserole

Your choice of *plan*over "Chili"
raw Jerusalem artichoke with Macadamia Nut Dressing

Lentil or Split Pea Soup with fresh side (uncured, unsmoked bacon) or *plan*over Roast Pork
zucchini slices (floated from Day 2)

Special Occasion Meals

Chili Feast–
Your choice of 1 or more of the following:
- –Mexican Medley Beans
- –Tomato-Free "Veggie" Chili
- –Tomato-Free Chili
- –Tomato-Free Vegetarian Chili

raw vegetable floated or moved from other days
Blueberry Tofu "Cheesecake"
Dacopa beverage

Company–
Shrimp Tofu Lasagna
Carob Buckwheat Brownies
Dacopa beverage

Recipes for Day 4

Creamy Buckwheat Cereal I

1/3 cup	buckwheat groats OR 1/3 cup purchased Cream of Buckwheat Cereal
1/4 teaspoon	sea salt
2 cups	water (room temperature)
1/4 cup	soy milk or Cashew Milk (page 243) OR additional water

1. Grind unroasted buckwheat groats in a blender just long enough to prepare a coarse meal. Omit this step if using purchased cereal.
2. Combine the above ingredients in the slow cooker.* Cook overnight and awake to enjoy this ready-to-eat, mouth-watering cereal.
3. Stir the cereal before serving. I eat this cereal plain or stir in 2 tablespoons of blueberries or a few grains of stevia for sweetness.

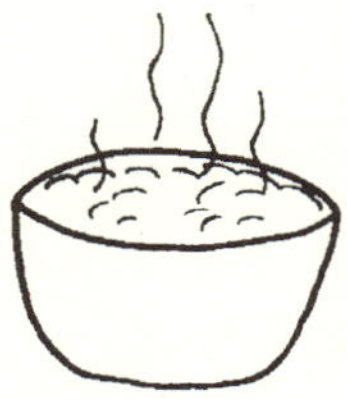

Yield: 2 cups

*This recipe is too small to cook in a standard-sized slow cooker, but can be easily doubled or tripled if desired. Cook on low if slow cooker has two settings. Also, see page 61 for more information on slow cooker.

Recipe idea is from Mastering Food Allergies newsletter, December-January 1988.

Creamy Buckwheat Cereal II

3 tablespoons	buckwheat groats OR 3 tablespoons purchased Cream of Buckwheat Cereal
1/8 teaspoon	sea salt
1 1/2 cups	water

1. If using buckwheat groats, prepare as in step 1 above for Creamy Buckwheat Cereal I.
2. Mix all ingredients with a whisk in a small saucepan.
3. Bring to boil. Cover and simmer 10 minutes. Serve same as above.

Yield: 1 cup

Cashew Milk

1/4 cup	cashews
1 cup	water

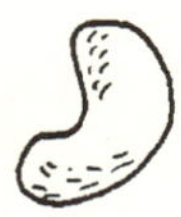

1. Blend cashews in blender on highest speed until they become a fine powder, approximately 1–2 minutes. Stop once or twice to scrape sides and bottom of blender jar.
2. Add water and blend on highest speed approximately 1 minute until well blended. Stop at least once to scrape sides and bottom of blender jar. Chill. Add salt if desired. Stir before serving. I love the rich flavor that Cashew Milk adds to buckwheat cereals.
3. Since I do not desire to make this nut milk each time I serve hot cereal, I prepare 1 or 2 cups at a time. After blending, pour immediately into ice cube trays. After frozen, remove the milk cubes and transfer to cellophane bags.

Yield: slightly more than 1 cup

Buckwheat Pancakes

7-8 Dollar-size	21-24 Dollar-size	YIELD
1/2 cup + 1 tablespoon	1 3/4 cups	White Buckwheat Flour (page 249)
1/2 teaspoon	1 1/2 teaspoons	baking soda
1/4 teaspoon	1/2 teaspoon	unbuffered, corn-free vitamin C crystals
2 pinches	scant 1/4 teaspoon	sea salt
1/2 cup	1 1/2 cups	water
2 teaspoons	2 tablespoons	safflower oil

1. Preheat griddle. I use a well-seasoned cast-iron griddle (see How to Season Cast Iron on page 63). Griddle is hot enough when water dances when sprinkled on the griddle. Spread 1 teaspoon of oil on griddle after preheating.
2. In mixing bowl, whisk together dry ingredients. Add water and oil. Stir with whisk for 15 seconds. Allow batter to set for up to 30 seconds to thicken. Batter will be a little thick. In fact, you may need to shake the spoon a little to remove the batter.
3. Dip batter onto the griddle using a tablespoon. Cook on first side until pancake bubbles, then smoothes out, and is slightly dry around edges, approximately 2 minutes. Turn. Cook until dry on second side, approximately 1 1/2 minutes. These pancakes do not bubble much. Most of the bubbles do not even break the surface of the pancake.
4. Serve with flaxseed oil and/or Rhubarb Jelly (page 281). You may freeze leftovers for future breakfasts and snacks.

Blueberry Buckwheat Pancakes

Add to above recipe:

7-8 Dollar-size	21-24 Dollar-size	YIELD
1/4 cup	3/4 cup	blueberries

Just before dipping batter onto the griddle, fold in thawed, drained blueberries. Cook as above.

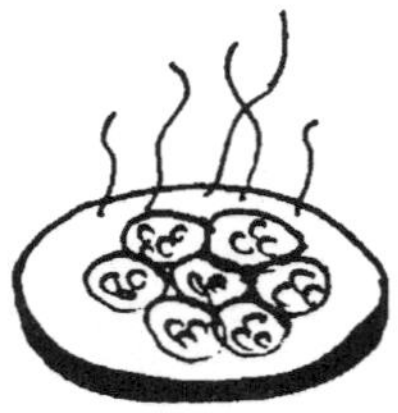

We should be patient with everyone, but above all with ourselves.

The smiles that count are those that shine when it rains.

Buckwheat Muffins

6 Muffins	12 Muffins	YIELD
1 cup	2 cups	White Buckwheat Flour (page 249)
1 teaspoon	2 teaspoons	baking soda
1/4 teaspoon	1/2 teaspoon	sea salt
1/4 teaspoon	1/2 teaspoon	unbuffered, corn-free vitamin C crystals
7/8 cup	1 3/4 cups	water (7/8 cup = 3/4 cup + 2 tablespoons)
1/2 teaspoon	1 teaspoon	guar gum
2 tablespoons	1/4 cup	safflower oil

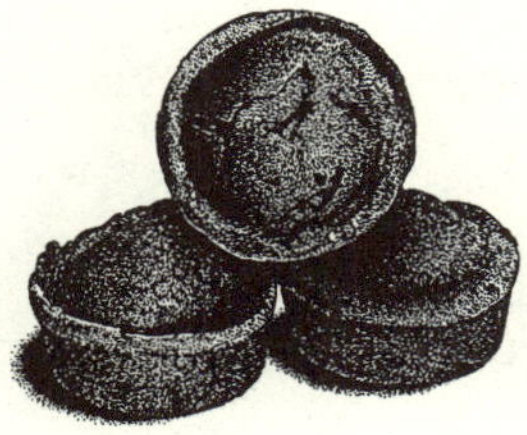

1. Preheat oven to 375°F.
2. Oil and flour bottom and sides of muffin cups.
3. In a mixing bowl, whisk together all dry ingredients except guar gum. Make a "well" in the center.
4. Add oil and guar gum to water. Mix. Add liquid mixture and stir just to moisten the dry ingredients. Batter will be rather sloppy at first. Also, batter will have some lumps. Mash the large lumps against sides of mixing bowl and gently stir to remove most of them.
5. Equally portion batter into prepared muffin cups, slightly more than 1/4 cup of batter each. Bake 20–22 minutes.
6. Cool muffins in the pan(s) on wire rack for 5 minutes. Then turn muffins out of pan(s). Sometimes you need to take a sharp thin knife around the edges of the muffins to loosen them from the sides. Muffins are best served warm. They freeze and reheat in microwave well.

Also, the 12 muffin recipe can be baked in 2 oiled and floured 8-inch square baking dishes for 23 minutes. The bread can be cut when warm. Cut into 6 or 8 pieces.

Variation: For a hint of orange flavor, add 2 teaspoons of alcohol-free orange extract with the liquid ingredients.

Blueberry Buckwheat Muffins

Add to above recipe:

6 Muffins	12 Muffins	YIELD
1/2 cup	1 cup	blueberries

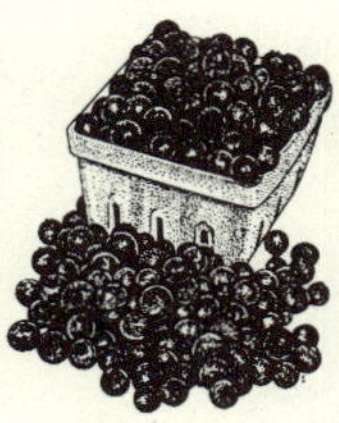

Just before portioning batter into muffin cups, fold in thawed, drained blueberries. Portion almost 1/3 cup of batter per muffin cup. Bake as above, except the blueberry muffins will usually take 24–25 minutes to bake.

Buckwheat Crackers*

1 1/4 cups	White Buckwheat Flour (page 249)
1 teaspoon	baking soda
1/2 teaspoon	guar gum
1/4 teaspoon	sea salt
1/4 teaspoon	unbuffered, corn-free vitamin C crystals
3 tablespoons	ground pumpkin seeds* (ground in food processor) OR 1 tablespoon additional White Buckwheat Flour
1/2 cup	water
3 tablespoons	safflower oil

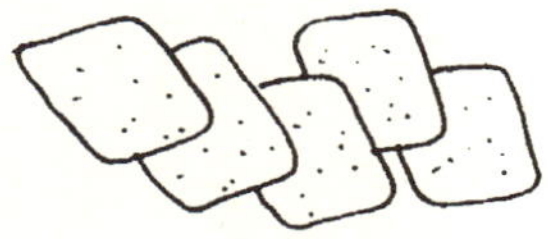

1. Preheat oven to 350°F.
2. Place 1 1/2 teaspoons of safflower oil on a 14 x 10-inch stainless steel baking sheet and set aside. (This amount of oil is in addition to the amount listed above.)
3. In large mixing bowl, whisk together dry ingredients and pumpkin seeds. Make "well" in center.
4. Add water and oil. Stir with rubber spatula or fork until dough clumps into a ball and flour is well mixed.
5. Spread oil on baking sheet with fingers to within two inches of the edge. As the dough is rolled out, it will push the oil to the edge of the baking sheet. In addition, using your fingers to spread the oil will lightly coat them and aid in working with the dough.
6. Transfer dough to center of the baking sheet. Use your hands to form dough so it has no rough edges. Press dough out evenly in all four directions until it cannot be further spread with your hands, making sure to maintain a rectangular shape.
7. If your baking sheet has sides on it, be sure the rolling pin will fit all the way down onto surface on both the width and length of the sheet and that its handles clear the edges.
8. Lightly dust rolling pin with flour and roll dough out from center to edges. Be sure to press in all four directions and to keep dough at a uniform thickness. Occasionally run your hand across the top of the dough to feel if there are any thick areas that need to be evened out.
9. As the dough gets thinner, use the dull back side of a table knife to press edges of dough to maintain rectangular shape. Continue rolling and shaping until dough is about 1/8–1/4 inch thick and fills baking sheet. To help reduce the possibility of extra-thin dough edge, use back side of a table knife to gently push all four edges of dough to make edge thickness uniform with remaining dough.
10. Using a pizza cutter, cut dough into squares as follows. Be sure to move pizza cutter slowly and with a back and forth motion to help avoid tearing dough if cutter goes directly across a pumpkin seed. Cut rectangle in half along dough length (see number 1 on diagram). Cut each half in half (see number 2), then cut each fourth in thirds (see number 3). This will create 12 strips.

continued on next page

Buckwheat Crackers (continued)

11. Next cut rectangle in half along dough width (see number 4). Cut each half in half (see number 5) and each fourth in half (see number 6). This will create 8 sections and 96 individual crackers. Next use a sharp knife to be sure each cut on the outer edge of the rectangle is completely separated.

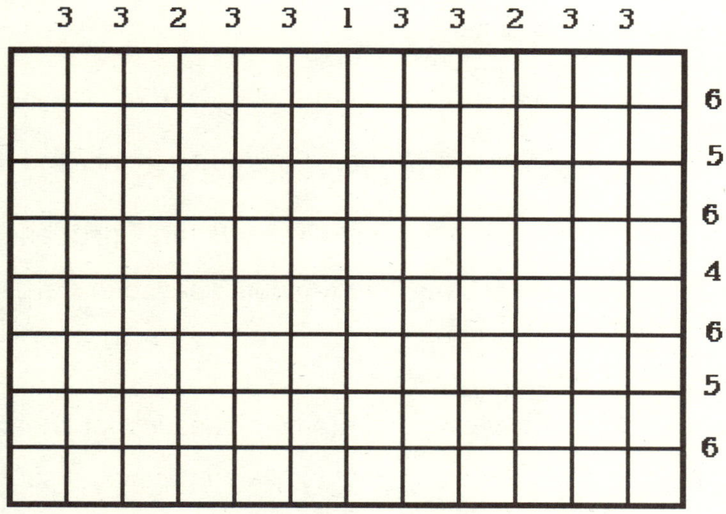

12. Prick holes in each square with fork. If you wish, you can salt the tops of the crackers with sea salt before baking.
13. Bake for 30 minutes. Remove baking sheet from oven and carefully remove outer circle of crackers if they are crispy. Return remaining crackers to oven for 5 minutes. To crisp crackers further, carefully loosen crackers from baking sheet and return them to oven for at least 15 minutes with oven turned off. Some Buckwheat Crackers will crack but for the most part they hold together.
14. Cool crackers on cooling rack by either leaving them on the baking sheet or removing and placing them directly on the cooling rack. After cool, store in the freezer. I prefer to use a wide-mouth quart jar. No need to thaw, eat straight from the freezer.

Yield: 96 crackers, approximately 3/4 quart.

*Realize that pumpkin is usually eaten on Day 2, so you need to avoid eating pumpkin on your Day 2 just before and after eating these crackers on your Day 4.

Every journey begins with a single step.

It never hurts to crack a smile.

Buckwheat Tortillas

1/2 cup	White Buckwheat Flour (amount needed to start) (page 249)
1/4 teaspoon	sea salt
1/2 teaspoon	guar gum
1/2 teaspoon	safflower oil
1/4 cup	water
1/2 cup	White Buckwheat Flour (amount needed for kneading & rolling)

Navy Bean Tortillas

1/2 cup	navy bean flour (amount needed to start)
1/4 teaspoon	sea salt
1/4 cup	water
1/2 teaspoon	safflower oil
1/2 cup	navy bean flour (amount needed for kneading and rolling)

Special Note: Before starting your tortilla preparation, I suggest you read Helpful Hints on Tortilla Preparation starting on page 79.

1. Preheat nonstick, unoiled griddle or skillet. I use a well-seasoned cast-iron griddle (see How to Season Cast Iron on page 63). Griddle is hot enough when water dances when sprinkled on the griddle.

2. In a curved-sided bowl, whisk together ingredients listed below. Make a "well" in the center.

For Buckwheat Tortillas	1/2 cup of flour and measurement of salt, and guar gum
For Navy Bean Tortillas	1/2 cup flour and measurement of salt

3. Add oil and water. Stir with rubber spatula or fork until dough clumps together into a moist ball. The dough ball is usually too sticky for kneading, so add up to 1 tablespoon more flour and mix in thoroughly.

4. Scatter flour on rolling surface (see amount in chart below). Transfer dough to floured rolling surface and knead to work in as much of this additional flour as possible. Dough texture should resemble Play Doh. Add more flour if needed. Form the dough into a ball and cut equal portions (see chart below). Flour the cut surfaces of each dough portion with remaining flour.

	Buckwheat	Navy Bean
flour on rolling surface	1 tablespoon	2 tablespoons
divide dough into portions	4 portions	3 portions

5. Lightly flour rolling pin and rolling surface. Pat dough portion into circular shape, then roll out tortilla by pressing evenly from the center out in all directions and working to keep tortilla as round as possible. Keep dough well floured on both sides (you will need approximate 1/2 tablespoon or less of flour per tortilla). Turn dough over often by loosening with a spatula before flipping. Feel dough surface occasionally to be sure it is evenly thin. Finished tortilla will be very thin and approximately 6–7 inches in diameter. Using a pastry brush, gently brush both sides of tortilla to remove excess flour.

continued on next page

Buckwheat or Navy Bean Tortillas (continued)

6. Cook each tortilla on preheated, unoiled griddle for cooking time indicated in chart below. Cool each tortilla on cooling rack as indicated (see chart below). Place the slightly cooled tortillas between two layers of a clean cotton towel.

	Buckwheat	Navy Bean
cooking time on each side	40 seconds	45 seconds
cooling time on cooling rack	1 minute	1–2 minutes

7. Serve either whole or cut in half. Use your imagination to create a simple deli-like sandwich—for example: roast pork, roast venison, sorrel, "Mayo," and sprouts are all good for Day 4. Also, use for Pork and Bean Burritos. Leftover tortillas may be frozen flat in a cellophane or plastic bag for future meals.

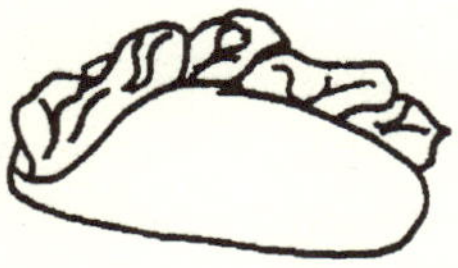

Yield: 4 buckwheat or 3 navy bean tortillas, 6–7 inches in diameter

Recipe idea for Buckwheat Tortillas from The Yeast Connection Cookbook by Crook & Jones, p. 159.

Attitudes are contagious! Is yours worth catching?

White Buckwheat Flour

(How to Prepare Using Raw Buckwheat Groats)

1. Before processing, sort through the buckwheat groats to remove any debris and immature grains which otherwise would float to the top when washing the groats. Also, you may place a small amount of buckwheat groats in a fine-mesh strainer over the sink and gently shake strainer to help remove any remaining debris.

2. Add groats to blender. Blend on highest speed until finely ground. For best results blend 2 cups of groats at a time for 1 1/2–2 minutes.

3. During the processing time leave the motor running, open the lid insert of the blender top, and use a narrow spatula to loosen the partially ground groats from the sides of the blender jar. Be careful not to get the spatula close to the blade. (This step is not necessary if using a KitchenAid blender.)

4. Continue to blend the groats until a fine flour is formed. To check your progress, stop the blender occasionally to feel the consistency of the flour with your fingers.

Yield: 2 cups of groats will yield about 2 1/2 cups of flour

Special Note: For best nutritional value, the flour should be used immediately, but you can store White Buckwheat Flour in a glass jar in the refrigerator or freezer for future needs.

Buckwheat Yeast-Free Bread and "Hamburger" Buns

2 cups	White Buckwheat Flour (page 249)
1 teaspoon	guar gum
1 teaspoon	sea salt
1 1/2 cups	water
1/3 cup	safflower oil
1/2 cup	White Buckwheat Flour
2 teaspoons	baking soda
1/2 teaspoon	unbuffered, corn-free vitamin C crystals
1 cup	frozen blueberries, thaw but do not need to drain (optional)

1. Preheat oven to 350°F.
2. Oil and flour needed baking dish(es):

For Bread	9x5-inch loaf pan
For "Hamburger" Buns	10–12 custard cups

3. In larger mixer bowl, whisk together first measurement of flour, guar gum, and salt. Set aside.
4. Measure amount of water and oil ready for use. In small bowl, whisk together second measurement of flour, baking soda, and vitamin C. Set aside.
5. Set up mixer with beaters. Add water and oil to the large bowl of flour mixture. Mix on low speed (stir speed) to moisten flour. Scrape sides with rubber spatula to assist in moistening the flour. Then beat on medium speed (mix speed) for 2 minutes. Scrape sides of bowl with rubber spatula throughout mixing process.
6. Without stopping mixer, add second measure of flour, soda, and vitamin C mixture. Continue to mix on medium or a little lower speed (scraping sides) until all flour is moistened. Then beat for 30 seconds on medium speed. If preparing with blueberries, add and stir them into batter.
7. <u>For bread</u>: Transfer batter to prepared loaf pan. Use a rubber spatula to spread batter evenly in pan and smooth on top. Bake 55–60 minutes or until toothpick comes out clean when inserted into center of loaf.

   <u>For "hamburger" buns</u>: Portion approximately 1/3 cup of batter into each custard cup. Spread batter evenly in dishes and smooth on top. Bake 40 minutes or until toothpick comes out dry when inserted into center of buns.

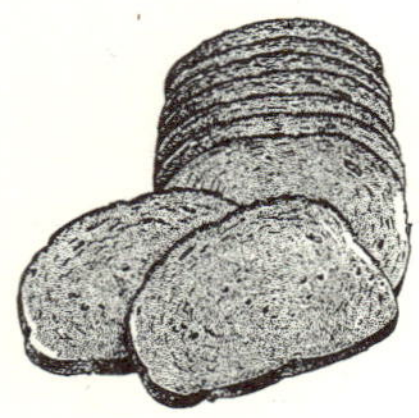

8. Immediately or at least within 5 minutes after baking, loosen bread or buns from sides of dish(es) and remove to cool on wire rack. Slice bread and buns when either slightly or completely cooled. Leftovers may be frozen. I prefer to freeze bread with sheets of cellophane in between the slices. Wax paper should also work if you can tolerate it.

Yield: 1 loaf of bread or 10–12 "hamburger" buns

Special Note: If I prepare the recipe without blueberries, I enjoy the bread toasted and served with a small amount of Rhubarb Jelly (page 281) for a quick breakfast.

Soy Lasagna Noodles*

3/4 cup	soy flour (amount of flour to start)
1/4 teaspoon	sea salt
1/4 teaspoon	garlic powder
1/2 teaspoon	leaf oregano
1/4 teaspoon	basil*
1/4 cup	water
1/2 cup	soy flour (amount needed for rolling)

1. In a bowl, whisk together 3/4 cup flour and seasonings.

2. Add water. Stir with rubber spatula or fork until dough clumps together into a moist ball.

<u>Noodles for circular baking dishes</u>:

3. Divide dough into eight (8) portions.

4. Lightly flour rolling pin and rolling surface. Pat dough portion into circular shape, then roll out noodle by pressing evenly from the center out in all directions and working to keep noodle as round as possible. Keep dough well floured on both sides. Approximately 1 tablespoon of flour is needed per noodle. When needed, turn dough over by loosening with a spatula before flipping. Finished noodle will be thin and 4 1/2 inches in diameter, the size of a Grab-It bowl. Using a pastry brush, gently brush both sides of noodle to remove excess flour.

OR

<u>Noodles for square or rectangular baking dishes</u>:

3. Divide dough into four (4) portions.

4. Lightly flour rolling pin and rolling surface. Pat dough portion into rectangular shape, then roll out noodle by pressing from the center out in all directions and working to keep noodle as rectangular as possible. Keep dough well floured on both sides. Approximately 2 tablespoons of flour is needed per noodle. When needed, turn dough over by loosening with a spatula before flipping. Finished noodle will be thin and approximately 5x10 inches, one half the size of a Corning 10-inch casserole dish.

5. Place each noodle between layers of cellophane wrap or wax paper. Store in a cellophane or plastic bag in the freezer until needed for lasagna recipes on both Day 2 and 4.

Yield: 8 noodles (each 4 1/2 inches in diameter) OR 4 noodles (each 5x10 inches)

*Basil is usually eaten on Day 2, so you need to avoid eating it on your Day 2 just before and after eating this recipe on Day 4.

Basic Buckwheat Groats

1 cup	buckwheat groats
2 cups	water
	OR Day 4 vegetable and/or meat broth
1/2 cup	leek, sliced (optional)
1/2 teaspoon	sea salt

1. Wash groats (page 36). Combine all ingredients in a 2 1/2 quart saucepan. Bring to boil on high. Cover. Reduce heat to between low and medium to allow the buckwheat to simmer. Simmer 15 minutes.
2. Serve immediately or remove from heat and allow to set up to 5 minutes.

Yield: 3 cups

Special Note: For best results, buckwheat should not be stirred or uncovered during the cooking process. If it is necessary to check the progress of the groats during the cooking time, do so quickly to minimize the loss of steam. Do not stir as this will disrupt the even cooking of the groats. If tasting for doneness, use a fork to gently remove a small amount from the surface of the groats. Different stoves and different pans may require adjustment in time, temperature, and amount of liquid used.

Buckwheat Groats—How to Roast

Many stores do not carry roasted buckwheat groats because they do not stay fresh as long as raw groats. You may roast and store your own groats or just roast the amount you wish to cook. Roasted buckwheat groats available for purchase in health-food or other grocery stores are usually called Kasha.

You should be aware that roasting raw buckwheat groats does intensify the flavor—perhaps more than you will enjoy.

1. First, measure out the amount of groats you want to roast. Wash (page 36). Remember that buckwheat groats are porous and should be washed quickly and gently so they do not soak up the washing water and affect the texture of your cooked groats.
2. Transfer the rinsed and drained buckwheat groats to a cold, heavy-bottomed pan. I prefer a well-seasoned cast-iron skillet (see How to Season Cast Iron on page 63). Place skillet on range. Turn burner to medium high. Roast on medium high, stirring almost continuously with a wooden spoon, until the groats are dry. Be sure to stir the groats so that each one gets turned.
3. You will need to stir more quickly toward the end of the roasting process. Also, you may prefer to turn down the heat to medium or lower toward the end of the process to help prevent burning the groats. This process may take up to 15 minutes. Continue with Basic Buckwheat Groats recipe.
4. If you desire to store the groats for later use, pour onto a large baking sheet to cool. Store the cooled groats in a glass jar with a tight-fitting lid in a cool, dry place. Use within 1 month. You can roast approximately 2 cups at one time in a 10-inch skillet.

Lentil or Split Pea Soup*

1 cup	lentils or green split peas
2–3	bay leaves* (optional)
2 cups	water
1/4 cup	leek, chopped
1/8 teaspoon	minced garlic (optional)
1/4 teaspoon	sea salt

Method 1

1. Rinse and drain lentils or green split peas. Cover more than double with water. Soak overnight in refrigerator (or for at least 8 hours).
2. Just before cooking, rinse lentils or peas thoroughly until rinsing water is clear. Drain.
3. Transfer lentils or peas to 1-quart size slow cooker (information on page 61) or double this recipe and cook in a standard-size slow cooker. Add rest of ingredients except salt. Cook on low for 5–7 hours or until tender but not mushy (see chart below).

Lentils	5–5 1/2 hours
Green split peas	6 1/2–7 hours

4. Add salt and remove bay leaves just before serving.

Yield: Lentil Soup, 3 cups Split Pea Soup, 3 1/2 cups

Method 2

1. Follow steps 1 and 2 from Method 1.
2. Combine all ingredients except salt with the prepared lentils or split peas in a 5-quart Dutch-oven Vision cookware kettle. Cook, covered, in a 700 watt microwave oven on full power for 7–10 minutes, or until boiling. Then cook on medium power for 5–7 minutes or until lentils or split peas are tender. Microwave cooking time will vary with different brands and wattage's of microwaves. After cooking, remove the bay leaves and add salt.

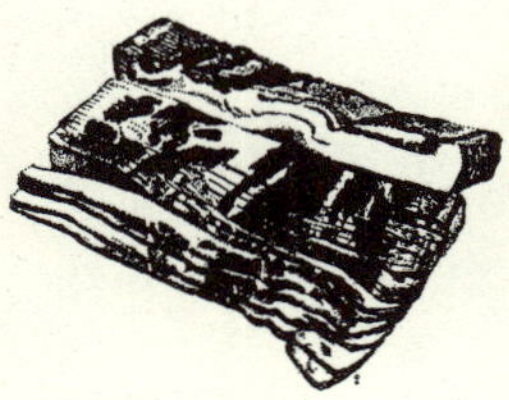

Serving Suggestion: Add cooked, crumbled fresh pork side (unsmoked and uncured bacon) to cooked lentils and serve as breakfast cereal. Add leftover cooked roast pork to split peas. You may add the cooked meat during the last hour of cooking or when reheating.

Special Note: If you do not have time to soak split peas, combine them with 4 cups of water in saucepan. Bring to boil and boil for 1 minute. Remove from heat and let stand, covered, for 1 hour. The lentils do not need to soak overnight, but I prefer it.

*Bay leaf belongs to the Laurel Family with avocado and cinnamon. Eating bay leaf on Day 2 breaks the rotation since cinnamon is used in many recipes on Day 3 and a few on Day 1. You can make your own decision about bay leaf. I personally use it without any concern regarding when I have or plan to consume cinnamon.

Tomato-Free Chili

1/2 cup	black turtle beans (these help with color)
1/2 cup	kidney beans
1/2 cup	pinto beans
1/2 cup	adzuki beans
1/2 cup	navy beans
	OR 2 1/2 cups of any combination of dried beans
5 cups	water
2 3-inch	kombu
1/2 cup	leek, diced
1/2 teaspoon	minced garlic
2 teaspoons	chili powder
1 teaspoon	Watkins Salsa Seasoning Blend or other Mexican blend spices
1 1/2 teaspoons	sea salt
1 pound	ground pork or venison

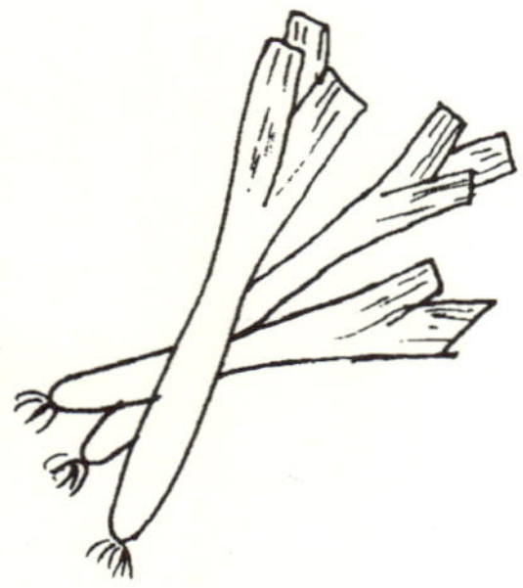

1. Rinse beans to remove dirt and dust. Soak beans 8–12 hours in refrigerator in 4 cups of water to allow beans to more than double in size.
2. Just before cooking, rinse beans thoroughly until rinsing water is clear. Drain.
3. Transfer beans to a standard-size slow cooker. Add all ingredients, except meat and salt. Cook on low for 10–12 hours or until beans are tender but not mushy.
4. In skillet, cook meat until done. Stir often to chop meat and brown evenly. Add cooked meat to the tender beans and cook on low for one additional hour. Just before serving, add salt and stir.

Special Note: The sauce thickens if allowed to cool in the refrigerator. You may need to add more water when reheating. After freezing and reheating the flavors are even better. Freeze the leftovers for many delicious meals to come.

Yield: 9 cups

Tomato-Free "Veggie" Chili*

1 cup	Tomato-Free Chili
1 pint	green beans, home canned, drained and reserve broth
1/2 cup	zucchini squash, peeled, cubed* (optional)
	OR 1/2 cup okra, sliced* (optional)

Combine ingredients in saucepan. Add green bean broth to get the consistency that you prefer. Simmer for 20 minutes to cook the squash and blend the flavors. Taste and add more seasonings if desired.

Yield: approximately 3 cups

*If you prepare this dish with zucchini squash or okra, you need to avoid eating them on your Day 2 just before and after eating this dish on Day 4.

Quick Bean Soup

1/2 cup	Navy Beans and Broth (page 263)
1 pint	green beans and broth, home canned or purchased
1/2 cup	cooked roast pork
1/2 cup	Pork Broth (page 260)

Combine and simmer to blend flavors and heat to serving temperature.

Yield: 3 cups

Special Note: Makes a complete meal with very little effort if you have planned and frozen *plan*overs in advance.

Italian Tofu*

1 cup	Muir Glen brand organic tomato puree*
1 cup	liquid (green bean broth and/or water)
2 cups	green beans, fresh, frozen, or drained canned (reserve liquid)
1/4 teaspoon	sea salt
1/4 teaspoon	minced garlic
1/4 teaspoon	basil*
1/2 teaspoon	leaf oregano
1 pinch	crushed cayenne (red) pepper*
8 ounces	tofu

1. In saucepan, combine all ingredients except tofu. Simmer until green beans are tender and flavors are blended. This mixture should yield approximately 2 1/2 cups.
2. Drain and dice tofu. Gently stir into hot tomato mixture. Heat just long enough to bring the tofu to serving temperature.

Yield: 2 servings

*These foods are usually eaten on Day 2 so you need to avoid eating tomatoes, basil, and cayenne pepper on your Day 2 just before and after serving this recipe on Day 4.

Tofu and Cucumber Salad Sandwich

1/2 pound	soft tofu, drained
2 cups	cucumber, diced
2 tablespoons	Macadamia* or Cashew "Mayo" (page 273)
1/8 teaspoon	sea salt
1/8 teaspoon	unbuffered, corn-free vitamin C crystals
1/4 teaspoon	tarragon

Mix all ingredients together. Chill. Serve on buckwheat or navy bean tortillas with sorrell leaves.

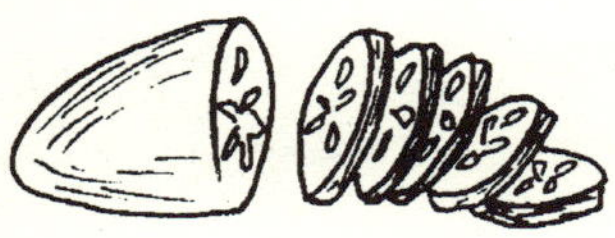

Yield: approximately 2 cups, ample amount for 4 tortillas

*Macadamia nuts are unassigned "Fun Foods" on this rotational diet, see explanation on pages 30–31.

Pork or Venison Fajita*

4	Buckwheat Tortillas (page 248)
2 3-ounce	tenderized pork or venison cutlets, cut into thin strips (approximately 1 cup)
1 cup	leek, thinly sliced
1 cup	green pepper strips*
1 1/2 cups	zucchini squash, cut into strips*
1–2 teaspoons	safflower oil
as needed	sea salt
as desired	fresh tomato*, diced, seasoned with a small amount of Watkins Salsa Seasoning Blend or other Mexican blend spices (optional)

1. Prepare or thaw tortillas.
2. Prepare tomato if desired. Chill.
3. Preheat well-seasoned cast-iron skillet on medium (see How to Season Cast Iron on page 63) or electric skillet to 300°F.
4. Prepare meat and vegetables as described above. Meat will cut into strips easier if partially frozen. Also, I recommend soaking venison strips in salted water for a few hours or overnight to remove most of the wild game taste.
5. Add oil to preheated skillet. Stir fry meat, stirring often to brown evenly. You may cover with splatter screen (information on page 60) when not stirring.
6. Add vegetables and sprinkle with salt. Stir often to cook meat and vegetables evenly. I prefer my vegetables crunchy.
7. Serve immediately. I have found the easiest way to serve fajitas is to begin with the tortilla on your plate. Spread approximately 3/4 cup of filling in the center of the tortilla lengthwise but about 1 inch from one side as Diagram A shows. Fold the 1-inch edge side over first, then fold the 1/3 side edges over the filling as Diagram B shows. Lift and hold with both hands. Eat and enjoy.

Yield: approximately 3 cups of filling, ample amount for 4 tortillas

*Tomato, green peppers, and zucchini are usually eaten on Day 2, so you need to avoid eating these foods on the Day 2 just before and after serving this recipe on Day 4.

Diagram A

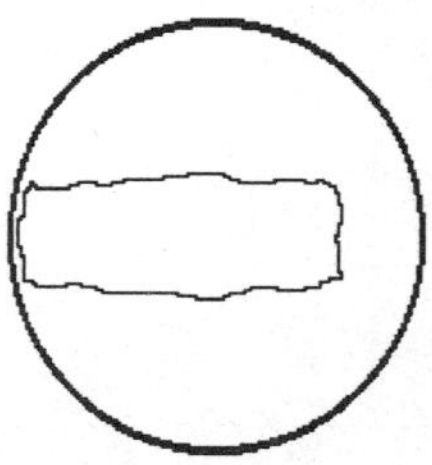

Diagram B

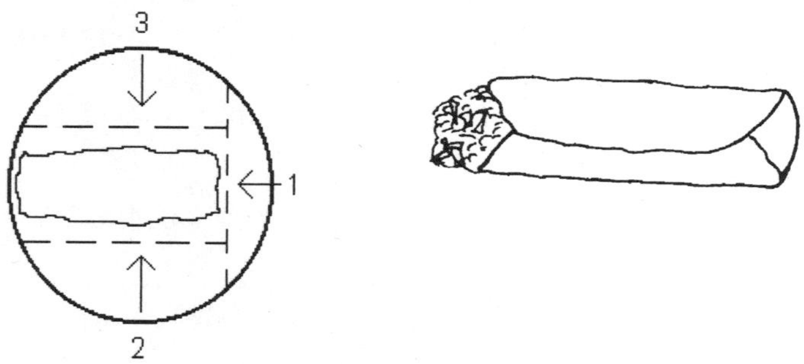

Venison and Buckwheat Pasta Casserole

1 pint	green beans, home canned, drained but reserve juice
1/2 cup	Venison Broth (page 260)
2 ounces	100% Buckwheat Soba Noodles
1/2 cup	cooked venison, leftover from venison roast
as needed	sea salt

1. In medium-size stainless steel saucepan, heat reserved green bean juice (add water to make 3/4 cup) and venison broth to boiling.
2. Break pasta into 2-inch lengths. Add noodles to boiling liquid. Turn heat down to medium high. Cook noodles for 10 minutes stirring often. Add up to 1/2 cup of water as needed when liquid is getting low or noodles begin to stick.
3. Add green beans and cooked venison (plus more water if needed). Reduce heat to medium. Cover and heat 5 minutes or longer until desired serving temperature. Stir often to prevent sticking. Taste and add salt as needed.

Yield: 2 1/2 cups

Special Note: I often prepare this casserole or the following one for a quick lunch and do not even thaw the cooked meat before preparing the recipe. Also, I enjoy these recipes when I need to travel away from home for lunch. Just cook the noodles only 8 minutes before continuing with the rest of the recipe. Pack in a wide-mouth stainless steel thermos. The noodles continue to cook in the thermos.

Pork and Buckwheat Pasta Casserole

Substitute cooked pork and Pork Broth (page 260) for venison in the above recipe.

If you have tried to do something and failed, you are vastly better off than if you had tried to do nothing and succeeded.

Just remember conditions are never "just right."

Pork Chop

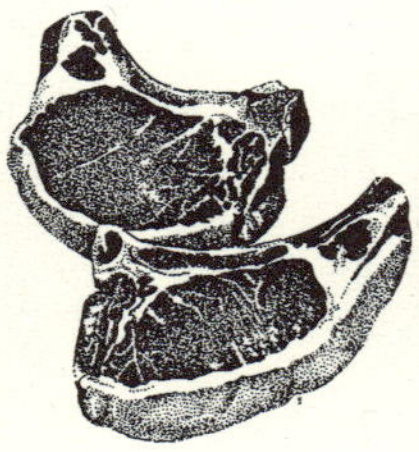

In skillet, brown pork chops for 2–3 minutes on each side in small amount of safflower oil at 400°F. or on medium high. Season with salt and/or garlic powder. Add 1 cup or more of water. Cover and simmer 15–20 minutes until tender. Do check from time to time and add more water if needed.

Breaded Pork Chop

1/4 cup	Jerusalem artichoke flour
1/4 teaspoon	paprika
1/4 teaspoon	sea salt
8	pork chops or boneless tenderized pork cutlet

1. Preheat oven to 450°F.
2. Trim excess fat off pork chops. Rinse and pat dry leaving them a little moist.
3. In a bowl, combine flour and seasonings. Place a small amount (approximately 1 tablespoon) in a container with a sealable lid (like Tupperware) that is also large enough to hold a pork chop.
4. Add 1 pork chop to container. Seal. Shake to coat. Place meat in unoiled stainless steel baking dish. Repeat to coat each chop. Add more flour mixture to container as needed.
5. Put baking dish in oven and reduce heat to 400°F. Bake for approximately 30–40 minutes or until internal meat temperature is 180°F. Baking time will depend upon thickness of pork.

Yield: 8 or more pork chops If you need to prepare less than 8 chops, simply use the amount of flour mixture that you need and freeze the rest for the next time.

Easy Meal Banquet

2 medium-size	sweet potatoes, peeled
2	pork chops, trim off excess fat
2 servings	asparagus spears, fresh or frozen

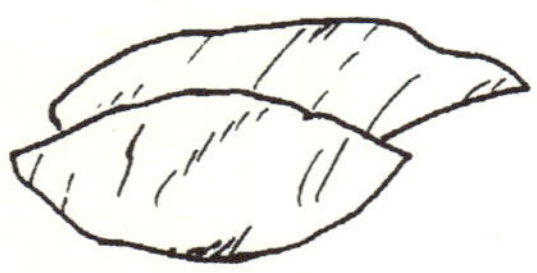

1. Fill bottom of a steamer pan with water to about 1/2 inch from the bottom of steamer insert. Heat water to boiling.
2. In the insert of steamer pan, lay peeled (whole) sweet potatoes and sprinkle with salt. Place pork chops on top of potatoes and sprinkle with salt. Place insert pan over boiling water. Cover. Steam on medium-high for 25 minutes.
3. Add asparagus spears and sprinkle with salt. Cover and continue to cook 10–15 minutes longer until pork chops and vegetables are tender. Dish onto plates arranging foods separately. This is not a stew.

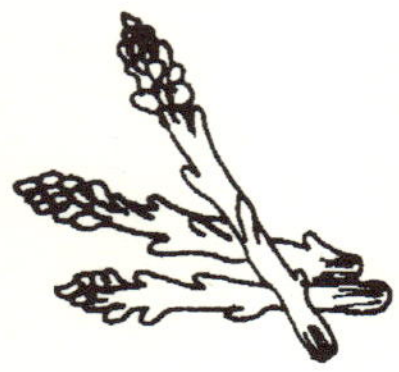

Yield: 2 complete easy meal servings

Recipe idea from The Yeast Connection Cookbook by Crook & Jones, p. 281.

Squash and Meatballs

1	acorn or butternut squash (1 3/4–2 pounds)
1 pound	ground pork
1/2 cup	leek, sliced
1/4 teaspoon	garlic powder
1/2 teaspoon	sea salt

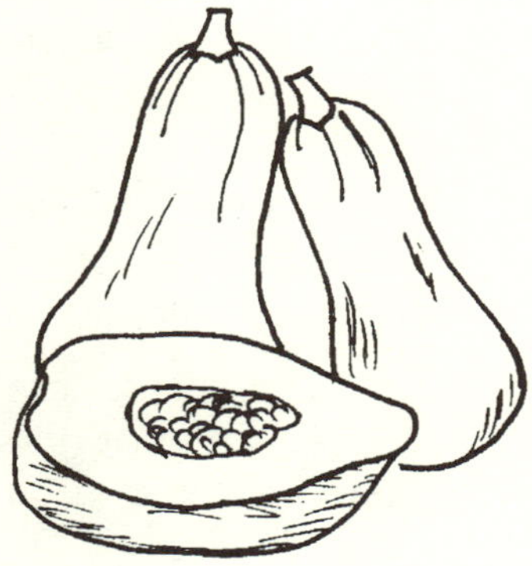

1. Oven temperature—350°F. Preheating not necessary.
2. Wash squash and cut in half lengthwise (core to core). Cut threads with scissors or with a serrated grapefruit knife which has a curved end. Then scoop out the seeds with a large spoon.
3. Rinse squash. Sprinkle a little salt inside the squash cavity. Place cut sides down in a casserole dish. (Use a covered casserole dish that is deep enough to hold a half squash with cavity filled with meatballs.) If needed, use two casserole dishes. Add approximately 1/4 cup of water to each casserole dish. Bake uncovered for 20 minutes.
4. While squash is baking, combine all other ingredients thoroughly. I prefer to mix with my hands while wearing disposable plastic gloves. Divide the meat into equal portions and form it into balls. This should yield around 16–20 meatballs.
5. Brown meatballs in skillet. Turn often to brown on all sides. Do not crowd in the skillet so you can roll each portion easily. Drain browned meatballs on paper towels.
6. Remove squash from oven. Turn squash over and fill each cavity with half of the meatballs. Cover and return to oven to bake another 30 minutes or until squash is tender and pork is at least 180°F.
7. To serve, remove porkballs and cut each squash portion in half crosswise. Serve each portion with 1/4 of the meatballs and baste with the delicious broth. To complete the meal, serve with green beans.

Yield: 4 servings

Special Notes: Leftovers may be frozen for future meals. Thaw and reheat, covered, in microwave (on medium power) or in slow oven (300°F.). When I reheat in the microwave, I prefer to heat the squash some before adding the pork.

This dish can also be prepared in the microwave. Cook squash with cut side down for 3 minutes. Turn squash over and add meatballs. Cook covered for 5 minutes or longer. Microwave cooking time will vary depending on the wattage of the oven. If you do prepare this dish in the microwave, I suggest you prepare the meatballs first and while they are browning start the squash.

Roast Pork and Broth

2–3 pounds	pork roast
1 teaspoon	sea salt
1 cup	leek, chopped large (optional)

Method 1

1. Sprinkle salt over meat on all sides. Place seasoned roast in standard-size slow cooker. If desired, add leek. Add water to cover roast or to within 1–inch of top of roast. Cook on low for 8–10 hours.
2. Serve with sweet potatoes or buckwheat noodles and Day 4 vegetables such as asparagus and/or green beans. You may serve some of the broth over the meat and vegetables.
3. After the meal, strain leftover broth through fine-meshed strainer and chill. After chilling, remove the fat that is solid on the top. Freeze broth in ice cube trays. After frozen, remove from the trays and keep frozen in a cellophane bag. Also, you may measure out specific amounts needed for recipes and freeze in glass jars. The broth is used in recipes such as Pork and Buckwheat Pasta Casserole, Ham and Bean Stew, and Quick Bean Soup as well as to cook 100% Buckwheat Soba Noodles. Also, freeze leftover meat in cellophane bags for future quick meals such as buckwheat tortilla sandwiches, Pork and Buckwheat Pasta Casserole, and Quick Bean Soup.

Method 2

Another way to prepare pork roast is to use Reynolds cooking bags. Just follow the directions provided with the bags. The package states that these bags may be used in the microwave, but I prefer to cook meat in the oven. Also, I do not shake flour in the bags, but do add more liquid than called for in the directions. Strain and freeze the leftover broth in the same manner as explained above in step

Roast Venison and Broth

2–3 pounds	venison roast
1 teaspoon	sea salt
1 cup	leek, chopped large (optional)

1. Soak venison roast in salted water overnight. This will assist in removing the strong wild game taste.
2. Follow steps 1 and 2 for Roast Port and Broth, Method 1.
3. After the meal, strain leftover broth through fine-meshed strainer and chill. After chilling, remove the fat that is solid on the top. Freeze broth in ice cube trays. After frozen, remove from the trays and keep frozen in a cellophane bag. Also, you may measure out specific amounts needed for recipes and freeze in glass jars. The broth is used in recipes such as Venison and Buckwheat Pasta Casserole and Mexican Venison and Bean Stew as well as to cook 100% Buckwheat Soba Noodles. Also, freeze leftover meat in cellophane bags for future quick meals such as buckwheat tortilla sandwiches and Venison and Buckwheat Pasta Casserole.

Pork Cutlet and Bean Gravy

2 servings	pork cutlet (approximately 1/3 pound each)
as needed	bean flour (both navy and pinto bean flour have been tested)
2 teaspoons	safflower oil
to season	sea salt

Ingredients for the gravy:

3 tablespoons	bean flour
2 cups	water
1/4 teaspoon	sea salt

1. Preheat electric skillet to 350°F. Add oil. This recipe was developed using a stainless steel electric skillet; others may require more oil.
2. Coat meat with flour and place in hot skillet. Sprinkle with salt as desired. Cover with a splatter screen (information on page 60). Brown the meat for 2 minutes—the browner the meat, the browner the gravy—but be careful not to dry the meat out or burn it. Turn meat, cover with splatter screen, and brown for another 2 minutes.
3. While the second side is browning, combine the gravy ingredients and blend with small whisk or fork. After meat has browned on second side, add the gravy mixture to skillet. Loosen any stuck meat pieces with a spatula. Cover and reduce heat to between simmer and 200°F. Simmer pork and gravy for 15–20 minutes. Do check on it from time to time.

Yield: 2 servings

Venison Steak and Bean Gravy

1 1/2 pounds	venison (round) steak
as needed	bean flour (both navy and pinto bean flour have been tested)
1 tablespoon	safflower oil
to season	sea salt

Ingredients for the gravy:

3 tablespoons	bean flour
2 cups	water
1/4 teaspoon	sea salt

1. Cut venison steak into small pieces. Cover with salted water and allow meat to soak for a few hours or overnight. This process helps remove excess blood and some of the wild taste.
2. Preheat electric skillet to 350°F. Add oil. This recipe was developed using a stainless steel electric skillet; others may require more oil.
3. Remove meat from water and drain or pat dry. If necessary, pound with a meat tenderizing hammer.
4. Continue with steps 2 & 3 from Pork Cutlet & Bean Gravy (recipe above).

Yield: at least 4 servings

Mexican Medley Beans

1/4 cup	black turtle beans (these help with color)
1/4 cup	kidney beans
1/4 cup	pinto beans
1/4 cup	adzuki beans
1/4 cup	navy beans
	OR 1 1/4 cups of any combination of dried beans
2 cups	water
1 3-inch	kombu
1/2 cup	leek, diced
1/4 teaspoon	minced garlic
1 teaspoon	chili powder
1/4 teaspoon	Watkins Salsa Seasoning Blend or other Mexican blend spices
1/2 teaspoon	sea salt

1. Rinse beans to remove dirt and dust. Soak beans 8–12 hours in refrigerator in 4 cups of water to allow beans to more than double in size.
2. Just before cooking, rinse beans thoroughly until rinsing water is clear. Drain.
3. Transfer beans to a 1-quart size slow cooker (information on page 61) or double this recipe and cook in a standard-size slow cooker. Add rest of ingredients except salt and cook on low for 10–12 hours or until beans are tender but not mushy.
4. Just before serving, add salt and stir.

Special Note: The sauce thickens if the cooked beans are allowed to cool in the refrigerator and then are reheated. After freezing and reheating the flavors are even better. Freeze the leftovers for many delicious meals to come.

Yield: 3 1/4 cups

Tomato-Free Vegetarian Chili*

3/4 cup	Mexican Medley Beans
1 pint	green beans, drain and reserve broth
1 cup	zucchini squash, peeled, cubed* (optional)
	OR 1 cup okra, sliced* (optional)

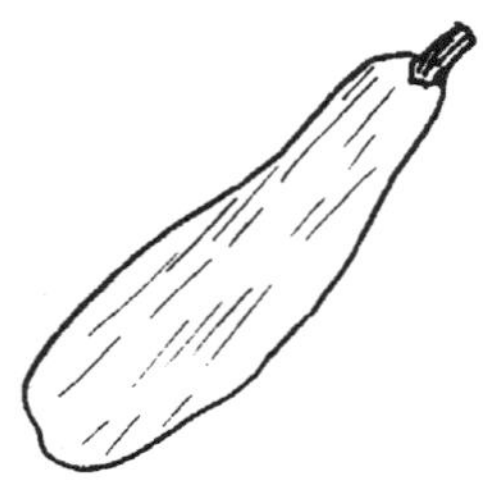

Combine ingredients in saucepan. Add green bean broth to get the consistency that you prefer. Simmer for 20 minutes to cook the squash and blend the flavors. Taste and add more seasonings if desired.

Yield: 2–2 1/2 cups

*If you prepare this dish with zucchini squash or okra, you need to avoid eating them on your Day 2 just before and after eating this dish on Day 4.

Navy Beans and Broth

2 cups	navy beans
3 1/2 cups	water
1 teaspoon	sea salt

1. Rinse beans to remove dirt and dust. Soak beans 8–12 hours or overnight in plenty of water so beans can more than double in size.
2. Just before cooking, rinse beans thoroughly until rinsing water is clear. Drain.
3. Transfer beans to standard-size slow cooker. Add water. Cook 2 1/2–3 hours on high or 6 1/2–7 hours on low, until beans are tender but not mushy.
4. Just before serving, add salt and stir.

Yield: 6 1/2 cups

Serving Suggestions: Serve as side dish or use them in Day 4 recipes such as Beans and Beans, Mexican Venison and Bean Stew, Ham and Bean Stew, and Quick Bean Soup. I prefer to plan ahead what recipes I may wish to use them for so I can freeze portions in glass jars ready to use in a jiffy.

Beans and Beans*

1 cup	Navy Beans and Broth (unsalted)
	OR 1 cup Garbanzo Beans and Broth* (unsalted) (page 161)
2 cups	green beans, cooked

Combine beans in saucepan. Simmer for 10 minutes to blend flavors. Add rounded 1/8 teaspoon salt, stir, and serve as a side dish or complete meal.

*If you use garbanzo beans, you need to avoid eating them on your Day 2 just before and after enjoying this simple recipe on Day 4.

Yield: 3 cups

A happy person is not a person in a certain set of circumstances, but rather a person with a certain set of attitudes.

Every survival kit should include a sense of humor.

Mexican Venison and Bean Stew

1 pound	venison stew meat or raw roast cut into 1/2-inch cubes
2 cloves	garlic, minced
1 tablespoon	safflower oil
1/2 teaspoon	sea salt
2 cups	Venison Broth (page 260) or water
1 cup	leek, sliced
4 cups	green beans, fresh or frozen
1/2 teaspoon	Watkins Salsa Seasoning Blend or other Mexican blend spices
1 teaspoon	chili powder
2 cups	Navy Beans and Broth (page 263)
1/3 cup	water
1/4 cup	navy bean flour

Ham and Bean Stew

1 pound	fresh ham steak, uncured, unsmoked, cut into 1/2-inch cubes
2 cloves	garlic, minced
1 tablespoon	safflower oil
1/2 teaspoon	sea salt
2 cups	Pork Broth (page 260) or water
1 cup	leek, sliced
4 cups	green beans, fresh or frozen*
2 cups	Navy Beans and Broth (page 263)
1/4 cup	water
2 tablespoons	navy bean flour

1. Trim excess fat off meat. Cut smaller, if needed, to be approximately 1/2-inch cubes. Soak venison in salted water for at least 2 hours or overnight. This will help to remove the wild game taste. Drain.

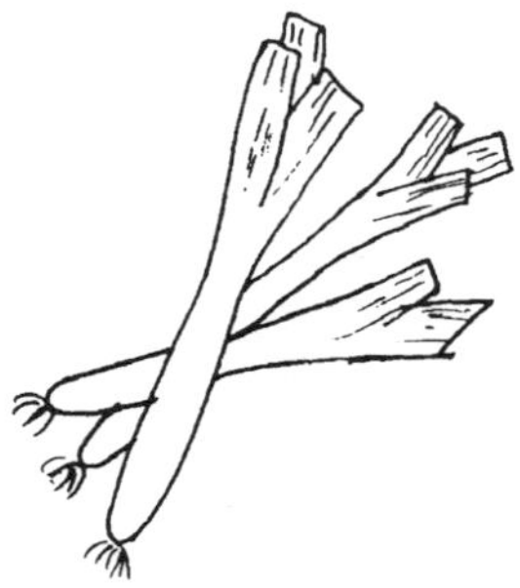

2. Brown stew meat and sauté garlic in oil in 5-quart Dutch-oven kettle. I prefer stainless steel. Stir often to brown meat evenly and prevent garlic from burning. Season with salt.

3. Add liquid, leeks, green beans, and rest of seasonings. Bring to boil. Reduce heat, cover, and simmer approximately 30 minutes until green beans are almost tender.

4. Add Navy Beans and Broth. Simmer about 5 minutes until all ingredients are tender and flavors are well blended. Taste and add more spices, if desired.

5. Whisk water and bean flour together and add to stew. Stir and cook stew to thicken broth. Leftover stew may be frozen, but thaw and reheat slowly.

Yield: about 6 1/2 cups, 4 servings

*May use canned green beans. Drain and reserve bean broth for use in 2 cups liquid measure (Venison/Pork Broth or water) or in thickener liquid measure (1/3 cup water). Canned green beans should be added in step 4 rather than step 3.

Meatballs and Gravy

1 pound	ground venison or pork
1/2 cup	leek, chopped or sliced
1/2 teaspoon	sea salt
1/4 teaspoon	garlic powder (optional)
1 1/2 cups	water
1/4 cup	navy or pinto bean flour

1. Combine ground meat, leeks, salt, and garlic thoroughly. I prefer to mix with my hands while wearing disposable plastic gloves.
2. Divide the meat into equal and form into balls. This should yield 16–20 meatballs.
3. Brown meatballs in skillet. Turn often to brown on all sides. Do not crowd in the skillet so you can roll each portion easily. Drain browned meatballs on paper towels if needed. Drain excess grease from skillet. Note: If meat is very lean you may need to brown meatballs in a small amount of safflower oil.
4. Return browned meatballs to skillet.
5. Combine water and bean flour and pour over meatballs. Cover and simmer 20 minutes. Serve gravy over peas for a creamed-peas taste and appearance.

Yield: 4 servings

Ham and Beans

1 pound	fresh ham hocks, uncured, unsmoked
2 cups	navy beans
4 cups	liquid (pork broth and/or water)
1/2 cup	leek, sliced
1 1/4 teaspoons	sea salt

1. In saucepan, simmer pork in 1–2 cups unsalted water for 2 hours or until meat is very tender. Remove meat and cool to touch. Strain broth through fine-meshed strainer and chill. After chilling, remove the fat that is solid on the top. Remove meat from bones and cut into bite-size pieces. Chill to use in step 4.
2. Rinse beans to remove dirt and dust. Soak beans 8–12 hours or overnight in plenty of water so beans can more than double in size.
3. Just before cooking, rinse beans thoroughly until rinsing water is clear. Drain.
4. Transfer beans to standard-size slow cooker. Add water. Cook 2 1/2–3 hours on high or 6 1/2–7 hours on low, until beans are tender but not mushy. Add cooked pork meat about midway through cooking of beans.
5. Just before serving, add salt and stir.

Yield: 7 cups

Stir-Fry Buckwheat and Vegetables

1 teaspoon	safflower oil
1 clove	garlic, minced
1/2	leek, sliced
1/4 teaspoon	chili powder
1/8 teaspoon	Watkins Salsa Seasoning Blend or other Mexican blend spices
2 cups	total Day 4 vegetables I prefer: 1 1/2 cups asparagus, blanched or frozen 1/2 cup edible pea pods, blanched or frozen OR frozen or fresh peas
1 1/2 cups	Basic Buckwheat Groats, chilled (page 252)
1/4 teaspoon	sea salt

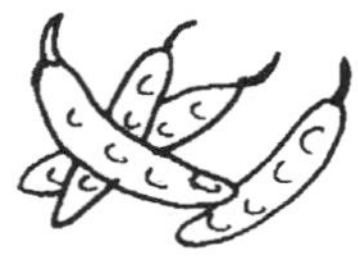

1. In large stainless steel skillet (I prefer an electric skillet), sauté garlic, leek, and seasonings in oil until soft.
2. Add vegetables and buckwheat. Sprinkle with salt. Cook at 300°F. or on medium until all ingredients are at serving temperature and vegetables are tender. Using a sharp-edged spatula, stir frequently and almost constantly during the end of cooking. This stirring is necessary to keep buckwheat from sticking to the skillet. Add more oil if desired.

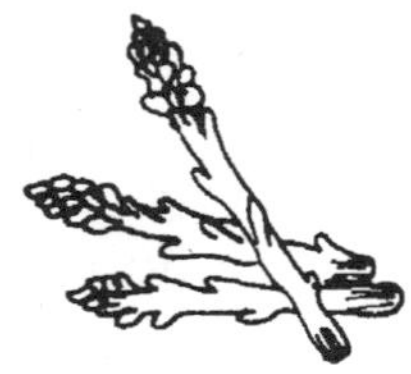

3. Serve as complete vegetarian meal or as side dish with meal.

Yield: 3 cups, 1 complete vegetarian meal or 3–4 side dish servings

Special Note: I enjoy this recipe for a quick lunch. If desired, you may omit the spices and/or adjust amounts of other ingredients. I often do not measure most of the ingredients, just dump and cook.

Stir-Fry Buckwheat and Vegetables with Shrimp*

Add desired amount of cooked, shelled, and deveined shrimp to above recipe.

*Shrimp is usually eaten on Day 2, so you need to avoid eating shrimp on your Day 2 just before and after eating this recipe on Day 4.

Stir-Fry Buckwheat and Vegetables with Venison or Pork

Add desired amount of leftover grilled venison steak or pork steak (cut into strips) to Stir-Fry Buckwheat and Vegetable recipe. Also, you can use raw tenderized venison steak or pork cutlet, cut into strips. If so, stir fry in needed amount of oil before adding the rest of the ingredients. Proceed with Stir-Fry Buckwheat and Vegetables (recipe above).

Suggestion: Raw meat will cut into strips easier if partially frozen. Also, I recommend soaking venison strips in salted water for a few hours or overnight to remove most of the wild game taste.

Stir-Fry Meal for Day 4

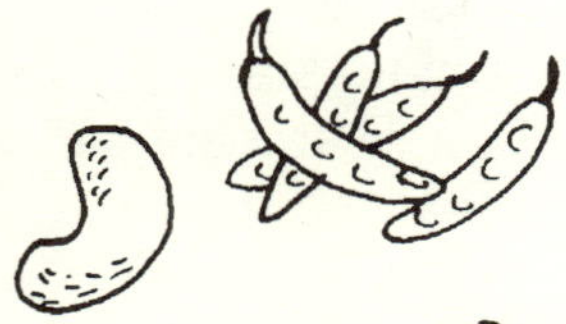

tenderized pork or venison cutlet
leek, thinly sliced
edible pea pods, blanched
asparagus, blanched
cashew pieces or toasted soybeans
safflower or soy oil
sea salt
paprika
garlic powder (optional)

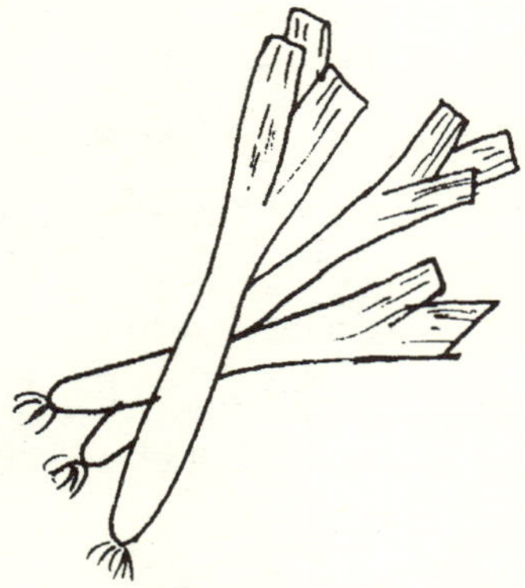

1. Preheat well-seasoned cast-iron on medium (see How to Season Cast Iron on page 63) or electric skillet to 300°F.
2. Prepare meat and vegetables in amounts desired. Meat will cut into strips easier if partially frozen. Also, I recommend soaking venison strips in salted water for a few hours or overnight to remove most of the wild game taste.
3. Add oil to preheated skillet. Stir fry meat, stirring often to brown evenly. When not stirring, cover with splatter screen (information on page 60).
4. Add vegetables and nuts. Sprinkle with seasonings. Stir often to cook meat and vegetables evenly. Serve immediately with Basic Buckwheat Groats (page 252).

Yield: I usually allow 3 ounces of meat, 2 cups of vegetables, and 1 teaspoon of oil per serving.

Life is a mixed bag of blessings and disaster. Living is the art of storing up enough joy to tide us over the rough spots.

Don't submit to being a prisoner of time. Learn to use your time. Don't let time use you.

Scalloped Potatoes and Ham*

1 pound	ham steak (unsmoked and uncured)
3 cups	potatoes,* peeled, thinly sliced, and rinsed
1 cup	leek, chopped or thinly sliced
3 tablespoons	potato starch*
1/4 cup	chopped cashew, macadamia or Brazil nuts*
1 teaspoon	sea salt
2 cups	water

1. Oven temperature—350°F. Preheating not necessary.
2. Trim excess fat off ham steak and dice.
3. Wash, peel, and thinly slice potatoes. I use my Black & Decker® Handy Shortcut™ Micro-Processor, using the slicer disk. Rinse and drain potatoes.

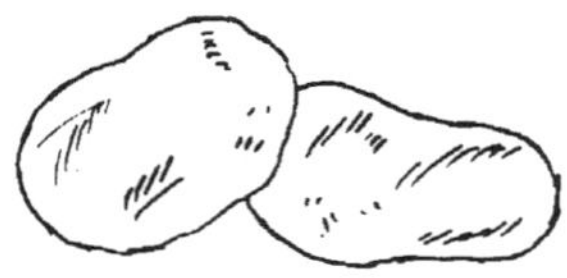

4. Layer potatoes, ham, and leeks in an oiled, covered, 2-quart casserole dish. I prefer to use a Corning 10-inch shallow casserole dish.
5. Combine potato starch, nuts, salt, and approximately 1/4 cup water in blender. Blend on high for approximately 1–2 minutes until well blended. Stop at least once to scrape sides and bottom of blender jar. Add rest of water to the blender and blend for a couple seconds. Pour liquid mixture over other ingredients in casserole dish. Lightly push any floating ingredients down into the mixture.
6. Cover and bake for 1 1/2 hours or until potatoes are tender. If you use a shallow casserole dish as described in step 4, the cooking time is reduced to 45–50 minutes.

Yield: approximately 3 cups

*Potatoes are usually eaten on Day 2, so you need to avoid eating potatoes on your Day 2 just before and after eating this recipe on Day 4. Also, Brazil and macadamia nuts are unassigned "Fun Foods" on this rotational diet, see explanation on pages 30–31.

> *Thorough preparation makes its own luck.*
>
> *Joe Poyer*

Easy Squirrel Dinner

1	squirrel, deboned and cut into strips, approximately 1 cup
2 tablespoons	navy bean flour
	OR 1 tablespoon kudzu starch
1/4 teaspoon	sea salt
1 cup	leek, sliced
2 cups	green bean cuts, fresh or frozen
1/4 teaspoon	sea salt
1/2 cup	water or broth from cooked navy beans

1. Prepare meat and vegetables as described above. Layer squirrel strips in bottom of standard-size slow cooker. Add flour and 1/4 teaspoon sea salt. Stir to coat meat with the flour.
2. Layer leeks and green beans on the top of the meat mixture. Sprinkle with another 1/4 teaspoon of salt. Do Not Stir. Pour water as evenly as possible over layered meat and vegetables. Again, Do Not Stir.
3. Cover and cook on high for 4–5 hours or on low for 8–10 hours. Serve over Navy Beans and Broth (page 263).

Yield: 2 servings

Special Note: I recommend that the squirrel be soaked for several hours or overnight in salt water to remove most of the wild game taste.

Pork and Bean Burritos

4	Buckwheat Tortillas (page 248)
3 cups	green beans, fresh, frozen, or canned
1/2 pound	ground pork
2 cups	Mexican Medley Beans (page 262)

1. Prepare or thaw tortillas.
2. If using fresh or frozen green beans, cook in saucepan until tender with sea salt and small amount of water.
3. In skillet, cook ground pork with 1/4 teaspoon of salt until done. Stir often to chop meat and brown evenly.
4. Add Mexican Medley Beans and cooked, drained green beans. (Sauce should be fairly thick. If too thick, a small amount of green bean liquid may be added.) Simmer 5 minutes to blend flavors. Taste and add more seasonings if needed. Sauce will yield 5 cups.
5. Spread 1/2 cup of bean mixture lengthwise on the center third of each tortilla. Fold tortilla from each side on top of bean mixture. Carefully transfer burrito to covered casserole dish and place folded side down. I prefer to use a 10-inch Corning shallow dish. Top with remaining bean mixture. Cover and bake at 350°F. until warm enough to serve.

Yield: 4 burritos

Shrimp Tofu Lasagna*

4 cloves	garlic, minced
1 cup	leaks, sliced
2 teaspoons	safflower oil
1/2 cup	chopped macadamia or Brazil nuts*
1/3 cup	kudzu starch
2 cups	liquid (water and/or green bean broth)
1 teaspoon	sea salt
1 1/2 teaspoons	basil**
1 tablespoon	leaf oregano
3 cups	Your choice of Day 4 vegetables: cooked green beans (fresh, frozen, or canned—drained) asparagus cuts and tips (fresh or frozen)—my preference
1 pound	Fresh Shelled Shrimp*, diced (2 cups) (page 181)
1 pound	soft packed tofu, drained, thinly sliced lengthwise (12 slices)
2 layers	Soy Lasagna Noodles (page 251)

<u>To Prepare Sauce</u>:

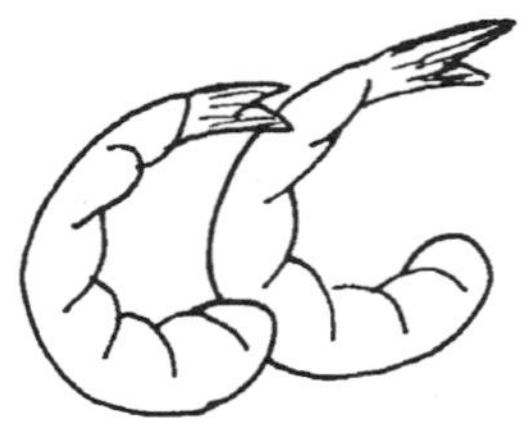

1. In medium saucepan, sauté garlic and leeks in oil until soft.
2. Combine nuts, kudzu, and small amount liquid in blender. Blend on highest speed for 1–2 minutes until well blended, stop at least once to scrape sides and bottom of blender jar. Add this mixture and rest of liquid to sautéd garlic and leeks. Cook on medium, stirring almost constantly, until thickened.
3. In large (8-cup) measure or bowl, combine thickened sauce, seasonings, vegetables, and shrimp. Sauce yields 5 1/2 cups.

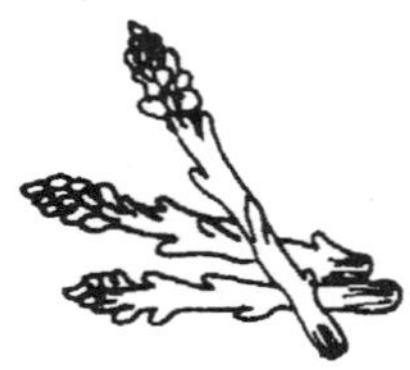

<u>To prepare Lasagna:</u>

4. Oven temperature—350°F. Preheating not necessary.
5. Layer ingredients in following order. (Amounts given are for Corning 10-inch square covered casserole dish. Recipe can also be prepared in 4 covered Corning Grab-It Bowls.)
   - 1 cup sauce, spread evenly
   - 1 layer of lasagna noodles
   - 6 slices of tofu
   - 1 1/2 cups sauce, spread evenly
   - 6 slices of tofu
   - 1 layer of lasagna noodles
   - 3 cups sauce, spread evenly
6. Cover and bake for 50–60 minutes until sauce is bubbling and all ingredients are fork tender. Remove from oven and allow to set approximately 5 minutes. Cut into desired serving portions and serve with a spatula. Leftovers may be frozen. For best quality, thaw and reheat leftovers slowly in a covered dish. If you prepare recipe in the individual bowls, you may freeze them unbaked. Thaw completely and bake as usual.

continued on next page

Shrimp Tofu Lasagna (continued)

Special Notes:

This recipe can be prepared using dry, uncooked whole-wheat or spelt noodles in place of Soy Noodles. However rotation is difficult to follow when you use this substitution.

I prefer to use an 8-cup measure to mix ingredients so I can check the yield of the sauce and evenly distribute it between layers, which is especially needed when preparing lasagna in individual dishes.

*Brazil and macadamia nuts are unassigned "Fun Foods" in this rotational diet, see explanation on pages 30–31.

**Realize that these foods are usually eaten on Day 2 so you need to avoid eating them on your Day 2 just before and after enjoying this recipe on your Day 4.

Yield: 4 servings

Baked Fish for Day 4

Your choice of Day 4 fish fillets	haddock, mahi mahi, ocean perch
Your choice of Day 4 seasonings	tarragon, garlic, oregano
Your choice of Day 4 foods	leeks, peas, lentils, or pea sprouts, macadamia nuts and/or cashews
Oil for Day 4	safflower or soy oil

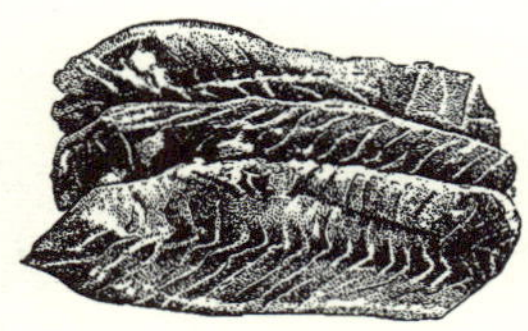

Place fish fillets in covered casserole dish. Sprinkle with salt and seasonings. Garnish with your choice of other foods. Drizzle with approximately 1/2 teaspoon of oil per serving. Also, I usually add 1–2 tablespoons of water to casserole dish. Cover and bake for approximately 30 minutes at 350ºF. until fish is flaky. Time will depend on thickness of fillet, whether fillet is frozen or thawed, and amount of other foods used.

Grilled Fish for Day 4

Day 4 fish fillet for grilling	mahi mahi
Your choice of Day 4 seasonings	tarragon, garlic, oregano
Oil for Day 4	safflower oil

Baste both sides of fish fillet with small amount of oil. Sprinkle both sides of fish fillet with salt and your choice of seasonings. Cook on small electric grill. Turn often to prevent burning. I use a grill which has a thermostat for better temperature control which is especially needed for fish.

Orange Roughy

Preheat electric skillet to 250ºF. Add small amount of safflower oil, Clarified butter, or butter and fish fillets. (Realize using butter or Clarified Butter does break rotation). Sprinkle with sea salt and tarragon. Cook until flaky. Turn often to prevent burning. Cooking time is approximately 5–8 minutes total. Time will depend on whether the fillets are frozen or thawed and also on the thickness of fillets. Cover with splatter screen (information on page 60) to prevent splattering of butter or oil. I enjoy Orange Roughy served with Cream of Asparagus Soup (page 276).

Yield: 1 pound of fish equals 3 servings

Black Beans and Sauce*

1 cup	black turtle beans
1 3-inch	kombu
2 cups	water
1/4 cup	fresh minced cilantro (optional)*
1/3 cup	green or red peppers, diced (optional)*
1/2 cup	leek, sliced or diced
1/2 teaspoon	sea salt

1. Rinse beans to remove dirt and dust. Soak beans 8–12 hours or overnight in plenty of water so beans can more than double in size.
2. Just before cooking, rinse beans thoroughly. Drain.
3. Transfer beans to 1-quart size slow cooker (information on page 61) or double this recipe and cook in a standard-size slow cooker. Add all ingredients except salt. Cook on low for 8 hours or until beans are tender but not mushy.
4. Add salt just before serving and stir. Serve as side dish or use as a sauce in the recipe below. Freeze leftovers for future quick meals.

Yield: 3 1/2 cups

Tofu and Asparagus in Black Bean Sauce*

1–1 1/2 cups	asparagus cuts and tips, fresh or frozen
1/2 teaspoon	safflower oil
1 clove	garlic, minced
7/8 cup	Black Beans and Sauce,* 1/4 of above recipe (7/8 cup = 3/4 cup + 2 Tbls.)
1/4 pound	tofu, soft or firm, drained, cubed

1. In saucepan, steam asparagus in small amount of salted water until almost tender. If needed, see cooking directions on page 274.
2. In skillet, sauté garlic in oil until soft. Add all ingredients to skillet, stir gently. Cover and heat to serving temperature. Stir gently occasionally during heating process.

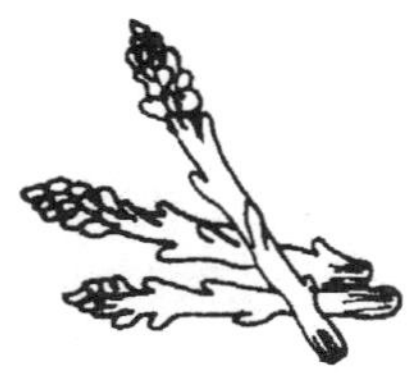

Yield: approximately 2 1/2 cups, complete vegetarian meal for 1

*Green peppers are usually eaten on Day 2, so you need to avoid eating green peppers on your Day 2 just before and after eating this recipe on Day 4. Also, I believe cilantro is in the Mustard Family which is eaten on Days 1 and 3. I personally do not concern myself with this minor break in rotation.

Special Note: I desire the combination of black turtle beans and asparagus more often that I can tolerate soy, so I often omit the tofu and serve the beans and asparagus with a pork chop.

Macadamia* or Cashew "Mayo"

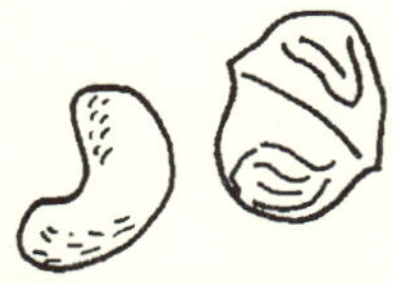

1/2 cup	chopped macadamia nuts* OR raw or dry roasted, unsalted cashew pieces
1 cup	water
1 teaspoon	unbuffered, corn-free vitamin C crystals
1 tablespoon	kudzu starch
1/4 teaspoon	sea salt

1. Blend nuts in blender on highest speed until they become a fine powder, approximately 1–2 minutes. Stop once or twice to scrape sides and bottom of blender jar.
2. Add rest of ingredients. Blend on highest speed for a minute longer, stop once or twice to scrape sides and bottom of blender jar.
3. Pour mixture into small saucepan. Cook over medium heat, stirring constantly, until mixture thickens. I prefer to stir with a whisk to keep mixture smooth.
4. Chill. You may store in a glass jar in the refrigerator for a week if necessary. You may add a tablespoon more water if too thick.

Yield: 1 1/3 cups

Recipe idea from The Yeast Connection Cookbook by Crook & Jones, p. 208.

Cucumber and Pea Salad

1 cup	peas, fresh or frozen, thawed and drained
1 cup	cucumber, sliced
1/2 cup	leek, sliced
1/8 teaspoon	sea salt
1/3 cup	Macadamia* or Cashew "Mayo" (page 273)
as desired	fresh sorrell

1. Prepare all ingredients as described above.
2. Gently toss together prepared vegetables.
3. Add "Mayo" of your choice and mix to coat vegetables. Chill.
4. Serve on a bed of sorrell leaves.

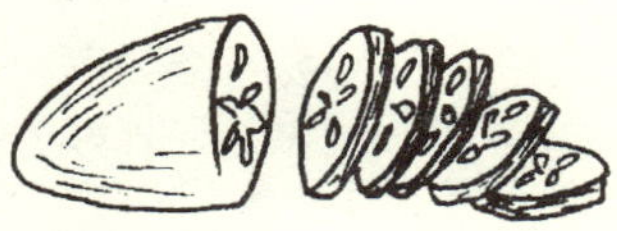

Yield: 2 cups

*Macadamia nuts are unassigned "Fun Foods" on this rotational diet, see explanation on pages 30–31.

Fresh Asparagus

Preparation of Asparagus Spears:

Asparagus spears are tender from the top down until they get close to the ground where they begin to develop a woody, fibrous texture. This woody portion of the spear is tough and tasteless and therefore should be removed before cooking. To remove this woody portion:

- Hold on to the spear at the top.
- With paring knife in other hand, place knife blade against "ground" end of asparagus on the side of the spear that is away from you and place your thumb on side of the spear toward you (opposite the blade).
- Apply gentle pressure with knife against spear as you move up the spear a small distance at a time. You will feel the difference in texture as you move past the woody part and into the tender part of the spear. This will happen when your knife blade cuts easily into the spear.

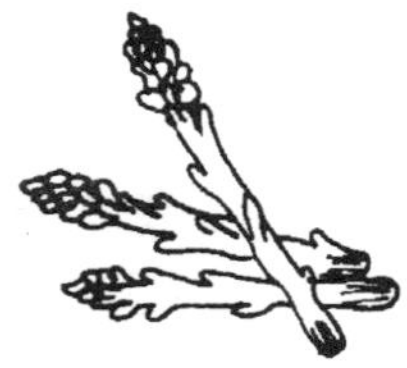

- Cut off and discard woody portion.
- Cut tender part of spear into approximately 6-inch lengths for spears and 1-inch lengths for cuts and tips.
- Wash pieces thoroughly to remove sand and dirt.

Cooking Asparagus:

Arrange asparagus spears in top portion of steamer pan or in a steamer basket. Sprinkle with salt as desired. Cook covered over steaming water for 10–15 minutes or until tender. Time will depend on diameter of spears. Cook cuts and tips as above or in saucepan with small amount of salted water for 10 minutes or until tender.

Tips on Freezing Asparagus

Prepare cuts or spears as described above.

To Blanch:

- Fill bottom of a steamer pan with water to about 1/2 inch from the bottom of steamer insert. Heat water to boiling.
- Add cuts or spears to insert of steamer pan. Cover and immediately begin timing. Cook over boiling water for 3–5 minutes. Time will depend upon diameter of asparagus spears.

3 minutes for small stalks	4 minutes for medium stalks	5 minutes for large stalks

- Immediately drain and chill in ice water until cold.

To Freeze:

- Drain well.
- Place in cellophane bag and freeze.

OR

Individually quick freeze on a baking sheet before placing in cellophane bag. See explanation on page 290 in the Canning and Freezing section of Chapter 12—Organics—The Only Way to Go!

Stir-Fry Vegetables for Day 4

asparagus cuts, blanched
leek, sliced
edible pea pods, blanched
green peas, fresh or frozen
roasted soy beans
cashews
safflower or soy oil
tarragon and/or garlic powder
sea salt
Jerusalem artichoke, sliced thin

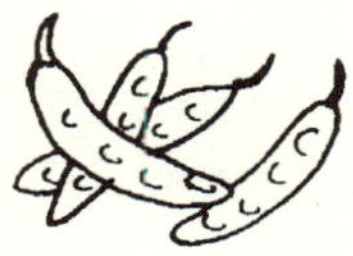

1. Preheat well-seasoned cast-iron skillet on medium (How to Season Cast Iron on page 63) or electric skillet to 300°F.

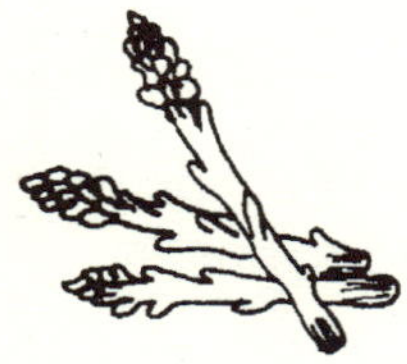

2. Prepare vegetables in amounts desired.
3. Add oil to preheated skillet (cast-iron skillet will require less oil). Add vegetables (except artichoke) and nuts. Sprinkle with seasonings. Stir often to cook vegetables evenly. Add artichoke near end of cooking time just prior to serving. I prefer my vegetables crunchy. Serve immediately.

Leeks—Lily Family

1. Remove and discard any wilted and dried portions from leek top and any portion that feels flabby.
2. Wash leek under running water to remove as much of the dust and sand as possible.
3. Cut the leek in half lengthwise. Wash each half thoroughly under running water or in basin of water. In order to wash out the sand and dirt that is trapped between the layers, you can carefully separate them since the root end is still intact.

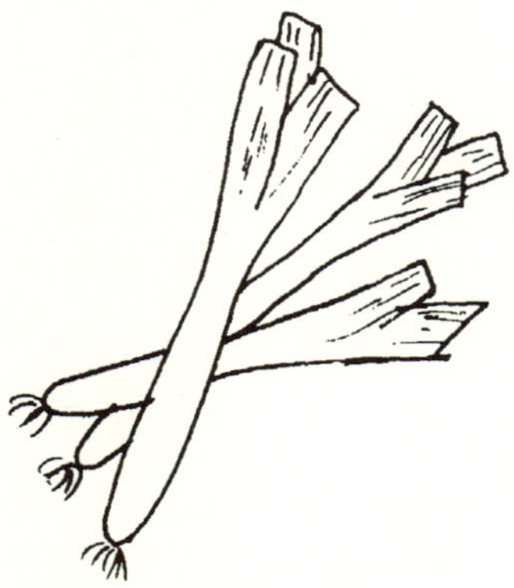

4. Cut off root end. Rinse cut end by carefully holding leek together.
5. Lay cut side of leak down on cutting board. Slice thin or thick depending on its use.
6. Freeze unneeded portion in cellophane bag for later use.

Yield: 1 medium leek yields approximately 1 cup sliced leek

Cream of Asparagus Soup*

2 cloves	garlic, minced
1/2 cup	leek, sliced or chopped
2 teaspoons	safflower oil
3 cups	asparagus cuts and tips, fresh or frozen (equivalent to 10 oz. package)
1 cup	water
1/2 teaspoon	sea salt
1/4 cup	chopped cashews macadamia nuts*
2 teaspoons	kudzu starch
1 cup	water
1/8 teaspoon	tarragon

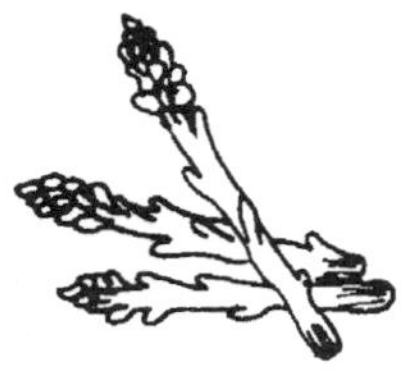

1. In medium-size saucepan, sauté garlic and leeks in oil until soft.
2. Add asparagus, 1 cup water, and salt. Bring to boil. Cover and reduce heat. Simmer for 15 minutes or until asparagus is tender.
3. While asparagus is cooking, combine nuts, kudzu, and approximately 1/4 cup water in blender. Blend on highest speed for 1–2 minutes until smooth and well blended. Add remaining water and approximately 1 cup of cooked asparagus mixture to blender. Blend about 20 seconds on lowest speed.
4. Pour blended mixture into saucepan. Add tarragon. Heat to serving temperature and to thicken. Stir almost constantly. This simple soup is delicious served with Orange Roughy for a complete light meal.

Yield: 3 cups

*Macadamia nuts are unassigned "Fun Foods" on this rotational diet, see explanation on pages 30–31.

Baked Beans

2 cups	navy beans
3 1/2 cups	water
1 cup	leek, chopped or sliced
1 1/2 teaspoons	basil
1 teaspoon	paprika
1 tablespoon	safflower oil
1 1/2 teaspoons	sea salt

1. Rinse beans to remove dirt and dust. Soak beans 8–12 hours or overnight in plenty of water so beans can more than double in size.
2. Just before cooking, rinse beans thoroughly until rinsing water is clear. Drain.
3. Add all ingredients except salt to standard-size slow cooker. Stir. Cook until beans are tender. Cooking time will be about 10–12 hours on low and 5–6 hours on high. You may desire to stir beans occasionally during cooking time. Add salt and stir just before serving.

Yield: 6 cups

Orange Buckwheat Cake

(Three Variations)

Stevia Sweetened

1 1/2 cups	White Buckwheat Flour (page 249)
1 1/2 teaspoons	baking soda
1/4 teaspoon	sea salt
1/16 teaspoon	stevia, white powder concentrate
1 1/4 cups	orange juice, freshly squeezed or made from concentrate
3/4 teaspoon	guar gum
2 tablespoons	safflower oil
1/2 teaspoon	alcohol-free orange flavoring

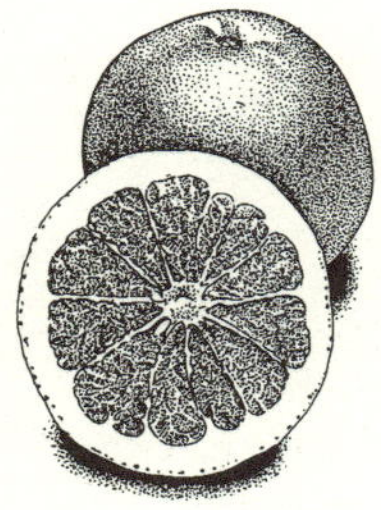

1. Preheat oven to 350°F.
2. Oil and flour 8-inch square baking dish. I use a stainless steel baking dish and therefore only need to oil the dish.
3. In a large mixing bowl, whisk together flour, soda, salt, and stevia. Make a "well" in the center.
4. To help eliminate lumps in the batter, whisk guar gum into orange juice. Add oil and orange flavoring. Mix.
5. Add liquids to dry ingredients. Stir to moisten evenly. Beat by hand for 20 strokes until you have a creamy, cake-like batter. Do not use an electric mixer.
6. Pour batter into prepared pan. Spread evenly in pan. Bake for 20–22 minutes until center bounces back when lightly tapped or toothpick comes out clean when inserted into the center of the cake.
7. Cool cake and serve plain or ice with Orange Glaze. Cut cake 4x4 to yield 16 small servings. May be frozen and thawed for future desserts. This cake is liked even by people who eat sweets and do not like buckwheat.

Lightly Honey Sweetened
Substitute 1 tablespoon of honey for stevia. Prepare as above, adding honey with other liquid ingredients. Bake 25–27 minutes.

Honey Sweetened
Substitute 2 tablespoons of honey for stevia. Prepare as above, adding honey with other liquid ingredients. Bake 28–30 minutes.

Orange Glaze for Cake (Stevia or Honey Sweetened)

3/4 cup	orange juice, freshly squeezed or made from concentrate
1/32 teaspoon	stevia (1/4 of 1/8 teaspoon)
	OR 1 tablespoon honey
1 tablespoon	kudzu starch
1/4 teaspoon	unbuffered, corn-free vitamin C crystals (optional)

1. In small saucepan, whisk together all ingredients except vitamin C. Cook over low to medium heat until mixture gently boils for 3–5 minutes. Stir almost constantly with whisk.
2. Add vitamin C crystals and stir to give the glaze a sweet-tart taste. I enjoy the tart taste to complement the cake.

Carob Cake Brownies
(Three Variations)

Stevia Sweetened

1 1/2 cups	White Buckwheat Flour (page 249)
1/3 cup	carob powder (after measuring, sift to remove lumps)
1 1/2 teaspoons	baking soda
1/4 teaspoon	sea salt
3/4 teaspoon	guar gum
1/2 teaspoon	unbuffered, corn-free vitamin C crystals
1/4 teaspoon	stevia, white powder concentrate
1 1/4 cups	water
1/4 cup	safflower oil
1/2 teaspoon	alcohol-free peppermint extract (optional)

1. Preheat oven to 350°F.
2. Oil and flour 8-inch square baking dish. I use a stainless steel baking dish and therefore only need to oil the dish.
3. In a large mixing bowl, whisk together dry ingredients. Make a "well" in the center.
4. Add water, oil, and peppermint. Using an electric mixer, mix on lowest speed until dry ingredients are moistened. Then blend on mix speed for 20 seconds until you have a creamy, cake-like batter. If you wish, you may also mix by hand. If so, first stir to moisten dry ingredients and then beat by hand for 30 seconds to make a creamy, cake-like batter.
5. Pour batter into prepared pan. Spread evenly in pan. Bake for 25–30 minutes until toothpick comes out clean when inserted into the center of the brownies. The top will be a little dry and cracked just like regular chocolate brownies.
6. Cool brownies in pan on a cooling rack. Also, cover with a towel so brownies will not dry out. If desired, spread with Carob Icing (page 279). Cut 4x4 to yield 16 small servings. Leftovers may be frozen and thawed for future desserts. These brownies are even liked by people who eat sweets and do not like buckwheat.

Special Note: My way of sifting the carob powder is to place the measurement of carob powder into a fine-mesh strainer. (Have a bowl under it.) Then stir the powder to work it through the mesh and into the bowl.

Lightly Honey Sweetened

Substitute 2 tablespoons of honey for stevia. Prepare as above, adding honey with other liquid ingredients.

Honey Sweetened

Substitute 1/4 cup of honey for stevia and use 1 tablespoon less water. Prepare as stevia-sweetened version, adding honey with other liquid ingredients. This version is the favorite of my family and friends who have not curbed their sweet tooth like I have.

Carob Icing
(Three Variations)

<u>Stevia Sweetened</u>

1/4 cup	carob powder, sifted
2 teaspoons	kudzu starch
1/16 teaspoon	stevia, white powder concentrate (1/2 of 1/8 teaspoon)
1/2 cup	water
1/4 teaspoon	alcohol-free peppermint extract (optional)

<u>Lightly Honey Sweetened</u>

1/4 cup	carob powder, sifted
2 teaspoons	kudzu starch
2 tablespoons	honey
3/8 cup	water (1/4 cup + 2 tablespoons)
1/4 teaspoon	alcohol-free peppermint extract (optional)

<u>Honey Sweetened</u>

1/4 cup	carob powder, sifted
2 teaspoons	kudzu starch
1/4 cup	honey
1/4 cup	water
1/4 teaspoon	alcohol-free peppermint extract (optional)

1. In small saucepan, whisk together dry ingredients. Add liquid ingredients and blend to dissolve dry ingredients.
2. Cook on medium heat until thickened. Stir with whisk almost constantly. Cool or spread warm on slightly cooled brownies.

Yield: 1/2 cup

> *When things start going your way,*
> *it's usually because you stopped going*
> *the wrong way down a one-way street.*
> *Los Angeles Times Syndicate*

Carob Pudding

1/2 cup	chopped macadamia or Brazil nuts*
1/4 cup	kudzu starch OR arrowroot starch **
2 cups	water
2 tablespoons	honey OR 1/8 teaspoon stevia, white powder concentrate
1/4 cup	carob powder (after measuring, sift to remove lumps)
1/4 teaspoon	alcohol-free peppermint extract (optional)

1. Blend chopped nuts, starch, and small amount of water in blender on highest speed for 1–2 minutes until well blended. Stop at least once to scrap sides and bottom of jar. Add rest of water, blend a few seconds longer.
2. Pour nut milk into saucepan, add rest of ingredients. Whisk to blend. Cook over medium heat, stirring almost constantly with whisk, until thickened. Pour into custard cups. Chill.

Yield: 2 1/4 cups

*Brazil and macadamia nuts are unassigned "Fun Foods" in this rotational diet, see explanation on pages 30–31.

**If you use arrowroot, you need to omit eating arrowroot on your Day 2 just before and after using arrowroot in this pudding on your Day 4.

Buckwheat Pie Crust

3/4 cup	White Buckwheat Flour (page 249)
3/4 teaspoon	guar gum
1/4 cup	cold water
3 tablespoons	safflower oil, cold
1/4 teaspoon	sea salt

1. Chill medium-size bowl and whisk.
2. Combine flour and guar gum in small unchilled bowl. Set aside.
3. Whisk water, oil, and salt in chilled bowl until opaque and slightly thick. (Oil which gets cloudy and thick in the refrigerator—such as olive and sesame—will become more opaque and thick, but for rotation I use safflower.)
4. Add flour mixture to liquids and stir with rubber spatula or fork until dough clumps together into a ball and is well mixed. Dough will be a little sloppy and soft at first. Continue stirring for a few seconds.
5. Transfer dough to an 8-inch pie pan. Press dough with oil-coated fingers to form pie shell, making sides and bottom as evenly thin as possible. Chill until filling is prepared and ready to bake.

Special Note: This crust recipe may also be pressed into the bottom of an 8-inch square baking dish to use with Tofu "Cheesecake" recipes (page 281).

Recipe idea from Mastering Food Allergies newsletter, September 1990.

Carob Tofu "Cheesecake"

2 pounds	soft tofu, drained
1/4 cup	carob powder (after measuring, sift to remove lumps)
3/8 cup	honey (3/8 cup = 1/4 cup + 2 tablespoons)
1/2 teaspoon	sea salt
2 tablespoons	dacopa (optional)

Blueberry Tofu "Cheesecake"

2 pounds	soft tofu, drained
1 cup	frozen blueberries, no need to thaw except to remove ice crystals
1/4 cup	honey
1/2 teaspoon	sea salt

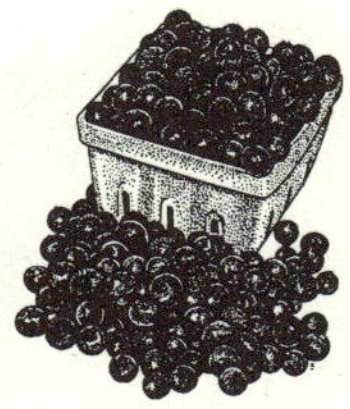

1. Preheat oven 350°F.
2. Combine your choice of ingredients in large mixing bowl. Using electric mixer or Braun hand mixer, blend ingredients until thoroughly mixed and tofu is smooth.
3. Pour into 8-inch square baking dish with unbaked Buckwheat Pie Crust pressed only in the bottom of the dish. Spread batter evenly.
4. Bake for 60–65 minutes or until filling is done and knife comes out clean when inserted into center. Chill. Cut 4x4 to yield 16 servings. Both versions may be frozen and thawed for future desserts. However, crust usually separates from cheesecake and is a little watery.

Special Note: My way of sifting the carob powder is to place measurement of carob powder into a fine-mesh strainer. (Have bowl under it.) Then stir the powder to work it through the mesh and into the bowl.

Rhubarb Jelly

2 cups	diced rhubarb
1/4 cup	honey
	OR 1/4 cup water and 1/4 teaspoon stevia, white powder concentrate
1/8 teaspoon	sea salt
1/2 teaspoon	kudzu starch

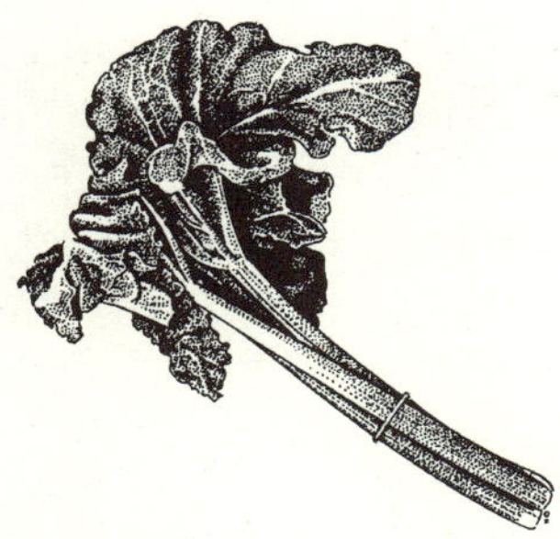

1. Combine all ingredients except kudzu in sauce pan. Cover and cook on low for 15 minutes or until rhubarb is very tender. Stir occasionally during cooking process.
2. Add kudzu and continue to cook, stirring constantly, until thickened. Cool. This jelly is delicious on toasted Buckwheat Yeast-Free Bread (page 250) for a quick breakfast or snack.
3. I freeze the stevia version in ice cube trays, 1 tablespoon per cube. When frozen, remove from trays and package in cellophane bags. Then thaw as needed. Usually 1/2 or 1 cube is perfect for one serving. The honey version may be frozen in a jar since it does not freeze as solid.

Yield: approximately 1 cup

Carob Shake

1/4 cup	Ener-G Pure Soy Quick
1/4 cup	carob powder
2 cups	water
1/16 teaspoon	stevia, white powder concentrated (1/16 tsp. = 1/2 of 1/8 tsp.)

Combine all ingredients in blender. Blend on highest speed until dissolved. Taste for desired sweetness. If needed, add more stevia (add only a few grains at a time) and blend a little longer. Chill. Shake or stir before drinking.

Yield: 1 cup

Cranberry Spritzer

1 bottle	carbonated, unflavored mineral water, chilled (12 ounces)
1/2 cup	unsweetened cranberry juice, chilled

Combine and serve immediately.

Yield: 2 cups

Orange Spritzer

1 bottle	carbonated, unflavored mineral water, chilled (12 ounces)
1/4 cup	unsweetened orange juice concentrate

Combine and serve immediately.

Yield: 1 3/4 cups

Cranberry-Orange Spritzer

1 bottle	carbonated, unflavored mineral water, chilled (12 ounces)
1/4 cup	unsweetened orange juice concentrate
1/2 cup	unsweetened cranberry juice, chilled

Combine and serve immediately.

Yield: 2 1/4 cups

Special Note: At publication the only brand of unsweetened 100% cranberry juice that I have used is R.W Knudsen. See Appendix C: Resources for another brand available from Walnut Acre Organic Farms. I prefer to mix in 1/4 teaspoon of stevia per quart of cranberry juice. Also, partially frozen cranberry juice added to the mineral water makes an interesting slush.

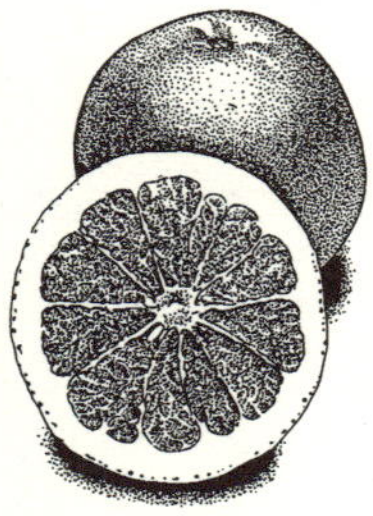

12. ORGANICS—THE ONLY WAY TO GO!

One of the most important considerations in incorporating a rotational diet and/or a healthier eating plan into your lifestyle is the quality of foods you use in creating meals. I cannot say enough in support of purchasing organic food products on an almost exclusive and consistent basis. Through the use of organic foods you decrease the chemical exposure that you experience with other commercially produced foods. In addition, you help support an environmentally sound, self-sustaining, and renewing method of food production that needs to be a priority if we are to avoid further damage to our environment and world. In truth, I emphatically believe that for these and many other reasons, organics is "The Only Way to Go."

If you have never before purchased organic foods or have purchased them only on a limited basis, the task of locating a convenient source(s) and changing your buying habits to incorporate an exclusive-as-possible organic format can seem formidable at first. Remember, as with all of the major changes recommended in this book, you can start gradually and work up to a higher level of organic food use. This will give you the opportunity to learn as you go—not only in locating the best sources for you, but also in acclimatizing your lifestyle to the difference in eating habits. Do as much or as little as you are able at first. Then gradually increase your commitment as you feel comfortable to do so. The goal is to help make your life healthier and easier, not to add more stress.

What Is Meant by "Organically Grown" Food?

Specific methods and standards are involved when you speak of "organically grown" food products. In general, organic growers use production methods which:

- maintain the long-term fertility of soils by fostering the creation of humus, replenishing organic matter, balancing mineral levels, and increasing microbial life.
- avoid materials which cause pollution or are known to be harmful to health, such as synthetic fertilizers, insecticides, fungicides, herbicides, hormones, or antibiotics.
- use local, renewable resources and allow farmers a decent return and healthy satisfaction from their work.

Organic foods are grown in nutrient-rich soil, are usually ripened before picking, and are some of the tastiest, most nourishing foods you will ever eat. They are produced without the use of pesticides, herbicides, or other chemicals and they are not artificially ripened using various chemical processes. Organic meats are obtained from animals raised on certified organic grains and hay and without added drugs such as hormones and antibiotics. In addition, organic food is processed and distributed using methods that retain freshness and nutritional quality without the use of synthetic or artificial fumigants, preservatives, additives, or irradiation.

The basic principle of organic agriculture is that a healthy plant grows from healthy soil and is more resistant to pests and diseases. If a problem does arise during the growth cycle, many times it is controlled by sophisticated biological technologies involving natural predators, biodegradable botanical sprays, resistant plant varieties, mechanical and pheromone traps, and other natural methods.

Many states have enacted organic food standards, which are used in the certification process for organic growers, processors, and vendors. On the next page is a listing of what these standards provide.

1. Control of the use of the word "organic" in advertising and labeling of food products.
2. Standards for methods of growing and processing products to be sold as organic, which restrict the use of synthetic fertilizers, pesticides, hormones, and antibiotics for a minimum of three years before a grower may apply for certification.
3. Record-keeping requirements for growers, processors, and vendors, including sworn statements to accompany products sold as organic.
4. Opportunity to obtain private certification for products that meet even higher quality standards than those established.
5. A means of enforcing the standards that will protect both consumers and growers.

The label "certified organic" on a food product involves a significant commitment on the part of organic producers to achieve and maintain organic certification for their products.

Since there are many phrasings used in labeling organic foods, you should be aware of the following definitions as you choose which product or produce to buy.

Biodynamically Grown Food. Biodynamically grown food is a special type of organically grown food that meets or exceeds all organic growing standards. The aim of this practice, which is more known in Europe than in the United States, is to produce the highest-quality nutrition for both humans and animals, while developing a self-contained farm ecosystem that regenerates land, plants, animals, and people.

"Certified Organically Grown." Grown by organic methods and certified by an independent organization or association of organic growers who verify that the farm meets particular criteria. The name of the certifying organization should accompany this label, and many have logos that are easy to recognize. This is the best assurance that the food is organically grown.

"Organically Grown" or "Organic." This label by itself is generally meaningless, unless the store has its own definition posted near the produce bin. Sometimes this term is used by stores that have signed statements from the grower, describing the precise growing practices. In these cases, the store must take the grower's word as truth, for there is neither time nor money to send knowledgeable people to inspect the farms, run pesticide tests, or perform all the other necessities to certify the produce.

"Represented" or "Claimed Organic." This label is generally used when the farmer has told the store that the produce is organic, but nobody has checked on it. Usually no signed statement of growing practices has been submitted.

"Transitional Organic." This usually means the farm is growing organically but hasn't been doing it for the required period to be able to meet state or private certification.

"Unsprayed." An "Unsprayed" label simply indicates that the food has not been sprayed with pesticides. It also usually means that the food has not been colored, gassed, or waxed, but it probably has not come from a farm with a soil-building program and may not be as carefully harvested or packaged. Artificial fertilizers have probably been used.

"IPM" (Integrated Pest Management) or "Ecologic." This indicates food grown on a farm that is using Integrated Pest Management (where they use a lesser amount of pesticides than nonorganic farmers) or that may be in the process of converting to organic methods.

Why Is It Important to Purchase Organic Food?

Stop and consider some of the procedures that have become a normal part of nonorganic agriculture over the past years. The consequences of these procedures, not only for the living beings that consume agricultural products, but also for the earth where they are produced, are alarming.

There are 1.5 billion pounds of pesticides used in this country each year on agricultural food products. This amounts to nearly 5 pounds of poisonous sprays for each person. About 45,000 different agricultural chemicals are used and 150 of these regularly show up as residue in food. About two dozen of them show up in amounts large enough to be toxic. Several of the chemicals used in these applications are known carcinogens (cancer causing agents). In addition, they have been linked to birth defects, miscarriages, mutations, Alzheimer's disease, and various degenerative diseases. Many crops of fruits and vegetables are sprayed twenty or more times a year with five or more of these active ingredients.

In addition, the use and overuse of agricultural chemicals is destroying our soils and poisoning our water supplies. These chemicals not only kill the destructive insects and weeds for which they are intended, they also kill beneficial insects, birds, fish, and animals. As a side effect, the destructive insects and weeds can develop resistance to these chemicals, which leaves chemical experts searching for ever stronger and more deadly remedies to use in this vicious cycle.

As a means to "protect" the general public from overexposure to the chemicals approved for use in the United States, the EPA (Environmental Protection Agency) is set up to regulate use levels and monitor the levels of residue found in foods. Unfortunately, due to possibly unreliable licensing safety tests for chemicals, untimely and inadequate laboratory processing, and a lack of adequate personnel, it is practically impossible for the EPA to adequately control the general public's exposure to these chemicals.

An added consideration when you are looking at the nonorganic fruits and vegetables in your local grocery store is that in January and February over 70% of the fresh produce in the United States comes from Mexico. Most of the rest comes from other foreign countries. Many times these countries do not have bans prohibiting the use of chemicals that have been tested and rejected in the United States. As an example, DDT has become a favorite chemical for foreign coffee growers. You were exposed to residues of this dangerous insecticide this morning if you did not drink organic coffee.

Why subject yourself and your family to the effects of these chemicals when there is a healthful, highly nutritious alternative in organic foods?

How and Where Do I Get Organic Foods?

Because of the set standards described above, it is relatively easy to identify organically grown and produced foods. Any product that is labeled "organically grown" or "certified organic" is done so in compliance with state laws that define and regulate organic products. Through the certification and documentation process, you can be assured of the organic quality of the food products you are purchasing.

You will probably find, as I have, that you will use a number of sources to purchase organic foods. Five of the most-used sources are discussed below, but keep your eyes and ears open for other possible organic food outlets in your area.

One of the best-known sources for organic foods is your local health-food store. It varies from store to store, but generally these businesses will carry a wide range of organic products, from flours, grains, oils, and packaged foods (such as cereals or pastas) to fresh produce and meats. Also, it may be the case that the store is a cooperative, where the purchase of a membership entitles you to lower prices for these quality products. Check your local telephone directory or yellow pages for headings such as grocers or health-food products or ask people in your neighborhood if they know of a local store that carries organic foods.

In Appendix E you will find a list of cooperative food warehouses located in the United States. By joining with others who are interested in purchasing organic food products and sharing time and energy, you could join or form a food-buying club that can purchase organic products at a savings from a wholesale warehouse. If you contact one of these warehouses in your area of the country, they more than likely will be able to send you information on what a buying club is and direct you to existing buying clubs in your area or provide information on how to start a new buying club. Since the required purchasing level for individual items for buying clubs is likely to be in case lots, forming or joining a club with participants having needs and interests similar to your own will greatly improve the club's effectiveness in saving money for all of its members.

If your locality has a seasonal farmer's market that has regularly scheduled sale days, go and check out the vendors. Many organic growers use this outlet to market their products. It may mean some extra planning ahead, but you could find some excellent sources of seasonal produce and may be able to purchase items to can or freeze for off-season use.

Mail-order sources are another option for the purchase of organic products. Ordering products by mail can be beneficial in two special ways. First, chemical exposure is likely to be lower when there are not several middle steps in the distribution process. And second, you expend less energy when you let the post office or UPS bring something to you rather than going to the store. In Appendix C: Resources, you will find a listing that will aid you in locating the mail-order companies that can supply the organic food products you wish to purchase. In addition, some of these companies will use special packaging for your order if you react to specific materials. Check with each company regarding their policy and options in this area.

Also, in Appendix F you will find a listing of Organizations Providing Information on Organic Food Production and Availability around the United States that can provide you with information on organically grown products and their availability in your area.

Having Your Own Organic Garden

By far, the best way to obtain organically grown produce is to grow it yourself. When this is possible for you, it can be a rewarding way to help guarantee that you are eating the safest and best quality food available.

Once again, be aware that organic gardening (just like any form of gardening) requires a time and energy commitment if it is to be worthwhile. If you do not have the energy or interest level that a garden would require, you may wish to ask friends or relatives to help by raising the organic produce for you. You might also consider hiring someone to do the garden work, possibly for a share of the produce.

If gardening is something you enjoy, remember that you do not necessarily have to raise a huge garden to reap the benefits of growing organic foods yourself. You can start small if you wish, maybe with one or two crops such as tomatoes and edible pea pods.

There are several excellent books available on organic gardening techniques and you will find at least a portion of them listed in Appendix D: Recommended Reading. They focus on such varied techniques as the use of compost, mulch, natural insect control, companion planting, and organic seed and gardening product sources. These techniques are briefly described below.

Compost

You can turn kitchen and yard wastes into a nutrient-rich soil supplement for your yard or garden through composting. By recycling organic waste such as grass clippings, leaves, vegetable peelings, apple cores, and other organic materials, you can decrease the amount that would normally go into a landfill. Yard waste and food scraps make up about one-fourth of the waste produced in the United States.

A compost pile should be at least four feet long by four feet wide by three feet tall to hold heat. The sides of the pile can be left unsupported or held by cinder-block or chicken-wire walls, built to allow air to pass through. It requires a good mixture of ingredients, such as dry leaves or straw (carbon-rich materials) and green grass clippings, certain kitchen wastes, and/or manure (nitrogen-rich material). By adding soil to the compost pile you introduce the microorganisms necessary for decomposition.

Moisture is also required in the decomposition process, and the compost pile should be as moist as a wrung sponge. If necessary, sprinkle it periodically with water during dry weather.

Air flow is important as well, so the pile should be prevented from collapsing or compacting under the weight of too much water or debris. By alternating layers of green material, dry material, and soil and turning the mixture every few weeks, you can achieve a faster rate of decomposition. A healthy compost pile will be warm because heat is released when organic material decomposes.

Chop or shred big items before adding them to the compost pile. This will help speed the rate of decomposition. Do not add meat, bones, cheese, or grease to the pile as they take a long time to decompose and will attract animals. Also, while horse, cow, or sheep manure is rich in nitrogen and beneficial to the compost pile, you should not use dog or cat droppings as they may carry diseases.

The compost pile will shrink as the materials decompose. The process may take a period of weeks or months, depending on the care the pile receives, but when the compost is dark and crumbly and has an earthy smell, it is ideal to use. Add a one- to three-inch layer of compost to your garden, spread it around individual plants, or use it as potting soil.

Mulch

To cut down on your garden maintenance by controlling weeds and moisture levels, you may wish to use a mulch. In fact, correctly applied mulch can totally eliminate weeding. Consisting of any material used to cover the ground, mulch comes in basically two categories—organic and nonorganic materials. Both are used in the organic garden.

Usually applied 2–6 inches deep, organic mulches function exceptionally well at holding moisture in the soil, especially if put down after a rain. The deeper the mulch, the more it cools the ground and retains moisture. Always wait until the soil is completely warm and always weed before putting down organic mulch. By placing a layer or two of newspaper first, holding it in place with a little soil, and then mulching 4 inches deep in organic material, you can really stop weeds. It is best to use newspaper printed with soybean ink. Don't use colored or glossy paper as it contains toxic ink. Since organic mulches decay and add nutrients to the soil, they can be tilled under in the fall which adds further organic matter to loosen and feed the soil.

If your garden does not drain well, organic mulch should be applied in a thin (2–4") layer or not at all to avoid creating a too-wet situation, which can damage plants. In addition, warmth-loving plants such as peppers, eggplant, and tomatoes should not be mulched too deep since this keeps their roots too cool.

Although they may not look quite as nice, nonorganic mulches stop all weeds until they are taken up in the fall. Black poly (plastic) mulch is beneficial for warmth-loving plants because it warms the soil. In addition, it can be laid early in the spring before any weeds get started. If any weeds have started, they will smother under the poly. The edges should be weighted down every 2–6 feet (depending on size) with heavy objects such as bricks, rocks, or logs. Mark an "X" on the poly to indicate proper spacing for plants, or cut small slits for seeds. For vining plants, it may be beneficial to put a very thin layer (1/2" to 1") of organic mulch on the poly to keep vines from burning in extremely hot weather. Poly mulch MUST be removed in the fall. If you use a 6 mil poly and store it inside (garage or shed) during the winter, you may be able to use it for 2–3 years.

The following examples of mulches may help you choose the best one for your garden.

A. Organic Mulches:
   * Grass Clippings—Make sure no pesticides or herbicides have been used on the grass as residues can kill your plants.
   * Leaves—It's best to let them set for 6–12 months. Never use walnut leaves as they contain juglone, a natural fungicide harmful to many garden plants.
   * Hay—The older the better because of weed seeds.
   * Straw—Same as hay.
   * Sawdust—Use sparingly or lime annually. Be sure it contains no sawdust from treated lumber as this is very toxic.
   * Cocoa Hulls—Wonderful mulch, but expensive.
   * Corn Husks and Cobs—Good for loosening hard ground.
   * Bark and Wood Chips—Nice mulch. Call electric companies as they often have truckloads available.

B. Nonorganic Mulches:
   * Black Poly—Six mil preferred. Available at lumber yards.
   * Carpet—Tends to fall apart rapidly and makes a mess.

Natural Insect Control

There are many steps an organic gardener can take to help prevent or control insect damage. Planting resistant varieties is an important first step. Maintaining a nutriently well-balanced soil in your garden helps produce healthy plants that are better able to withstand insect damage. You can also help reduce insect and disease problems by keeping weed growth to a minimum. Many destructive insects that carry diseases thrive in weed-infested areas.

Rotating crops on a three-year cycle is also an essential part of insect control. Keep crops of the same family (such as broccoli, cabbage, and cauliflower or tomato and potato) away from plots where they were grown the past two seasons. This will help prevent damage from pests that may have wintered over in the soil and are waiting for a new crop to destroy.

By placing natural deterrent plants such as marigold, onion, garlic, shallots, mint, tansy, nasturtium, and radish throughout the garden, you can help keep a fairly wide variety of detrimental insects away.

Taking steps to encourage "beneficials" to inhabit your organic garden is a positive measure in pest control. Some important beneficial insects are ladybugs, spiders, ground beetles, assassin bugs, damsel flies, green lacewing, praying mantis, and a wide variety of wasps and flies. These bugs are avid hunters of the insects that eat garden plants.

The first and most important step to encourage beneficial insects is to use NO poison chemicals. By incorporating plants such as flowers and herbs that supply nectar, pollen, rest stops, and breeding grounds you can encourage beneficial insects to inhabit your organic garden. Important helpful plants include those in the carrot family—for example, dill, parsley, fennel, angelica, and Queen Anne's lace. Other plants that attract these insects are yarrow, petunia, cosmos, zinnia, nasturtium, marigold, and sunflower.

Other beneficial creatures such as toads, birds, and bats offer assistance in controlling detrimental insects. You can provide a small moist shelter that will attract toads by placing a shallow dish of water inside a flower pot on its side near your garden. The main diet of birds such as bluebirds, swallows, martins, wrens, phoebes, warblers, and the titmouse consists of insects. By providing birdhouses and baths you can help attract them to your area. Bats are also important insect consumers. Bat houses have been popular in Europe for 60 years and are becoming more readily available at garden centers here in the United States.

Organic gardening is dependent upon a healthy balance of these beneficial techniques. By maintaining a naturally balanced system, you can greatly improve your ability to control the amount of insect damage to your crops.

If a major insect problem arises, intervene with caution. Remember you are altering the natural process. Never use diatomaceous earth on your garden* as it is an indiscriminate killer of all soft-bodied insects, including beneficial ones. Rotenone is deadly to fish and other aquatic life. If intervention is absolutely necessary, insecticidal soaps, traps, and microorganisms, such as Bt, are probably the safest and have the least negative impact. Keep in mind that such measures are only a shortcut and that the best long-term solution is a healthy balance of beneficial plants, insects, and animals.

Companion Planting

By intercropping a mixture of plants that benefit one another, you can help attract beneficial insects, birds, and animals; prevent insect destruction and disease; and improve plant health and yield.

You can ease your garden workload by using a common location for plants that share similar nutritional needs. In the summer heat, sun-loving plants, such as corn or tomatoes, serve as natural shade for the cool weather plants, such as lettuce or spinach. Plants with deep root systems are good companions to shallow-rooted plants. This enables both plants to thrive since they are not competing for space or moisture.

Research on companion planting can also help you avoid such practices as planting onions with peas or tomatoes with fennel which can actually reduce plant yield and vigor. Consult books such as Country Woman: A Handbook for the New Farmer and Carrots Love Tomatoes (see Appendix D: Recommended Reading) for additional information on companion planting and how you can use it to improve your organic garden.

Organic Seed and Gardening Product Sources

For a good resource for organic seeds and garden supplies, check with your local health-food store or warehouse for possible product sources in your area. Gardening centers may also stock or be able to direct you to a resource for the seeds and products you need for your organic garden.

A good mail-order source for organic seeds is Seeds of Change in Santa Fe, NM (see Appendix C: Resources for address and phone). A free catalog is available upon request.

By raising your own organic produce you have a low-cost and need-specific source for the foods you want to use regularly. You can plan ahead to can or freeze your garden abundance so that you can enjoy these foods year round.

* For chemically sensitive persons, diatomaceous earth is the most appropriate insect control substance to use around your home. But do not use it in your garden.

Canning and Freezing—Creating Your Own Organic Storehouse

Having my own organic storehouse helps me stay on my rotational diet throughout the winter, especially with regard to vegetables. Several books on canning and freezing are available at your local library. However, I do recommend that you contact the local office of your state's Department of Agriculture Extension Service. They have low-cost booklets containing the most up-to-date methods for canning and freezing.

Because there are many books available on standard canning and freezing procedures, I will not go into great detail on the process. Instead, the following is a list of tips that I have learned through my years of canning and freezing.

Use Proper Equipment. Purchase helpful tools to do your canning and freezing.

- A large food processor is helpful if you are going to slice vegetables such as beets.
- Purchase a juicer if you are going to make tomato sauce, beet juice, apple or pear sauce, etc.
- If you are going to do canning, purchase a good large pressure canner. This does not need to be stainless steel because the food will not touch it directly. I like my aluminum pressure canner which is tall enough to hold one layer of quarts or two layers of pints.
- Some large stainless steel kettles for washing large amounts of food, blanching tomatoes and removing the skins, or cooking beets are essential.
- Another good helpful tool to have is a spare refrigerator. Some people have one in their basement or in their heated garage.

Follow Updated Procedures. Due to the recent development of lower-acidity tomato hybrids, the canning procedures for tomatoes have changed. If you have an older canning book, you will need to acquire the tomato update information (available from the Extension Service). The basic change with the tomato procedure involves adding some sort of acetic acid to your tomatoes. Citric acid is recommended in many of the available guidelines, however lemon juice is a better choice for those with *Candida* Related Complex. I use freshly squeezed lemon juice by squeezing several at a time and then freezing the juice so that I can thaw and use it when I am canning tomatoes. I use one tablespoon of lemon juice per one pint of tomatoes or tomato sauce. If your sauce is very, very thick (more like paste than thick juice), you may need to use an additional amount of lemon juice.

Start Simple. Concentrate on foods that are relatively quick and easy to process. For example, you simply wash green peppers; remove the seeds and inside membranes; cut them into strips or dice them; package; and place in freezer. Other vegetables such as zucchini and eggplant are also very easy to process. Simply peel, slice or dice, package, and place in freezer.

Include those foods that you cannot purchase locally or through the mail (especially through the winter). For me this list includes eggplant, parsnips, green pepper, peapods, zucchini, and asparagus.

Individually Quick Freeze. One method I use when freezing several foods such as green peppers, zucchini, eggplant, peapods, asparagus, broccoli, cauliflower, and parsnips is to freeze them in single layers on baking sheets so that they are individually frozen. After freezing, simply package in cellophane bags. By using this method, I can pour out just the amount I need to use and return the unused portion to the freezer. This is the type of freezing procedure used for vegetables such as corn or peas sold in plastic bags in the grocery store.

Blanching. To blanch you apply high heat and steam to vegetables for a short amount of time. You can use a steamer pan, steamer basket, or microwave to blanch vegetables. I prefer a steamer. Time varies depending on type of vegetable, size of vegetable, method used, amount blanched at one time, and to some degree personal preference.

Immediately following steaming time, place vegetables in ice water for about twice the amount of time that you applied heat. Drain. Freeze on baking sheets. After freezing, package and store in freezer until ready to cook them.

The blanching process stops the ripening of the vegetables to prevent them from acquiring a strong green grass-like taste. Most freezing charts will recommend blanching all vegetables including green peppers, zucchini, and eggplant. These are three vegetables for which I omit the blanching process without noticing any distorted flavor. You may have different tastes and may choose to blanch them.

Divide Process into Several Steps. Whenever possible, split big canning jobs into stages with rest breaks in between. My method for green beans is to:

1. Stem the green beans while relaxing in my recliner watching television.
2. Wash, drain, and put beans in a large kettle in spare refrigerator.
3. The next morning, rinse them one more time, fill jars, pour boiling water on them, adjust the lids, and start the pressure canning process.

This way I have broken the task into two or more steps and successfully preserved 20 pints of green beans without overexertion.

Do Small Amount Each Day. Some preserving, such as freezing beet juice, is a long messy project so I prefer to prepare and freeze my full year's supply in 1–2 days. (I hire help for this job.) However, with vegetables such as green peppers, zucchini, eggplant, peapods, and asparagus I prefer to freeze a small amount each day. These vegetables are easy to freeze and use very little equipment. (Special Note: I do blanch my peapods and asparagus before freezing.) Many times I can prepare these vegetables to blanch and/or freeze during other meal preparation. By freezing them on baking sheets, I can go back later and spend a little time packaging for the freezer. I can freeze in small amounts as they become available in the garden. Before I know it I have spent very little energy and very little noticeable time throughout the summer to have a storehouse of various vegetables in my freezer ready for easy use during the winter.

Sit Down Whenever Possible. To save my energy, I do as much of the process as possible while sitting down. For example, I sit in my recliner when I stem my green beans and edible pea pods.

Delegate. Hire someone or recruit family members to assist you. I have done this for the past few years and it has worked very well.

Estimate Needs. Study the recipes that you use often or want to prepare during the winter time. Think about how often you would want to prepare them and begin to work out how much of the individual food items you will need to preserve to do this.

You can begin this process with the fact that you are on a 4–day rotation. By dividing 365 days per year by 4, you will have 91 days on which you will eat Day 1 foods, 91 days on which you will eat Day 2 foods, etc. This helps me to determine the quantity of foods needed such as green beans. I usually consume 2–3 pints every 8 days (or 1–2 pints every 4 days). Also, I subtract the number of rotations that green beans are in season and can be prepared fresh.

Another estimating method may begin with the factor that you prepare a certain casserole, such as Millet or Quinoa Turkey Vegetable Stew, once a month. Reviewing the recipe, you will notice that you need 1 1/2 cups of sliced parsnips. By multiplying 1 1/2 cups by the number of times you anticipate making the recipe (12 times), you have the minimum amount of sliced parsnips you will want to put in your freezer for preparing these casseroles.

Sometimes estimating is difficult, especially when you learn to cook new foods or recipes during the year or find new favorite recipes. You may find that you need to cut back on the number of times you prepare the new dishes (e.g., every eight days instead of every four) so that you won't run short of the foods needed to prepare them.

As you begin using a rotational diet, you may need to cook "regular" foods for your family as well as cooking your own foods. Gradually, your family members may work with you and start eating more and more of the foods you prepare for yourself. This will add to the amount of foods you need to preserve for use throughout the year.

Do not expect your estimates to come out exactly right at the end of the year. It will take you a while to learn all of the different factors that influence the specific needs for you and your family. However, by at least attempting to make an estimate of the amounts you will need, you have a useful guideline for knowing how much to process and store. This will help you avoid running short of foods or preserving too much and having to discard some because of freezer burn.

Save Time, Money, and Energy. Canning and freezing may take you a little time in the summer or late fall, but later it will save you time, money, and energy. You will be able to fix several meals in the off-season much faster including pizza and spaghetti sauce, stews and casseroles, and stir fries. All of these things will help you make quick and easy meals and have more freedom in your time schedule.

In Conclusion

As a final thought, organic agriculture is not only important for you and for me, it is essential to the well-being of the earth and <u>all</u> the creatures of the air, land, and water. So the next time you consider purchasing one of those "picture perfect" vegetables that has been sprayed with chemicals multiple times to keep away the bugs, just remember—

IF THE BUGS WON'T EAT IT, WHY SHOULD YOU?

Don't wait for a crisis
to discover what is
important in your life.

BIBLIOGRAPHY

"About Amaranth." Pamphlet from Nu-World Amaranth, Inc., P.O. Box 2202, Naperville, IL 60567.

"About Amaranth—and Us." Pamphlet from Nu-World Amaranth, Inc., P.O. Box 2202, Naperville, IL 60567.

"Amaranth." Pamphlet from Nu-World Amaranth, Inc., P.O. Box 2202, Naperville, IL 60567.

"Amaranth—The Grain with a Future." Pamphlet from Nu-World Amaranth, Inc., P.O. Box 2202, Naperville, IL 60567.

Beaman, Chris. Flax Oil Recipe Booklet. Colorado Springs, CO: Omega Logic Books, 1988. *(Available from Allergy Resources, Inc., P.O. Box 888, 264 Brookridge, Palmer Lake, CO 80133.)*

Bell, Louise, M.Sc., R.P.Dt., Miriam Hoffer, R.P.Dt., and J. Richard Hamilton, M.D., F.R.C.P. "Recommendations for Foods of Questionable Acceptance for Patients with Celiac Disease," Journal of the Canadian Dietetic Association, 42, no. 2 (April 1981). Abstract. *(Available from The National Buckwheat Institute, P.O. Box 440, Penn Yan, NY 14527.)*

"Buckwheat Backgrounder." Pamphlet from The National Buckwheat Institute, P.O. Box 364, Penn Yan, NY 14527.

Burton, Gail. The *Candida* Control Cookbook. New York, NY: New American Library Books, a Division of Penguin Books USA, Inc., 1989.

Campbell, J.A., Ph.D. "Diet Therapy of Celiac Disease and *Dermatitis herpetiformis*," World Review Nutritional Dietetics, 51: 189-233. *(Available from The National Buckwheat Institute, P.O. Box 440, Penn Yan, NY 14527.)*

________. "Food for Celiacs," Journal of the Canadian Dietetic Association, 43, no 1 (January 1982). Abstract. *(Available from The National Buckwheat Institute, P.O. Box 440, Penn Yan, NY 14527.)*

Candida Albicans - Booklet of Reprints. San Diego, CA: Price-Pottenger Nutrition Foundation. *(Price-Pottenger Nutrition Foundation, P.O. Box 2614, LaMesa, CA 91943-2614)*

Chevalier, Denise (Ed.) Growing and Marketing Your Organic Produce. Iowa City, IA: Iowa Organic Growers and Buyers Association, P.O. Box 2935, Iowa City, IA 52244-2935.

Collier's Encyclopedia, 1963 ed. S.v. "Arrowroot," 2: 704.

Collier's Encyclopedia, 1963 ed. S.v. "Tapioca," 22: 66.

"Composting." Information sheet from Earth Day 1990, P.O. Box AA, Stanford, CA 94309.

Connolly, Pat and Associates of the Price-Pottenger Nutrition Foundation. The *Candida Albicans* Yeast-Free Cookbook. New Canaan, CT: Keats Publishing, Inc., 1985. *(Keats Publishing, Inc., 27 Pine Street [Box 876], New Canaan, CT 06840)*

"A Consumers Guide to Organically Grown Produce." Pamphlet from Albert's Organics, Inc., Los Angeles, CA.

Crook, William G., M.D. Chronic Fatigue Syndrome and the Yeast Connection. Jackson, TN: Professional Books, Inc., 1992. *(Professional Books, Inc., 681 Skyline Drive, Jackson, TN 38301)*

________. The Yeast Connection. New York, NY: Vintage Books, a Division of Random House, 1986. *(Available from Professional Books, Inc., 681 Skyline Drive, Jackson, TN 38301.)*

________ and Marjorie Hurt Jones, R.N. The Yeast Connection Cookbook. Jackson, TN: Professional Books, 1989. *(Professional Books, Inc., 681 Skyline Drive, Jackson, TN 38301)*

Dadd, Debra Lynn. Nontoxic, Natural, and Earthwise. Los Angeles, CA: Jeremy P. Tarcher, Inc., 1990.

Donovan, Ann, C.N. "Spelt." Colorado Springs, CO: By the author, 1991. *(Ann Donovan, C.N., 627 N. Weber, Colorado Springs, CO 80903)*

Dumke, Nicolette M. Allergy Cooking with Ease. Lancaster, PA: Starburst Publishers, 1992. *(Available from Allergy Adapt, Inc., 1877 Polk Avenue, Louisville, CO 80027.)*

________. "Stevia the Herbal Sweetener," Mastering Food Allergies, VI, no. 4, issue #54 (April 1991): 1. *(See Mastering Food Allergies address in Appendix D, Newsletter section.)*

Eibensteiner, Karl E. "Dinkle (Spelt) Rediscovered." Port Coquitlam, B.C., Canada: Lentia Enterprises, Ltd. *(Available from Nature Farm Foods, Inc., 328 E. Second Street, Sumner, IA 50674.)*

Erasmus, Udo. Fats and Oils. Vancouver, B.C., Canada: Alive Books, 1986.

"Flours." Information sheet from Blooming Prairie Warehouse, 2340 Heinz Road, Iowa City, IA 52240.

"Fresh Flax Oil." Pamphlet from Allergy Resources, Inc., P.O. Box 888, 264 Brookridge, Palmer Lake, CO 80133.

Friedman, Harold M., M.D., Robert E. Tortolani, M.D., John Glick, M.D., and Richard T. Burtis, M.D. "Spelt is Wheat," Allergy Proceedings, 15, no. 4 (July-August 1994): 217-218.

"From the Cradle of Civilization to Your Table in Only 6000 Years!" Information sheet from the Kamut® Association of North America, 295 Distribution Street, San Marcos, CA 92069 (September, 1992).

Fukuyasu, T., T. Oshida, and K. Ashida. "Effect of Oligosaccharides on Growth of Piglets and on Bacterial Flora, Putrefactive Substances and Volatile Fatty Acids in Their Feces," Bulletin of Animal Hygiene, 26 (1987): 15-22. Abstract. *(Copy available from Canary Connect, see Appendix G.)*

Futrell, Sue. "Farming Sustainably: Where Farmers and Producers Can Go for Answers," Blooming Prairie Prairie News, 2340 Heinz Road, Iowa City, IA 52240 (May/June 1992): A-97.

Golos, Natalie and Frances Golos Golbitz. Coping with Your Allergies. New York, NY: A Fireside Book, Published by Simon and Schuster, Inc., 1986.

________. If This Is Tuesday, It Must Be Chicken. New Canaan, CT: Keats Publishing, Inc., 1983. *(Keats Publishing, Inc., 27 Pine Street [Box 876], New Canaan, CT 06840)*

Golos, Natalie and William J. Rea, M.D. Success in the Clean Bedroom. Rochester, NY: Pinnacle Publishers, 1992.

Goulart, Frances Sheridan. Cooking with Carob: The Healthful Alternative to Chocolate. Charlotte, VT: Garden Way Associates, Inc., 1980. *(Garden Way Associates, Inc., Dept. F157, Charlotte, VT 05445)*

"Grains." Information sheet from Blooming Prairie Warehouse, 2340 Heinz Road, Iowa City, IA 52240.

Greenberg, Ron, M.D. and Angela Nori. Freedom from Allergy Cookbook. Vancouver, B.C., Canada: Blue Poppy Press, 1988.

Grimmett, Charlene. Beat the Yeast Cookbook. Aurora, IL: By the author, 1985. *(Charlene Grimmett, P.O. Box 1971, Aurora, IL 60507)*

Harris, Gardiner. "Low Stomach Acidity," Medical Nutrition (Spring 1989): 39-40.

Hayes, Stephanie, R.D. and Barbara Maynard, R.D. Rotational Bon Appetite! Dallas, TX: WJR and Associates, P.A. dba Environmental Health Center-Dallas, 1986. *(Environmental Health Center–Dallas, 8345 Walnut Hill Lane, Suite 205, Dallas, TX 75231)*

Hidaka, H., T. Eida, T. Takizawa, T. Tokunaga, and Y. Tahiro. "Effects of Fructooligosaccharides on Intestinal Flora and Human Health," *Bifidobacteria* Microflora, 5, no. 1 (1986): 37-50. Abstract. *(Copy available from Canary Connect, see Appendix G.)*

"A History of Buckwheat." Pamphlet from Birkett Mills, P.O. Box 440A, Penn Yan, NY 14527.

Hoff, Dena. "Why Organic?" Information sheet from Blooming Prairie Warehouse, 2340 Heinz Road, Iowa City, IA 52240.

"Honey: From Nature's Food Industry." Information packet from the National Honey Board, 421 21st Avenue, Suite #203, Longmont, CO 80501.

Hosoya, N., D. Dhorranintra, and H. Hidaka. "Utilization of [U-^{14}C] Fructooligosaccharides in Man as Energy Resources," Journal of Clinical Biochemical Nutrition, 5 (1988): 67-74. Abstract. *(Copy available from Canary Connect, see Appendix G.)*

"I Just Don't Have Time for Stress!" Perpetual calendar. Marshalltown, IA: Thoughtful Books Sta-Kris, Inc., 1991. *(Thoughtful Books Sta-Kris, Inc., P.O. Box 1131, Marshalltown, IA 50158)*

"IOFS: Iowans for Organic Food Standards." Pamphlet from Iowans for Organic Food Standards, P.O. Box 2935, Iowa City, IA 52244-2935.

Johnston, Ingeborg M., C.N., and James R. Johnston, Ph.D. Flaxseed (Linseed) Oil and the Power of Omega-3: How to Make Nature's Cholesterol Fighters Work for You. New Canaan, CT: A Good Health Guide, Keats Publishing, Inc., 1990. *(Keats Publishing, Inc., 27 Pine Street [Box 876], New Canaan, CT 06840)*

Jones, Marjorie Hurt, R.N. The Allergy Self-Help Cookbook. Emmaus, PA: Rodale Press, 1984. *(Available from MAST Enterprises, Inc., 2615 N. Fourth Street #616, Coeur d'Alene, ID 83814.)*

________. "Balance in Your Diet: Tough But Possible," Mastering Food Allergies, V, no. 9, issue #49 (October 1990): 1. *(See Mastering Food Allergies address in Appendix D, Newsletter section.)*

________. "Bean Cookery," Mastering Food Allergies, IV, no. 3, issue #33 (March 1989): 1.

________. "Between Us: Leavening Agents," Mastering Food Allergies, VII, no. 2, issue #62 (February 1992): 5.

________. "Buckwheat Basics: Rediscovering an Old Treasure," Mastering Food Allergies, VIII, no. 2, issue #72 (March-April 1993): 1.

________. "*Candida*—A Different Approach," Mastering Food Allergies, IV, no. 7, issue #37 (July-August 1989): 3.

________. "FOS—A 'Good for You' Sweetener," Mastering Food Allergies, VII, no. 10, issue #70 (November 1992): 1.

________. "Kamut®—Another Ancient Grain," Mastering Food Allergies, VII, no. 1, issue #61 (December-January 1992): 1.

________. "Leaky Gut: A Common Problem with Food Allergies," Mastering Food Allergies, VIII, no. 5, issue #75 (September-October, 1993): 1.

________. "New Foods and How to Use Them," The Human Ecologist, no. 52 (Winter 1991): 1. *(The Human Ecologist, P.O. Box 49126, Atlanta, GA 30359-1126)*

________. "Spelt, Wonderful Spelt," Mastering Food Allergies, V, no. 7, issue #47 (July-August 1990): 1.

________. "Superfood #5: Spelt," Mastering Food Allergies, V, no. 3, issue #43 (March 1990): 1.

________. Super Foods. Coeur d'Alene, ID: Mast Enterprises, Inc., 1990. *(Mast Enterprists, Inc., 2615 N. Fourth Street #616, Coeur d'Alene, ID 83814)*

Jordan, C.L., M.D. and Associates. "The Total Person: The Concept of Health-Chiropractic," Allergy Connections, 1, no. 4 (Winter 1992): 1. *(Allergy Connections, P.O. Box 154, Pewaukee, WI 53072)*

Kamen, Betty, Ph.D. "FOS: A Healthful Sweetener (No Kidding!)," Let's Live Magazine, 60, no. 10 (October 1992): 32-34. *(Let's Live Magazine, P.O. Box 74908, Los Angeles, CA 90004)*

Kamut®'s Effectiveness for People with Wheat Allergies Scientifically Confirmed. Press release from the Kamut® Association of America, 295 Distribution Street, San Marcos, CA 92069 (November 15, 1991).

Lee, William H., R.Ph., Ph.D. The Friendly Bacteria. New Canaan, CT: A Good Health Guide, Keats Publishing, Inc., 1988. *(Keats Publishing, Inc., 27 Pine Street [Box 876], New Canaan, CT 06840)*

Levin, Alan Scott, M.D. and Merla Zellerbach. The Type 1/Type 2 Allergy Relief Program. Los Angeles, CA: Jeremy P. Tarcher, Inc., 1983.

Mandell, Marshall, Ph.D. and Lynne Waller Scanlon. 5-Day Allergy Relief System. New York, NY: Pocket Books, a Division of Simon and Schuster, Inc., 1979.

"Manitok Wild Rice," Blooming Prairie Price Guide Supplement and Prairie News, 2340 Heinz Road, Iowa City, IA 52240 (November-December 1991): 70.

McCormick, Angela. "How to Start a Food Buying Club," Allergy Connections, 1, no. 3 (Fall 1991): 9. *(Allergy Connections, P.O. Box 154, Pewaukee, WI 53072)*

McKellar, R.C. and H.W. Modler. "Metabolism of Fructooligosaccharides by *Bifidobacterium sp.*," Applied Microbiology Biotechnology, 31 (1989): 537-541. Abstract. *(Copy available from Canary Connect, see Appendix G.)*

Meehan, Beth Ann. "Linus Pauling's Rehab," Discover Magazine, 14, no. I (January 1993): 54.

Mitsuoka, T. "*Bifidobacteria* and Their Role in Human Health," Journal of Industrial Microbiology, 6 (1990): 263-268. *(Copy available from Canary Connect, see Appendix G.)*

________. "Effects of Long-term Intake of Neosugar (Fructooligosaccharides) on Intestinal Flora and Serum Lipids," Proceedings of the 3rd Neosugar Conference, Tokyo (1986). Abstract. *(Copy available from Canary Connect, see Appendix G.)*

________, H. Hidaka, and T. Eida. "Effect of Fructooligosaccharides on Intestinal Microflora," Die Nahrung, 31, no. 5-6 (1987): 427-436. Abstract. *(Copy available from Canary Connect, see Appendix G.)*

Modler, H.W., R.C. McKellar, and M. Yaguchi. "*Bifidobacteria* and *Bifidogenic* Factors," Journal of Canadian Institute of Food Science and Technology, 21, no. 1 (1990): 29-41. *(Copy available from Canary Connect, see Appendix G.)*

Morse, Roger A., Ph.D. "Honey Fact Sheets." Information sheets from the National Honey Board, 420 21st Avenue, Suite #203, Longmont, CO 80501.

The New Encyclopaedia Britannica, 1990 ed. S.v. "Arrowroot," 1: 589.

The New Encyclopaedia Britannica, 1990 ed. S.v. "Tapioca," 11: 554.

The 1994 National Organic Directory: A Guide to Organic Information and Resources. Davis, CA: CAFF, 1994: 150–164. *(Community Alliance with Family Farmers, P.O. Box 464, Davis, CA 95617)*

"Nutritional Analysis of Kamut® Brand Grain." Information sheet from the Kamut® Association of North America, 295 Distribution Street, San Marco, CA 92069 (September, 1992).

Oku, T, T. Tkunaga, and N. Hosoya. "Nondigestibility of a New Sweetener, 'Neosugar', in the Rat," Journal of Nutrition, 114 (1984): 1574-1581. Abstract. *(Copy available from Canary Connect, see Appendix G.)*

"Organically Grown Food: Answers to Some Common Questions." Pamphlet from Organic Farms, Inc., 10714 Hanna Street, Beltsville, MD 20705.

"Organically Grown Wild Rice." Pamphlet from Manitok Wild Rice, P.O. Box 97, Callaway, MN 56521.

Perna, Peter J., Ph.D., Manager. "Fructooligosaccharides (FOS): An All Natural Food which Promotes *Bifidobacteria* and *Lactobacillus*." Broomfield, CO: Center for Applied Nutrition, ZeaGen, Inc., 530 Interlocken Boulevard, 80021. (Available from Canary Connect, see Appendix G.)

Phillips, Sheila. "Natural Foods Primer: Grains." Information sheet from Blooming Prairie Warehouse, 2340 Heinz Road, Iowa City, IA 52240.

________. "Oils." Information sheet from Blooming Prairie Warehouse, 2340 Heinz Road, Iowa City, IA 52240.

________. "Sweeteners." Information sheet from Blooming Prairie Warehouse, 2340 Heinz Road, Iowa City, IA 52240.

Pomeranz, Yeshajahu and George S. Robbins. "Amino Acid Composition of Buckwheat," Agricultural and Food Chemistry, 20, no. 2 (March/April 1972): 270. *(Available from The National Buckwheat Institute, P.O. Box 440, Penn Yan, NY 14527.)*

"Purity Farms Clarified Butter." Pamphlet from Purity Farms, Inc., 14635 Westcreek Road, Sedalia, CO 80135.

Randolph, Theron G., M.D. and Ralph W. Moss, Ph.D. An Alternative Approach to Allergies. New York, NY: Bantam Books, Inc., 1980.

Rinkel, Herbert John, Theron G. Randolph, and Michael Zeller. Food Allergy. Springfield, IL: Thomas, 1951.

Rockwell, Sally, Nutritionist. Coping with *Candida* Cookbook (Revised). Seattle, WA: By the author, 1986. *(Sally J. Rockwell, P.O. Box 31065, Seattle, WA 98103)*

Rogers, Sherry A., M.D. The E.I. Syndrome. Syracuse, NY: Prestige Publishers, 1986. *(Prestige Publishers, Box 3161, 3502 Brewerton Road, Syracuse, NY 13220)*

Saltzman, Joanne. Amazing Grains. Tiburon, CA: H.J. Kramer, Inc., 1990. *(H.J. Kramer, Inc., P.O. Box 1082, Tiburon, CA 94920)*

Sano, T. "Effect of Neosugar (Fructooligosaccharides) on Constipation, Intestinal Microflora and Gallbladder Contraction in Diabetics," Proceedings of the 3rd Neosugar Conference, Tokyo (1986). Abstract. *(Copy available from Canary Connect, see Appendix G.)*

Semon, Bruce, M.D., Ph.D. "Understanding the Yeast Problem," Allergy Connections, 1, no. 4 (Winter 1992): 8. *(Allergy Connections, P.O. Box 154, Pewaukee, WI 53072)*

Skerritt, J.H. "Molecular Comparison of Alcohol-Soluble Wheat and Buckwheat Proteins," Cereal Chemistry, 63, no. 4: 365-369. *(Available from The National Buckwheat Institute, P.O. Box 440, Penn Yan, NY 14527.)*

Spiegel, J.E., R. Rose, P. Karabell, V.H. Frankos, and D.F. Schmitt. "Safety and Benefits of Fructooligosaccharides as Food Ingredients," Food Technology (January 1994): 85-89. *(Copy available from Canary Connect, see Appendix G.)*

Springer, Jerry. Allergies - Making Kids Crazy. Interview with Doris Rapp, M.D. Air Date: December 17, 1992. 45 min., Multimedia Entertainment, Inc., 1994. Videocassette. *(Available from Video Archives, Inc., 41 Paoli Plaza #3D, Paoli, PA 19301.)*

"Stevia Rebaudiana." Information sheet from Allergy Resources, Inc., P.O. Box 888, 264 Brookridge, Palmer Lake, CO 80133.

Strehlow, Wighard, M.D. The Wonder Food Spelt. Konstanz, Germany: By the author, 1989. *(Available from Purity Foods, Inc., 2871 W. Jolly Road, Okemos, MI 48864.)*

Takahashi, Y. "Effects of Neosugar (Fructooligoaccharides) in the Chronic Renal-Failure Patient," Proceedings of the 3rd Neosugar Conference, Tokyo (1986). Abstract. *(Copy available from Canary Connect, see Appendix G.)*

"Thickeners and Binders for Non-Gluten Recipes." Information sheet from FoodCare, Inc., P.O. Box 40, Seymour, IL 61875. *(FoodCare is no longer in business.)*

Tokunaga, T, T. Oku, and N. Hosoya. "Utilization and Excretion of a New Sweetener, Fructooligosaccharides (Neosugar), in Rats," Journal of Nutrition, 119 (1989): 553-559. Abstract. *(Copy available from Canary Connect, see Appendix G.)*

Truss, C. Orian, M.D. The Missing Diagnosis. Birmingham, AL: By the author, 1982. *(The Missing Diagnosis, P.O. Box 26508, Birmingham, AL 35226)*

U.S. Department of Agriculture. Food Guide Pyramid: A Guide to Daily Food Choices. Washington, DC: Government Printing Office, 1992. (Provided by the Iowa State University Extension Service.)

Waters, Jim. "Why Organic Agriculture?" Information sheet from Blooming Prairie Warehouse, 2340 Heinz Road, Iowa City, IA 52240.

Webster's New Universal Unabridged Dictionary. Deluxe Second Edition. New York, NY: Simon and Schuster, 1983.

"What Is a Coop Food Buying Club?," An Organizers' Manual for Cooperative Food Buying Clubs. Iowa City, IA: Central States Cooperative: 2. *(Central States Cooperative, 2340 Heinz Road, Iowa City, IA 52240)*

Williams, C.H., S.W. Witherly, and R.K. Buddington. "Influence of Dietary Neosugar on Selected Bacterial Groups of the Human Faecal Flora," Microbial Ecology in Health and Disease, 7 (1994): (accepted for publication). *(Copy available from Canary Connect, see Appendix G.)*

Wood, Rebecca. "The Incredible 'New' Wheat," Men's Fitness, 5 (November 1989).

Yamashita, K., K. Kawai, and M. Itakura. "Effects of Fructo-oligosaccharides on Blood Glucose and Serum Lipids in Diabetic Subjects," Nutrition Research, 4 (1984): 961-966.9. *(Copy available from Canary Connect, see Appendix G.)*

Yunginger, John W., M.D. "Food Ingredient Labeling: How Many Ways Can Wheat Be Spelt?" Allergy Proceedings, 15, no. 4 (July-August 1994): 219-220.

APPENDIX A
FOOD FAMILIES

Foods are grouped into botanical families based on their biological origin. Each food family is assigned a name and a number for identification. List 1 provides an alphabetical listing of foods along with their assigned number. List 2 categorizes the same foods in numerical groupings called food families. These lists are used to construct a Rotary Diversified Diet. List 2 is especially helpful in enabling the reader to avoid eating foods from the same family group in a repetitive way. The lists also include nonedible plants because persons who are allergic to a weed or plant included in a family group may need to avoid foods in that family. For more information on how to use these lists to construct a Rotary Diversified Diet or to revise the diet contained in this cookbook, see Chapter 3—Rotational Diet.

These lists were compiled from various sources, which include the following books. (See bibliography for compete information regarding these books.)

Coping with Your Allergies by Golos and Golbitz
An Alternative Approach to Allergies by Randolph and Moss
Rotational Bon Appetite! by Hayes and Maynard
If This Is Tuesday, It Must Be Chicken by Golos and Golbitz

List 1: Food Families (Alphabetical)

A

81	abalone
80	absinthe
41	acacia (gum)
46	acerola
79	acorn squash
41	adzuki beans
1	agar agar
12	agave
98	albacore
41	alfalfa
1	Algae Family
63	allspice
40b	almond
11	*Aloe vera*
54	althea root
30	amaranth
12	Amaryllis Family
94	amberjack
86	American eel
64	American Ginseng
68	American persimmon
117	Amphibians
41	anasazi beans
85	anchovy
85	Anchovy Family
65	angelica
65	anise
38	annatto
136	antelope
40a	apple
73	apple mint
40b	apricot
47	arrowroot, Brazilian (tapioca)
9	arrowroot (*Colocasia*)
17	arrowroot, East Indian (*Curcuma*)
19	Arrowroot Family
13	arrowroot, Fiji (*Tacca*)
4	arrowroot, Florida (*Zamia*)
19	arrowroot (*Maranta* starch)
16	arrowroot (*Musa*)
18	arrowroot, Queensland
80	artichoke flour
80	artichoke, globe
80	artichoke, Jerusalem
9	Arum Family
11	asparagus
2	*Aspergillus*
34	avocado

B

C

65 celery
65 celery leaf
65 celery seed
80 celtuce
81 Cephalopod
9 ceriman
80 chamomile
52 champagne
28 chard
79 chayote
137 cheese, goat
137 cheese, milk
40b cherry
65 chervil
24 chestnut
73 chia seed
124 chicken
41 chickpea
67 chicle
80 chicory
80 chicory, witloof
74 chili pepper
36 Chinese cabbage
64 Chinese Ginseng
56 Chinese gooseberry
14 Chinese potato (yam)
79 Chinese preserving melon
7 Chinese water chestnut
24 chinquapin
11 chives
55 chocolate
111 chub
7 chufa
40b cider
34 cinnamon
2 citric acid
45 citron
6 citronella
45 Citrus Family (Rue)
81 clam
73 clary
63 clove
41 clover
81 cockle
55 cocoa
55 cocoa butter
8 coconut
8 coconut meal
8 coconut oil
79 cocozelle
87 cod (scrod)
87 Codfish Family
76 coffee
55 cola nut
36 collards
80 coltsfoot
36 colza shoots
71 comfrey
80 Composite Family
5 Conifer Family
65 coriander
6 corn
124 cornish hen
6 corn meal
6 corn oil
6 corn products
78 corn salad
6 cornstarch
6 corn sugar
6 corn syrup
80 costmary
54 cottonseed oil
41 coumarin
36 couve tronchuda
41 cowpea
82 crab
40a crabapple
66 cranberry
114 crappie
82 crayfish
52 cream of tartar
79 Crenshaw melon
96 croaker
96 Croaker Family
79 crookneck squash
82 Crustaceans
79 cucumber
65 cumin
36 curly cress
39 currant
79 cushaw squash
87 cusk
32 custard-apple
32 Custard-Apple Family
4 Cycad Family

D

103 dab
80 Dacopa beverage (dahlia)
80 dahlia (Dacopa beverage)
80 dandelion
9 dasheen
8 date
8 date sugar
135 deer
135 Deer Family
40c dewberry

T

List 2: Food Families (Numerical)

Plant

1 **Algae**
- agar-agar
- carrageen (Irish moss)
- dulse*
- kelp (seaweed)

2 **Fungi**
- baker's yeast ("Red Star")
- brewer's or nutritional yeast
- mold (in certain cheeses)
  - citric acid (*Aspergillus*)
- morel
- mushroom
- puffball
- truffle

3 **Horsetail Family,** *Equisetaceae*
- shavegrass (horsetail)*

4 **Cycad Family,** *Cycadaceae*
- Florida arrowroot (*Zamia*)

5 **Conifer Family,** *Coniferae*
- juniper (gin)*
- pine nut (piñon, pinyon)

6 **Grass Family,** *Gramineae*
- barley
  - malt
  - maltose
- bamboo shoots
- corn (mature)
  - corn meal
  - corn oil
  - cornstarch
  - corn sugar
  - corn syrup
  - hominy
  - hominy grits
  - popcorn
- Job's tears
- Kamut®
- lemon grass
  - citronella
- millet
- oat
  - oat bran
  - oatmeal
- rice
  - rice bran
  - rice flour
- rye
- sorghum grain
  - syrup
- spelt
- sugar cane
  - cane sugar
  - molasses
  - raw sugar
- sweet corn
- teff
- triticale
- wheat
  - bran
  - bulgur
  - flour
    - gluten
    - graham
    - patent
    - whole wheat
  - wheat germ
- wild rice

7 **Sedge Family,** *Cyperaceae*
- Chinese water chestnut
- chufa (groundnut)

8 **Palm Family,** *Palmaceae*
- coconut
  - coconut meal
  - coconut oil
- date
  - date sugar
- palm cabbage
- sago starch (*Metroxylon*)

9 **Arum Family,** *Araceae*
- ceriman (*Monstera*)
- dasheen (*Colocasia*)
  - arrowroot
- taro (*Colocasia*)
  - arrowroot
  - poi
- malanga (*Xanthosoma*)
- yautia (*Xanthosoma*)

10 **Pineapple Family,** *Bromeliaceae*
- pineapple

11 **Lily Family,** *Liliaceae*
- *Aloe vera*
- asparagus
- chives
- garlic
- leek

*One or more plant parts (leaf, root, seed, etc.) used as a beverage.

onion
ramp
sarsaparilla*
shallot
yucca (soap plant)

12 **Amaryllis Family,** *Amaryllidaceae*
agave
mescal, pulque, and tequila

13 **Tacca Family,** *Taccaceae*
Fiji arrowroot (*Tacca*)

14 **Yam Family,** *Dioscoreaceae*
Chinese potato (yam)
ñame (yampi)

15 **Iris Family,** *Iridaceae*
orris root (scent)
saffron (*Crocus*)

16 **Banana Family,** *Musaceae*
arrowroot (*Musa*)
banana
plantain

17 **Ginger Family,** *Zingiberaceae*
cardamon
East Indian arrowroot, (*Curcuma*)
ginger
tumeric

18 **Canna Family,** *Cannaceae*
Queensland arrowroot

19 **Arrowroot Family,** *Marantaceae*
arrowroot (*Maranta* starch)

20 **Orchid Family,** *Orchidaceae*
vanilla

21 **Pepper Family,** *Piperaceae*
peppercorn (*Piper*)
black pepper
white pepper

22 **Walnut Family,** *Juglandaceae*
black walnut
butternut
English walnut
heartnut
hickory nut
pecan

23 **Birch Family,** *Betulaceae*
filbert (hazelnut)
oil of birch (wintergreen)
(some wintergreen flavor is methyl salicylate)
xylitol

24 **Beech Family,** *Fagaceae*
chestnut
chinquapin

25 **Mulberry Family,** *Moraceae*
breadfruit
fig
hop*
mulberry

26 **Protea Family,** *Proteaceae*
macadamia (Queensland nut)

27 **Buckwheat Family,** *Polygonaceae*
buckwheat
garden sorrel
rhubarb
sea grape

28 **Goosefoot Family,** *Cheopodiaceae*
beet
chard
lamb's-quarters
quinoa
spinach
sugar beet
tampala

29 **Carpetweed Family,** *Aizoaceae*
New Zealand spinach

30 **Purslane Family,** *Portulacaceae*
amaranth
pigweed (purslane)

31 **Buttercup Family,** *Ranunculaceae*
golden seal*

32 **Custard-Apple Family,**
Annona species
custard-apple
papaw (pawpaw)

33 **Nutmeg Family,** *Myristicacae*
nutmeg
mace

*One or more plant parts (leaf, root, seed, etc.) used as a beverage.

34 Laurel Family, *Lauraceae*
- avocado
- bay leaf
- cassia bark
- cinnamon
- sassafras*
  - filé (powdered leaves)

35 Poppy Family, *Papaveraceae*
- poppyseed

36 Mustard Family, *Cruciferae*
- broccoli
- Brussels sprouts
- cabbage
- cauliflower
- Chinese cabbage
- collards
- colza shoots
- couve tronchuda
- curly cress
- horseradish
- kale
- kohlrabi
- mustard greens
- mustard seed
- radish
- rape
- canola oil
- rutabaga (swede)
- turnip and turnip greens
- upland cress
- watercress

37 Caper Family, *Capparidaceae*
- caper

38 Bixa Family, *Bixaceae*
- annatto (natural yellow dye)

39 Saxifrage Family, *Saxifragaceae*
- currant
- gooseberry

40 Rose Family, *Rosaceae*
- a. pomes
  - apple
    - cider
    - vinegar
    - pectin
  - crabapple
  - loquat
  - pear
  - quince
  - rosehips*
- b. *stone fruits*
  - almond
  - apricot
  - cherry
  - peach (nectarine)
  - plum (prune)
  - sloe
- c. *berries*
  - blackberry
    - boysenberry
    - dewberry
    - loganberry
    - longberry
    - youngberry
  - raspberry (leaf)*
    - black raspberry
    - red raspberry
    - purple raspberry
    - wineberry
  - strawberry (leaf)*
- d. herb
  - burnet (cucumber flavor)

41 Legume Family, *Leguminoseae*
- alfalfa (sprouts)*
- beans
  - adzuki
  - anasazi
  - black turtle
  - fava
  - lima
  - mung (sprouts)
  - navy
  - northern
  - pinto
  - string (kidney)
- black-eyed pea (cowpea)
- carob*
  - carob syrup
- chickpea (garbanzo)
- cloves
- fenugreek*
- garbanzo (chickpea)
- guar gum
- gum acacia
- gum tragacanth
- jicama
- kudzu (kuzu)
- lentil
- licorice*
- pea
- peanut
  - peanut oil
- red clover*

*One or more plant parts (leaf, root, seed, etc.) used as a beverage.

senna*
soybean
  lecithin
  soy flour
  soy grits
  soy milk
  soy oil
  tempeh
  tofu
tamarind
tonka bean
coumarin

42 **Oxalis Family**, *Oxalidaceae*
carambola
oxalis

43 **Nasturtium Family**, *Tropaeolaceae*
nasturtium

44 **Flax Family**, *Linacaea*
flaxseed*
linseed oil

45 **Rue (Citrus) Family**, *Rutaceae*
citron
grapefruit
kumquat
lemon
lime
murcot
orange
pummelo
tangelo
tangerine

46 **Malpighia Family**, *Malpighiaceae*
acerola (Barbados cherry)

47 **Spurge Family**, *Euphorbiaceae*
cassava or yuca (*Manihot*)
  cassava meal
  tapioca (Brazilian arrowroot)
castor bean
  castor oil

48 **Cashew Family**, *Anacardiaceae*
cashew
mango
pistachio
poison ivy
poison oak
poison sumac

49 **Holly Family**, *Aquifoliaceae*
maté (yerba maté)

50 **Maple Family**
maple sugar
maple syrup

51 **Soapberry Family**, *Sapindaceae*
litchi (lychee)

52 **Grape Family**, *Vitaceae*
grape
  brandy
  champagne
  cream of tartar
  dried "currant"
  raisin
  wine
  wine vinegar
muscadine

53 **Linden Family**, *Tiliaceae*
basswood (linden)*

54 **Mallow Family**, *Malvaceae*
althea root*
cottonseed oil
hibiscus (roselle)*
okra

55 **Sterculia Family**, *Sterculiaceae*
chocolate (cacao)*
cocoa*
  cocoa butter
cola nut

56 **Dillenia Family**, *Dilleniaceae*
Chinese gooseberry (kiwi berry)

57 **Tea Family**, *Theaceae*
tea*

58 **Passion Flower Family**, *Passifloraceae*
granadilla (passion fruit)

59 **Papaya Family**, *Caricaceae*
papaya

60 **Cactus Family**, *Cactaceae*
maguey (Aguamiel)
prickly pear

61 **Pomegranate Family**, *Puniceae*
pomegranate
  grenadine

62 **Sapucaya Family**, *Lecythidaceae*
Brazil nut
sapucaya nut (paradise nut)

*One or more plant parts (leaf, root, seed, etc.) used as a beverage.

63 Myrtle Family, *Myrtaceae*
- allspice (*Pimenta*)
- clove
- eucalyptus*
- guava

64 Ginseng Family, *Araliaceae*
- American Ginseng*
- Chinese Ginseng*

65 Carrot Family, *Umbelliferae*
- angelica
- anise
- caraway
- carrot
  - carrot syrup
- celeriac (celery root)
- celery
  - seed & leaf*
- chervil
- coriander
- cumin
- dill
  - dill seed
- fennel*
  - finocchio
    - Florence fennel
- gotu kola*
- lovage*
- parsley*
- parsnip
- sweet cecily

66 Heath Family, *Ericaceae*
- bearberry*
- blueberry*
- cranberry
- huckleberry*

67 Sapodilla Family, *Sapotaceae*
- chicle (chewing gum)

68 Ebony Family, *Ebonaceae*
- American persimmon
- kaki (Japanese persimmon)

69 Olive Family, *Oleaceae*
- olive (green or ripe)
  - olive oil

70 Morning-Glory Family, *Convolvulacea*
- sweet potato

71 Borage Family, *Boraginaceae* (Herbs)
- borage
- comfrey (leaf & root)*

72 Verbena Family, *Verbenaceae*
- lemon verbena*

73 Mint Family, *Labiatae* (Herbs)
- apple mint
- basil
- bergamot
- catnip*
- chia seed*
- clary
- dittany*
- horehound*
- hyssop*
- lavender
- lemon balm*
- marjoram
- oregano
- pennyroyal*
- peppermint*
- rosemary
- sage
- spearmint*
- summer savory
- thyme
- winter savory

74 Nightshade (Potato) Family, *Solanaceae*
- eggplant
- ground cherry
- pepino (melon pear)
- pepper (Capsicum)
  - bell, sweet (all colors)
  - cayenne (red)
  - chili
  - paprika
  - pimiento
- potato
- tobacco
- tomatillo
- tomato
- tree tomato

75 Pedalium Family, *Pedaliaceae*
- sesame seed
  - sesame oil
  - tahini

76 Madder Family, *Rubiaceae*
- coffee*
- woodruff

77 Honeysuckle Family, *Caprifoliaceae*
- elderberry
  - elderberry flowers

*One or more plant parts (leaf, root, seed, etc.) used as a beverage.

78 **Valerian Family,** *Valerianaceae*
- corn salad (fetticus)

79 **Gourd Family,** *Cucurbitaceae*
- chayote
- Chinese preserving melon
- cucumber
- gherkin
- loofah (*Luffa*) (vegetable sponge)
- muskmelons
  - cantaloupe
  - casaba
  - crenshaw
  - honeydew
  - Persian melon
- pumpkin
  - pumpkin seed & meal
- squashes
  - acorn
  - buttercup
  - butternut
  - Boston marrow
  - caserta
  - cocozelle
  - crookneck & straightneck
  - cushaw
  - golden nugget
  - Hubbard varieties
  - pattypan
  - turban
  - vegetable spaghetti
  - zucchini
- watermelon

80 **Composite Family,** *Compositae*
- absinthe
- boneset*
- burdock root*
- cardoon
- chamomile
- chicory*
- coltsfoot
- costmary
- dahlia (Dacopa beverage)
- dandelion
- endive
- escarole
- globe artichoke
- goldenrod*
- Jerusalem artichoke
  - artichoke flour
- lettuce
  - celtuce
- pyrethrum
- romaine
- safflower oil
- salsify (oyster plant)
- santolina (herb)
- scolymus (Spanish oyster plant)
- scorzonera
- southernwood
- stevia (sweet herb)
- sunflower
  - sunflower seed, meal, and oil
- tansy (herb)
- tarragon (herb)
- witloof chicory (French endive)
- wormwood (absinthe)
- yarrow*

Animal

81 ***Mollusks***
- Gastropods
  - abalone
  - snail
- Cephalopod
  - squid
- Pelecypods
  - clam
  - cockle
  - mussel
  - oyster
  - scallop

82 ***Crustaceans***
- crab
- crayfish
- lobster
- prawn
- shrimp

83 *Fishes* (*Saltwater*)

84 **Herring Family**
- menhaden
- pilchard (sardine)
- sea herring

85 **Anchovy Family**
- anchovy

86 **Eel Family**
- American eel

87 **Codfish Family**
- cod (scrod)
- cusk
- haddock
- hake
- pollack

*One or more plant parts (leaf, root, seed, etc.) used as a beverage.

88 Sea Catfish Family
ocean catfish

89 Mullet Family
mullet

90 Silverside Family
silverside (whitebait)

91 Sea Bass Family
grouper
sea bass

92 Tilefish Family
tilefish

93 Bluefish Family
bluefish

94 Jack Family
amberjack
pompano
yellow jack

95 Dolphin Family
dolphin

96 Croaker Family
croaker
drum
sea trout
silver perch
spot
weakfish (spotted sea trout)

97 Porgy Family
northern scup (porgy)

98 Mackerel Family
albacore
bonito
mackerel
skipjack
tuna

99 Marlin Family
marlin
sailfish

100 Swordfish Family
swordfish

101 Harvestfish Family
butterfish
harvestfish

102 Scorpionfish Family
rosefish (ocean perch)

103 Flounder Family
dab
flounder
halibut
plaice
sole
turbot

104 *Fishes (freshwater)*

104 Sturgeon Family
sturgeon (caviar)

105 Herring Family
shad (roe)

106 Salmon Family
salmon species
trout species

107 Whitefish Family
whitefish

108 Smelt Family
smelt

109 Pike Family
muskellunge
pickerel
pike

110 Sucker Family
buffalofish
sucker

111 Minnow Family
carp
chub

112 Catfish Family
catfish species

113 Bass Family
white perch
yellow bass

114 Sunfish Family
black bass species
sunfish species
  pumpkinseed
crappie

115 Perch Family
sauger
walleye
yellow perch

116 Croaker Family
freshwater drum

117 *Amphibians*

117 Frog Family
- frog (frogs' legs)

118 Reptiles

119 Snake Family
- rattlesnake

120 Turtle Family
- terrapin
- turtle species

121 Birds

121 Duck Family
- duck
  - eggs
- goose
  - eggs

122 Dove Family
- dove
- pigeon (squab)

123 Grouse Family
- ruffed grouse (partridge)

124 Pheasant Family
- chicken
  - eggs
- cornish hen
- peafowl
- pheasant
- quail

125 Guinea Fowl Family
- guinea fowl
  - eggs

126 Turkey Family
- turkey
  - eggs

127 Mammals

128 Opossum Family
- opossum

129 Hare Family
- rabbit

130 Squirrel Family
- squirrel

131 Whale Family
- whale

132 Bear Family
- bear

133 Horse Family
- horse

134 Swine Family
- hog (pork)
- bacon
- ham
- lard
- pork gelatin
- sausage
- scrapple

135 Deer Family
- caribou
- deer (venison)
- elk
- moose
- reindeer

136 Pronghorn Family
- antelope

137 Bovine Family
- beef cattle
  - beef
  - beef by-products
    - gelatin
    - oleomargarine
    - rennin (rennet)
    - sausage casings
    - suet
  - milk products
    - butter
    - cheese
    - ice cream
    - lactose
    - spray dried milk
    - yogurt
  - veal
- buffalo (bison)
- goat (kid)
  - cheese
  - ice cream
  - milk
- sheep (domestic)
  - lamb
  - mutton
  - Rocky Mountain sheep

Appendix B
Candida Questionnaire and Score Sheet*

This questionnaire lists factors in your medical history that promote the growth of the common yeast, *Candida Albicans* (Section A), and symptoms commonly found in individuals with yeast-connected illness (Sections B and C).

For each yes answer in Section A, circle the Point Score in that section. Total your score, and record it in the box at the end of the section. Then move on to Sections B and C, and score as directed.

Section A: History

		Point Score
1. Have you taken tetracyclines or other antibiotics for acne for 1 month (or longer)?		**35**
2. Have you at any time in your life taken "broad spectrum" antibiotics or other antibacterial medication for respiratory, urinary, or other infections for 2 months or longer, or in shorter courses 4 or more times in a 1-year period?		**35**
3. Have you taken a broad spectrum antibiotic drug—even in a single dose?		**6**
4. Have you, at any time in your life, been bothered by persistent prostatitis, vaginitis, or other problems affecting your reproductive organs?		**25**
5. Are you bothered by memory or concentration problems?		**20**
Do you sometimes feel spaced out?		**20**
6. Do you feel "sick all over" yet, in spite of visits to many different physicians, the causes haven't been found?		**20**
7. Have you been pregnant...	2 or more times?	**5**
	1 time?	**3**
8. Have you taken birth control pills...	For more than 2 years?	**15**
	For 6 months to 2 years?	**8**
9. Have you taken steroids orally, by injection or inhalation?	For more than 2 weeks?	**15**
	For 2 weeks or less?	**6**
10. Does exposure to perfumes, insecticides, fabric shop odors and other chemicals provoke...	Moderate to severe symptoms?	**20**
	Mild symptoms?	**5**
11. Does tobacco smoke really bother you?		**10**
12. Are your symptoms worse on damp, muggy days or in moldy places?		**20**
13. Have you had athlete's foot, ring worm, "jock itch," or other chronic fungous infections of the skin or nails? Have such infections been..	Severe or persistent?	**20**
	Mild to moderate?	**10**
14. Do you crave sugar?		**10**
	Total Score, Section A	

*Filling out and scoring this questionnaire should help you and your physician evaluate how Candida Albicans may be contributing to your health problems. Yet it will not provide an automatic yes or no answer. A comprehensive history and physical examination are important.

* Adapted by William G. Crook, M.D., from The Yeast Connection and used with his permission. (New York, NY: Vintage Books, a Division of Random House, 1986.)

Section B: Major Symptoms

For each of your symptoms, enter the appropriate number in the Point Score column:
If a symptom is **occasional or mild** . . . . 3 points
If a symptom is **frequent and/or moderately severe** . . . . 6 points
If a symptom is **severe and/or disabling** . . . . 9 points
Add total score and record it in the box at the end of this section.

	Point Score
1. Fatigue or lethargy	
2. Feeling of being "drained"	
3. Depression or manic depression	
4. Numbness, burning, or tingling	
5. Headache	
6. Muscle aches	
7. Muscle weakness or paralysis	
8. Pain and/or swelling in joints	
9. Abdominal pain	
10. Constipation and/or diarrhea	
11. Bloating, belching, or intestinal gas	
12. Troublesome vaginal burning, itching, or discharge	
13. Prostatitis	
14. Impotence	
15. Loss of sexual desire or feeling	
16. Endometriosis or infertility	
17. Cramps and/or other menstrual irregularities	
18. Premenstrual tension	
19. Attacks of anxiety or crying	
20. Cold hands or feet, low body temperature	
21. Hypothyroidism	
22. Shaking or irritable when hungry	
23. Cystitis or interstitial cystitis	
Total Score, Section B	

Section C: Other Symptoms*

For each of your symptoms, enter the appropriate number in the Point Score column:

If a symptom is **occasional or mild** . . . . 1 point
If a symptom is **frequent and/or moderately severe** . . . . 2 points
If a symptom is **severe and/or disabling** . . . . 3 points

Add total score and record it in the box at the end of this section.

	Point Score
1. Drowsiness, including inappropriate drowsiness	
2. Irritability or jitteryness	
3. Incoordination	
4. Frequent mood swings	
5. Insomnia	
6. Dizziness/loss of balance	
7. Pressure above ears...feeling of head swelling	
8. Sinus problems...tenderness of cheekbones or forehead	
9. Tendency to bruise easily	
10. Eczema, itching eyes	
11. Psoriasis	
12. Numbness, tingling	
13. Indigestion or heartburn	
14. Sensitivity to milk, wheat, corn, or other common foods	
15. Mucus in stools	
16. Rectal itching	
17. Dry mouth or throat	
18. Mouth rashes, including "white" tongue	
19. Bad breath	
20. Foot, hair, or body odor not relieved by washing	
21. Nasal congestion or post nasal drip	
22. Nasal itching	
23. Sore throat	
24. Laryngitis, loss of voice	
25. Cough or recurrent bronchitis	

(This section is continued on the next page.)

*While the symptoms in this section occur commonly in patients with yeast-connected illness, they also occur commonly in patients who do not have *Candida*.

Section C: Other Symptoms* (continued)

For each of your symptoms, enter the appropriate number in the Point Score column:

If a symptom is **occasional or mild** . . . . 1 point
If a symptom is **frequent and/or moderately severe** . . . . 2 points
If a symptom is **severe and/or disabling** . . . . 3 points

Add total score and record it in the box at the end of this section.

	Point Score
26. Pain or tightness in chest	
27. Wheezing or shortness of breath	
28. Urinary frequency or urgency	
29. Burning on urination	
30. Spots in front of eyes or erratic vision	
31. Burning or tearing eyes	
32. Recurrent infections or fluid in ears	
33. Ear pain or deafness	

Total Score, Section C	
Total Score, Section A	
Total Score, Section B	

GRAND TOTAL SCORE (Add totals from Sections A, B, and C)	

*While the symptoms in this section occur commonly in patients with yeast-connected illness, they also occur commonly in patients who do not have *Candida*.

The Grand Total Score will help you and your physician decide if your health problems are yeast-connected. Scores in women will run higher as 7 items in the questionnaire apply exclusively to women, while only 2 apply exclusively to men.

Yeast-connected health problems are almost certainly present in women with scores **over 180**, and in men with scores **over 140**.

Yeast-connected health problems are probably present in women with scores **over 120**, and in men with scores **over 90**.

Yeast-connected health problems are possibly present in women with scores **over 60**, and in men with scores **over 40**.

With scores of less than 60 in women and 40 in men, yeasts are less apt to cause health problems.

APPENDIX C
RESOURCES

This resource appendix is for the reader's information only. At publication date, to the best of our knowledge all of the companies listed in this appendix are reputable mail-order sources for the indicated products. As an individual, it is your responsibility to ask the appropriate questions to ensure that the products you order meet your specific needs. None of the listed companies have paid to be listed in this book. When you contact them for information or to place an order, please mention where you learned of their service.

The appendix is divided in the following four sections.

- Section 1: Resources for Food and Non-Food Products
- Section 2: Resource Guides
- Section 3: Resources for Personalized Assistance for Food Allergy and Rotational Diet Planning
- Section 4: Resources for Locating a Physician

Section 1: Resources for Food and Non-Food Products

This section contains two separate lists. List A: Products is divided into Food Products and Non-food Products listed in alphabetical order with the names of nationwide companies who supply the products by mail-order. List B: Addresses gives the name, address, and phone number of each company that is mentioned in List A.

List A: Products

Food Products

Adzuki beans, *organic*
Jaffe Brothers, Inc.
Gold Mine Natural Food Co.
Mountain Ark Trader

Agar-agar powder
Now Natural Foods

Almond butter, *organic*
Jaffe Brothers, Inc.
Allergy Resources
Walnut Acres Organic Farms

Almond oil, *organic*
Flora, Inc.

Almonds, *organic*
Allergy Resources
Jaffe Brothers, Inc.
Mountain Ark Trader

Amaranth flour
Nu-World Amaranth
Arrowhead Mills (*organic*)
Jaffe Brothers, Inc. (*organic*)
Now Natural Foods (*organic*)
Allergy Resources (*organic*)

Amaranth garden seed
Nu-World Amaranth
Seeds of Change (*organic*)

Amaranth, puffed
Nu-World Amaranth
Allergy Resources

Amaranth, whole seed
Nu-World Amaranth
Arrowhead Mills (*organic*)
Jaffe Brothers, Inc. (*organic*)
Now Natural Foods (*organic*)
Gold Mine Natural Food Co. (*organic*)
Mountain Ark Trader (*organic*)
Allergy Resources (*organic*)

Apple juice, *organic*
Jaffe Brothers, Inc.
Mountain Sun

Applesauce, *organic*
Mountain Ark Trader
Jaffe Brothers, Inc.

Arrowroot starch
Now Natural Foods
Mountain Ark Trader
Allergy Resources
Walnut Acres Organic Farms

Baking powder, Featherweight Brand
Ener-G Foods, Inc.

Barley flour, *organic*
Arrowhead Mills
Mountain Ark Trader
Allergy Resources

Barley, pearled, *organic*
Arrowhead Mills
Allergy Resources
Gold Mine Natural Food Co.
Mountain Ark Trader

Beans *(see individual listings)*
Adzuki beans
Black turtle beans
Garbanzo beans
Kidney beans
Lentils
Navy beans
Peas, green split
Pinto beans

Beef, *natural/organic*
Walnut Acres Organic Farms

Bits of Barley cereal
Arrowhead Mills

Black turtle beans, *organic*
Arrowhead Mills
Mountain Ark Trader
Gold Mine Natural Food Co.
Jaffe Brothers, Inc.
Allergy Resources

Brazil nuts
Jaffe Brothers, Inc.

Breads (see individual listings)
Kamut®, sourdough
Rice, yeast-free
Rye, sourdough
Spelt, sourdough

Brown rice products *(see Rice, brown)*

Buckwheat cereal, *Pocono brand*
Birkett Mills

Buckwheat flour, light & dark
Birkett Mills

Buckwheat groats, *organic*
Birkett Mills
Mountain Ark Trader
Gold Mine Natural Food Co.
Jaffe Brothers, Inc.
Allergy Resources

Buckwheat groats, roasted, *organic*
Birkett Mills,
(available in 4 granulations)
Arrowhead Mills
Gold Mine Natural Food Co.
Mountain Ark Trader
Allergy Resources

Buckwheat soba noodles, 100%, *organic*
Mountain Ark Trader
Gold Mine Natural Food Co.

Buffalo
D'Angelo Brother Products
Family Pride Meats
Czimer Foods, Inc.
Game Sales International, Inc.
Allergy Resources, canned (*organic*)

Butter *(see individual listings)*
Almond
Clarified (Ghee)
Sunflower

Canola oil, *organic*
Flora, Inc.
Gold Mine Natural Food Co.

Caraway seed
Frontier Herbs Cooperative

Carob chunks
Now Natural Foods
Allergy Resources

Carob powder
Mountain Ark Trader
Jaffe Brothers, Inc.
Heartland Foods

Cashews, raw
Now Natural Foods
Jaffe Brothers, Inc.

Chicken, *natural/organic*
D'Angelo Brother Products
Walnut Acres Organic Farms

Chickpea *(see Garbanzo)*

Citrus pectin
Now Natural Foods
Allergy Resources

Clarified butter (Ghee)
Allergy Resources

Cranberry juice
Walnut Acres Organic Farms

Dacopa (beverage from dahlia tubers)
An Ounce of Prevention
California Natural Products
Allergy Resources

Egg replacer, Ener-G brand
Ener-G Foods, Inc.

Exotic meats *(see Wild game)*

Extracts & flavorings, alcohol-free
Frontier Herbs Cooperative
An Ounce of Prevention

Filberts (hazelnuts), *organic*
Jaffe Brothers, Inc.

Flavorings *(see Extracts)*

Flaxseed, *organic*
Arrowhead Mills
Allergy Resources
Now Natural Foods

Flaxseed meal, *organic*
Allergy Resources
Now Natural Foods

Flaxseed oil, *organic*
Flora, Inc.
Gold Mine Natural Food Co.
Allergy Resources

Flours *(see also individual grains/nongrains or beans)*

Flours, freshly ground
Special Foods
Gold Mine Natural Food Co.
Allergy Resources

Fish/shellfish *(see Salmon, Shrimp, Tuna)*

FOS (Fructo-oligo saccharides)
Canary Connect

Garbanzo bean flour
Arrowhead Mills
Allergy Resources

Garbanzo beans (chickpea), *organic*
Mountain Ark Trader
Gold Mine Natural Food Co.
Allergy Resources
Jaffe Brothers, Inc.

Garlic *(some organic)*
Walnut Acres Organic Farms
Watkins
Frontier Herbs Cooperative

Ghee *(see Clarified butter)*

Green split peas *(see Peas, green split)*

Guar gum
Now Natural Foods
Allergy Resources

Hazelnuts *(see Filberts)*

Herbs & spices
Walnut Acres Organic Farms
Frontier Herbs Cooperative
Watkins
Heartland Foods

Honey
Walnut Acres Organic Farms

Jam/jelly, all fruit spreads
Walnut Acres Organic Farms
Mountain Ark Trader

Jerusalem artichoke flour
Now Natural Foods
Allergy Resources

Kamut® bread, sourdough, *organic*
Nokomis

Kamut® flakes, quick cooking, *organic*
Allergy Resources

Kamut® flour, *organic*
Arrowhead Mills
Jaffe Brothers, Inc.
Allergy Resources

Kamut® grain, *organic*
Arrowhead Mills
Mountain Ark Trader
Gold Mine Natural Food Co.
Jaffe Brothers, Inc.
Allergy Resources

Kamut® pasta, *organic*
Mountain Ark Trader
Gold Mine Natural Food Co.
Allergy Resources

Kamut®, puffed, *organic*
Arrowhead Mills

Kasha *(see Buckwheat, roasted)*

Kidney beans, *organic*
Arrowhead Mills
Jaffe Brothers, Inc.
Gold Mine Natural Food Co.
Mountain Ark Trader
Allergy Resources

Kombu
Gold Mine Natural Food Co.
Mountain Ark Trader

Kudzu (Kuzu)
Gold Mine Natural Food Co. (*organic*)
Mountain Ark Trader
Allergy Resources

Lamb, organic
Game Sales International, Inc.
Walnut Acres Organic Farms

Lemonade, Mountain Sun brand, *organic*
Mountain Sun

Lentils, *organic*
Arrowhead Mills
Mountain Ark Trader
Gold Mine Natural Food Co.
Jaffe Brothers, Inc.
Allergy Resources

Macadamia nuts, *organic*
Jaffe Brothers, Inc.

Maple granules
Walnut Acres Organic Farms (*organic*)
Jaffe Brothers, Inc. (*organic*)
Allergy Resources

Meats *(see individual listings)*
Beef
Buffalo
Chicken
Lamb
Pheasant
Rabbit
Turkey
Venison
Wild game and exotic meats

Millet, hulled, *organic*
Arrowhead Mills
Now Natural Foods
Gold Mine Natural Food Co.
Mountain Ark Trader
Jaffe Brothers, Inc.
Allergy Resources

Millet, puffed
Arrowhead Mills

Navy bean flour
Allergy Resources

Navy beans, *organic*
Allergy Resources
Gold Mine Natural Food Co.
Jaffe Brothers, Inc.

Nuts *(see individual listings)*
Almonds
Brazil nuts
Cashews
Filberts
Macadamia nuts
Pecans
Walnuts

Oat bran, *organic*
Allergy Resources
Jaffe Brothers, Inc.

Oat flour, *organic*
Arrowhead Mills
Allergy Resources

Oats, old fashioned rolled, *organic*
Walnut Acres Organic Farms
Gold Mine Natural Food Co.
Jaffe Brothers, Inc.

Oil *(see individual listings)*
Almond
Canola
Olive
Safflower
Sesame
Sunflower
Walnut

Olive oil, *organic*
Flora, Inc.
Gold Mine Natural Food Co.

Orsa real salt
Allergy Resources

Pastry poppers, wheat-free
Mountain Ark Trader
Heartland Foods

Pau D'Arco tea (Argentinian La Pacho/Taheebo Bark)
Allergy Resources

Peas, green split, *organic*
Arrowhead Mills
Gold Mine Natural Food Co.
Mountain Ark Trader
Jaffe Brothers, Inc.

Pecans, *organic*
Jaffe Brothers, Inc.

Pheasant
Czimer Foods, Inc.
Games Sales International, Inc.

Pinto beans, *organic*
Arrowhead Mills
Mountain Ark Trader
Gold Mine Natural Food Co.
Allergy Resources
Jaffe Brothers, Inc.

Potato starch flour
Now Natural Foods
Mountain Ark Trader
Heartland Foods

Poultry *(see Chicken, Pheasant, and Turkey))*

Produce, organic *(mail-order)*
Diamond Organics
Mountain People's Warehouse
Walnut Acres Organic Farms
Your area food-buying cooperative warehouse (See Appendix E)

Pumpkin seeds
Mountain Ark Trader
Gold Mine Natural Food Co.
Jaffe Brothers, Inc.

Quinoa flour, *organic*
Quinoa Corporation
Allergy Resources

Quinoa pasta *(also contains corn & sesame)*
Quinoa Corporation
Allergy Resources

Quinoa, whole seed, *organic*
Quinoa Corporation
Arrowhead Mills
Now Natural Foods
Mountain Ark Trader
Allergy Resources
Gold Mine Natural Food Co.
Jaffe Brothers, Inc.

Rabbit
D'Angelo Brother Products
Game Sales International, Inc.

Rice & Shine Cereal
Arrowhead Mills

Rice Dream Beverage, Original-Lite
Mountain Ark Trader (*organic*)

Rice bread, yeast-free
Allergy Resources
Ener-G Foods, Inc.

Rice, brown basmati, *organic*
Mountain Ark Trader
Gold Mine Natural Food Co.
Walnut Acres Organic Farms

Rice cakes, *organic*
Mountain Ark Trader

Rice cereal, brown, *organic*
Walnut Acres Organic Farms

Rice—Creamy Rice™ Cereal
Lundberg Family Farms

Rice—Organic Brown Rice Crunchies
Lundberg Family Farms

Rice flakes, brown, *organic*
Allergy Resources

Rice flour, brown, *organic*
Arrowhead Mills
Now Natural Foods
Mountain Ark Trader
Jaffe Brothers, Inc.
Allergy Resources

Rice, long-grain, brown, *organic*
Arrowhead Mills
Mountain Ark Trader
Gold Mine Natural Food Co.
Walnut Acres Organic Farms
Jaffe Brothers, Inc.

Rice, medium-grain, brown, *organic*
Arrowhead Mills
Mountain Ark Trader
Gold Mine Natural Food Co.

Rice, short-grain, brown, *organic*
Arrowhead Mills
Mountain Ark Trader
Gold Mine Natural Food Co.
Walnut Acres Organic Farms
Jaffe Brothers, Inc.

Rice pasta
Jaffe Brothers, Inc. (*brown, organic)*
Allergy Resources
Mountain Ark Trader

Rice, puffed
Arrowhead Mills

Rice syrup, brown, *organic*
Lundberg Family Farms
Mountain Ark Trader

Rice, white basmati, *organic*
Arrowhead Mills
Gold Mine Natural Food Co.
Jaffe Brothers, Inc.
Mountain Ark Trader

Rock salt (*see Orsa real salt*)

Rye bread, sourdough, yeast-free
Allergy Resources
Nokomis

Rye pasta
Allergy Resources

Safflower oil, *organic*
Flora, Inc.

Salmon *(packed in glass jars)*
Chuck's Seafood Products
(sold by 12/case)
Canary Connect
(Chuck's brand, sold by individual jar)
Walnut Acres Organic Farms

Salt *(see Orsa real salt and Sea salt)*

Salsa Seasoning Blend, Watkins brand
Watkins (product number 1401)

Sea salt
Gold Mine Natural Food Co.
Mountain Ark Trader

Seeds *(see individual listings)*
Caraway
Flax
Pumpkin
Sesame
Sunflower

Sesame oil, *organic*
Flora, Inc.
Gold Mine Natural Food Co.

Sesame seeds, *organic*
Arrowhead Mills
Gold Mine Natural Food Co.
Mountain Ark Trader
Jaffe Brothers, Inc.

Shrimp
Schwan's Sales Enterprises
(Seafarer's Choice medium peeled and deveined shrimp.)

Soy Quick, Ener-G brand Pure
Ener-G Foods, Inc.

Soy, flour (also other soy products)
Arrowhead Mills
Now Natural Foods (*organic*)

Spelt bread, sourdough, *organic*
Nokomis
Allergy Resources
Mountain Ark Trader

Spelt flakes, quick cooking, *organic*
Allergy Resources

Spelt flour, *organic*
Arrowhead Mills
Allergy Resources
Brumwell Flour Mill, Inc.
Mountain Ark Trader

Spelt grain, *organic*
Mountain Ark Trader
Gold Mine Natural Food Co.
Allergy Resources
Jaffe Brothers, Inc.

Spelt pasta, *organic*
Allergy Resources
Mountain Ark Trader

Spices *(see Herbs)*

Starches *(see individual listings)*
Arrowroot
Kudzu (Kuzu)
Potato
Tapioca

Stevia, white powder concentrate
Body Ecology Diet

Sunflower oil, *organic*
Flora, Inc.

Sunflower seeds, raw
Arrowhead Mills
Gold Mine Natural Food Co. *(organic)*
Mountain Ark Trader *(organic)*
Now Natural Foods *(organic)*

Tahini, *organic*
Arrowhead Mills
Walnut Acres Organic Farms
Mountain Ark Trader
Jaffe Brothers, Inc.

Tapioca starch flour
Now Natural Foods
Allergy Resources

Teff grain, brown and ivory
The Teff Company
Arrowhead Mills *(brown only)*
Gold Mine Natural Food Co.
Mountain Ark Trader

Teff flour, brown and ivory
The Teff Company
Arrowhead Mills *(brown only)*

Tomato products, Muir Glen, *organic*
Mountain Ark Trader

Tuna *(packed in glass jars)*
Chuck's Seafood Products
(sold by 12/case)
Canary Connect
(Chuck's brand, sold by individual jar)
Walnut Acres Organic Farms

Turkey
D'Angelo Brother Products

Venison
D'Angelo Brother Products
Czimer Foods, Inc.

Vitamin C crystals, unbuffered, corn-free (use with baking soda for leavening and to replace vinegar in salad dressings)
Freeda Vitamins (product #0150)
Bronson Pharmaceuticals (product #49)
An Ounce of Prevention (Vital Life Brand)

Walnut oil, *organic*
Flora, Inc.

Walnuts, *organic*
Jaffe Brothers, Inc.
Allergy Resources

Wild game and exotic meat
D'Angelo Brother Products
Czimer Foods, Inc.
Family Pride Meats
Game Sales International, Inc.

Wild rice, *organic*
Gold Mine Natural Food Co.
Walnut Acres Organic Farms
Jaffe Brothers, Inc.

Wild-rice pasta, *organic*
Allergy Resources

Non-food Products

Books
Allergy Alternative
Allergy Resources
The Cotton Place
E.L. Foust Co., Inc.
Environment Health Shopper™
Gold Mine Natural Foods Co.
Mountain Ark Trader

Cellophane bags
Pak-Sel
Janice Corporation
The Living Source
Seventh Generation

Cookware, stainless steel
Saladmaster
Estia Corporation
Walnut Acres Organic Farms
Gold Mine Natural Food Co.
Miracle Exclusives, Inc.
Mountain Ark Trader

Filtered water systems
R. H. of Texas
An Ounce of Prevention
N.E.E.D.S.
Nigra Enterprises

Food supplements
Allergy Alternative
An Ounce of Prevention
Canary Connect (FOS)
Freeda Vitamins
Klaire Laboratories, Inc.
N.E.E.D.S.
The Living Source

Garden seeds, *organic*
Seeds of Change

Granny's Old Fashioned Products
(household and personal care products)
Canary Connect

Juicer, Champion
Pak-Sel

Knives (cutlery)
Cutco Cutlery Corporation

List B: Addresses

Arrowhead Mills
P.O. Box 2059
Hereford, TX 79045
(800) 749-0730
FAX (806) 364-8242
(Product list available.)

Allergy Alternative
440 Godfrey Drive
Windsor, CA 95492
(707) 838-1514
Orders: 1-800-838-1514
(Catalog available.)

Allergy Resources
P.O. Box 888
264 Brookridge
Palmer Lake, CO 80133
Order line: (800) 873-3529
Customer service line: (719) 488–3630
FAX: (719) 481-3737
(Catalog available.)

An Ounce of Prevention
8200 E. Phillips Place
Englewood, CO 80112
(303) 770-8808
(Products for the chemically sensitive, catalog available, personal attention.)

Birkett Mills
P.O. Box 440A
Penn Yan, NY 14527
(315) 536-3311
(Product list available.)

Body Ecology Diet
1266 W. Paces Ferry Road
Suite 505-B
Atlanta, GA 30327
(404) 352-8048
FAX: (404) 352-3409

Bronson Pharmaceuticals
1945 Craig Road
St. Louis, MO 63146
1-800-235-3200

Brumwell Flour Mill, Inc.
328 East 2nd Street
Sumner, IA 50674
(319) 578-8106
FAX: (319) 578-3207
(Product list available.)

California Natural Products
P.O. Box 1219
Lathrop, CA 95330
(209) 858-2525

Canary Connect
P.O. Box 5317
Coralville, IA 52241–0317
(319) 351-2317
FAX: (319) 351-2317
(See Appendix G for more details.)

Chuck's Seafood Products
P.O. Box 5488
Charleston, OR 97420–0613
(503) 888-4600
FAX: (503) 888-2121
(Product list available.)

The Cotton Place
P.O. Box 59721
Dallas, TX 75229
Local: (214) 243-4149
Outside Dallas area: 1-800-451-8866
(Catalog available.)

Cutco Cutlery Corporation
1116 East State Street
Olean, NY 14760
1-800-828-0448

Czimer Foods, Inc.
13136 W. 159th Street
Lockport, IL 60441
(708) 301-0500
(Several exotic meats including buffalo, venison, quail, pheasant, duck. Grass-fed animals, no antibiotics or steriods. Product list available.)

D'Angelo Brother Products
909 South 9th Street
Philadelphia, PA 19147
(215) 923-5637
(Widest selection—50 or more—of organic farm feed exotic animals including buffalo, venison, rabbit, goose, wild turkey, ostrich, moose. No antibiotics or steriods, not hunted. Free-range. Quality care! Product list available.)

Diamond Organics
P.O. Box 2159
Freedom, CA 95019
1-800-922-2396
(Product list available.)

E.L. Foust Co. , Inc.
P.O. Box 105
Elmhurst, IL 60126
Illinois: (312) 834-4952
Outside Illinois: 1-800-225-9549
(Catalog available.)

Ener-G Foods, Inc.
P.O. Box 84487
Seattle, WA 98124–5787
1-800-331-5222
In WA state 1-800-325-9788
(Contact your local health-food stores or the above address for Ener-G brand bread and baking products.)

Environmental Health Shopper™
P.O. Box 239
Fate, TX 75132
1-800-447-1100
(Catalog available.)

Estia Corporation
155 Park Avenue
Lyndhurst, NJ 07071
(201) 939-7077
(Catalog available.)

Family Pride Meats
19 Main Street
Ipswich, SD 57451
(605) 426-6343 or
(605) 426-6288
(Buffalo with no antibiotics or steriods. Also ask about availability of other exotic meats. Product list available.)

Flora, Inc.
Box 950
East Badger Road
Lynden, WA 98264
1-800-446-2110
FAX: (206) 354-5355
(Product list available.)

Freeda Vitamins
36 E. 41st Street
New York, NY 10017
In NY state: (212) 685-4980
Out of NY state: 1-800-777-3737
(Catalog available.)

Frontier Herbs Cooperative
3021 78th Street
P.O. Box 299
Norway, IA 52318
1-800-786-1388
(Catalog available.)

Game Sales International, Inc.
P.O. Box 5314
444 Washington Street
Loveland, CO 80538
Local (303) 667-4090
1-800-729-2090
(Exotic animals including buffalo, venison, rabbit, pheasant, duck, partridge. Product list available.)

Gold Mine Natural Food Co.
3419 Hancock Street
San Diego, CA 92110–4307
Order line: (800) 475-3663
Customer service line: (619) 296-8536
FAX: (619) 296-9756
(Catalog available.)

Heartland Foods
Lucy Wilson Sherman
R.R. 2 Box 189-B
Susquehanna, PA 18847
(717) 879-8790
(Catalog available.)

Jaffe Brothers, Inc.
P.O. Box 636
Valley Center, CA 92082–0636
(619) 749-1133
FAX: (619) 749-1282
(Catalog available.)

Janice Corporation
198 US Highway 46
Budd Lake, NJ 07828–3001
1-800-526-4237
(Catalog available.)

Klaire Laboratories, Inc.
1573 West Seminole
San Marcos, CA 92069
(619) 744-9680
(Catalog available.)

The Living Source
3500 MacArthur Drive
Waco, TX 76708
(817) 756-6341
(Catalog available.)

Lundberg Family Farms
P.O. Box 369
Richvale, CA 95974
(916) 882-4551
(Product list available.)

Miracle Exclusives, Inc.
3 Elm Street
P.O. Box 349
Locust Valley, NY 11560
(516) 676-0220
1-800-645-6360
FAX: (516) 671-2774
(Catalog available.)

Mountain Ark Trader Co.
P.O. Box 3170
Fayetteville, AR 72702
1-800-643-8909
(Catalog available.)

Mountain People's Warehouse
110 Springhill Drive
Grass Valley, CA 95945
1-800-679-8735
(Product list available.)

Mountain Sun
18390 Hwy 145
Delores, CO 81323
(303) 882-2283
(Ask for your geographic distributor.)

N.E.E.D.S.
527 Charles Avenue 12-A
Syracuse, NY 13209
1-800-634-1380
FAX: 1-800-295-NEED (6333)
(Catalog available.)

Nigra Enterprises
5699 Kanan Road
Agoura, CA 91301
(818) 889-6877

Nokomis
W2 495 County Road E.S.
East Troy, WI 53120
1-800-367-0358
(Request information packet.)

Now Natural Foods
550 Mitchell Road
Glendale Heights, IL 60139
(708) 545-9000
FAX: (708) 545-9075
(Catalog available.)

Nu-World Amaranth, Inc.
Attention: Larry Waters
P.O. Box 2202
Naperville, Illinois 60567
(708) 369-6819
(Product list available.)

Pak Sel
7524 S.W. Macadam Avenue
Portland, Oregon 97219
1-800-635-BAGS (2247)
(503) 244-9661
(Product list available.)

Quinoa Corporation
P.O. 1039
Torrance, California 90505
(310) 530-8666

R. H. of Texas
Box 780392
Dallas, TX 75378
(214) 351-6681
(Specializes in designing water purification systems for the chemically sensitive.)

Saladmaster International Headquarters
912 113th Street
Arlington, TX 76011
(817) 633-3555

Schwan's Sales Enterprises
Corporate Office *(home delivery company)*
115 W. College Drive
Marshall, MN 56258
1-800-533-5290
(Quality assurance extension #8144.)

Seeds of Change
P.O. Box 15700
Santa Fe, NM 87506–5700
(505) 438-8080
(Catalog available.)

Seventh Generation
Colchester, VT 05446–1672
(800) 456-1177
(Catalog available.)

Special Foods
9207 Shotgun Court
Springfield, VA 22153
(703) 644-0991
(Very specialized flours, baking powders, baked products, pastas, and lip balms. Ask for product list.)

The Teff Company
P. O. Box A
Caldwell, Idaho 83606
(208) 454-3330
(Product list available.)

Walnut Acres Organic Farms
Penns Creek, PA 17862
1-800-433-3998
(Catalog available.)

Watkins, Inc.
P. O. 5570
Winona, MN 55987-0570
Credit card order: 1-800-247-5907
FAX: (507) 452-6723
ID Number 00201
(Catalog available.)

This space is available to write in other resource companies that you use. Please write me about additional companies and what you purchase from them so I may share the information with others through Canary Connect News newsletter (see AppendixG).

Section 2: Resource Guides

This section gives four guides/books that I recommend you acquire for additional resources on locating organic food, clothing, bedding, cleaning products, and more for the chemically sensitive and environmentally aware.

Consumer's Organic Mail-order Directory
Published by California Action Network
P.O. Box 464
Davis, CA 95617
(916) 756-8518
FAX: (916) 756-7857

Home Grown Green
Rich Kimball
105 Franklin
Roseville, CA 95678
(916) 773-5751
Resource directory for environment/health. Published quarterly. For latest prices, quotes, info, contact Rich Kimball at above address.
(Reasonable price, good value.)

Highways to Health
The S.T.A.T.E. Foundation
(Sensitive to a Toxic Environment)
P.O. Box 834
Orchard Park, NY 14127
(716) 675-1164
Donations very helpful.

Nontoxic, Natural, and Earthwise: How to Protect Yourself and Your Family from Harmful Products and Live in Harmony with the Earth.
Book by Debra Lynn Dadd in collaboration with Steve Lett and Judy Collins. Los Angeles, CA: Jeremy P. Tarcher, Inc., 1990. Contains an excellent resource section.

Section 3: Resources for Personalized Assistance for Food Allergy and Rotational Diet Planning

This section lists resources which offer personalized assistance in rotational diet planning and specialized recipes.

Allerdiet, Inc.
Mary Beth Hughes
4903 Creek Shadows
Kingwood, TX 77339
(713) 360-6655
(Also has computer software for rotational diets available for use by physicians and/or labatories.)

Immuno Laboratories
1620 W. Oakland Park Blvd.
Ft. Lauderdale, FL 33311
(305) 486-4500
1-800-231-9197
FAX (305) 739-6563

Allergy Adapt, Inc.
Nicolette Dumke
1877 Polk Avenue
Louisville, CO 80027
(303) 666-8253

Canary Connect
P. O. Box 5317
Coralville, IA 52241-0317
(319) 351-2317
(See Appendix G for more information on how to receive help with specialized recipes.)

* *

Section 4: Resources for Locating a Physician

The following sources may be contacted for information on physicians who treat CRC in your geographical area. These organizations may require a small monetary donation for their list. Also, for the fastest service, I would suggest you include a #10, self-addressed, stamped envelope with your request.

Price-Pottenger Nutrition Foundation (PPNF)
P.O. Box 2614
LaMesa, CA 91943–2614
Enclose a $6 donation.

Human Ecology Action League (HEAL)
P.O. Box 49126
Atlanta, GA 30359–1126
(Also, an excellent resource for local HEAL support groups. Donations very helpful.)

American Academy of Environmental Medicine
P.O. Box 16106
Denver, Colorado 80216
Enclose a $5 donation and state the geographic area in which you are interested.

World Research Foundation
15300 Ventura Blvd. #405
Sherman Oak, CA 91403
(818) 907-5483
(Donations very helpful.)

APPENDIX D
RECOMMENDED READING

Books

Candida Albicans - Booklet of Reprints. San Diego, CA: Price-Pottenger Nutrition Foundation. *(Price-Pottenger Nutrition Foundation, P.O. Box 2614, LaMesa, CA 91943-2614)*

Crook, William G., M.D. Chronic Fatigue Syndrome and the Yeast Connection. Jackson, TN: Professional Books, Inc., 1992. *(Professional Books, Inc., 681 Skyline Drive, Jackson, TN 38301)*

________. Detecting Your Hidden Allergies. Jackson, TN: Professional Books, Inc., 1988. *(Professional Books, Inc., 681 Skyline Drive, Jackson, TN 38301)*

________. The Yeast Connection. New York, NY: Vintage Books, a Division of Random House, 1986. *(Professional Books, Inc., 681 Skyline Drive, Jackson, TN 38301)*

________ and Marjorie Hurt Jones, R.N. The Yeast Connection Cookbook. Jackson, TN: Professional Books, 1989. *(Available from Professional Books, Inc., 681 Skyline Drive, Jackson, TN 38301 or Mast Enterprises, Inc., 2615 N. Fourth Street #616, Coeur d'Alene, ID 83814.)*

Dadd, Debra Lynn. Nontoxic, Natural, and Earthwise. Los Angeles, CA: Jeremy P. Tarcher, Inc., 1990.

"Fresh Flax Oil." Pamphlet from Allergy Resources, Inc., P.O. Box 888, 264 Brookridge, Palmer Lake, CO 80133.

Golos, Natalie and Frances Golos Golbitz. Coping with Your Allergies. New York, NY: A Fireside Book, Published by Simon and Schuster, Inc., 1986.

Golos, Natalie and William J. Rea, M.D. Success in the Clean Bedroom. Rochester, NY: Pinnacle Publishers, 1992.

Levin, Alan Scott, M.D. and Merla Zellerbach. The Type 1/Type 2 Allergy Relief Program. Los Angeles, CA: Jeremy P. Tarcher, Inc., 1983.

Mandell, Marshall, Ph.D. and Lynne Waller Scanlon. 5-Day Allergy Relief System. New York, NY: Pocket Books, a Division of Simon and Schuster, Inc., 1979.

Randolph, Theron G., M.D. and Ralph W. Moss, Ph.D. An Alternative Approach to Allergies. New York, NY: Bantam Books, Inc., 1980.

Riotte, Louise. Carrots Love Tomatoes: Secrets of Companion Planting for Successful Gardening. Pownal, VT: Garden Way Publishing, a division of Storey Communications, Inc., 1975.

Rogers, Sherry A., M.D. The E.I. Syndrome. Syracuse, NY: Prestige Publishers, 1986. *(Prestige Publishers, Box 3161, 3502 Brewerton Road, Syracuse, NY 13220)*

Saltzman, Joanne. Amazing Grains. Tiburon, CA: H.J. Kramer, Inc., 1990. *(H.J. Kramer, Inc., P.O. Box 1082, Tiburon, CA 94920)*

Springer, Jerry. Allergies - Making Kids Crazy. Interview with Doris Rapp, M.D. Air Date: December 17, 1992. 45 min., Multimedia Entertainment, Inc., 1994. Videocassette. *(Available from Video Archives, Inc., 41 Paoli Plaza #3D, Paoli, PA 19301.)*

Thomas, Sherry and Jeanne Tetrault. Country Woman: A Handbook for the New Farmer. San Angelo, TX: Anchor Press, 1976. This book is currently out of print, but you should be able to find it in your local library.

Truss, C. Orian, M.D. The Missing Diagnosis. Birmingham, AL: By the author, 2614 Highland Avenue, 1982. *(The Missing Diagnosis, P.O. Box 26508, Birmingham, AL 35226)*

Cookbooks

Crook, William G., M.D. and Marjorie Hurt Jones, R.N. The Yeast Connection Cookbook. Jackson, TN: Professional Books, 1989. *Especially for vegetable cookery and salad dressings, as well as helpful ideas. (Available from Professional Books, Inc., 681 Skyline Drive, Jackson, TN 38301 or Mast Enterprises, Inc., 2615 N. Fourth Street #616, Coeur d'Alene, ID 83814.)*

Dumke, Nicolette M. Allergy Cooking with Ease. Lancaster, PA: Starburst Publishers, 1992. *Especially for alternative meats and gluten-free bread and pastas. (Available from Allergy Adapt, Inc., 1877 Polk Avenue, Louisville, CO 80027, (303) 666-8253.)*

________. More Allergy Cooking with Ease #1. Louisville, CO: Allergy Adapt, Inc., 1993. *Especially for yeasted wheat-free bread prepared in programmable bread machines and specialized recipes needed for EPD diet. (EPD is Enzyme Potentiated Desensitization allergy treatment.) (Allergy Adapt, Inc., 1877 Polk Avenue, Louisville, CO 80027, (303) 666-8253)*

Gates, Donna with Linda Schatz. The Body Ecology Diet: Recovering Your Health and Rebuilding Your Immunity. Atlanta, GA: B.E.D. Publications, 1993. *Especially for meat-free recipes. (B.E.D. Publications, 1266 West Paces Ferry Road, Suite 505, Atlanta, GA 30327)*

Golos, Natalie and Frances Golos Golbitz. If This Is Tuesday, It Must Be Chicken. New Canaan, CT: Keats Publishing, Inc., 1983. *Especially for information on rotation. (Keats Publishing, Inc., 27 Pine Street [Box 876], New Canaan, CT 06840)*

Grimmett, Charlene. Beat the Yeast Cookbook. Aurora, IL: By the author, 1985. *Especially for low carbohydrate recipes. (Charlene Grimmett, P.O. Box 1971, Aurora, IL 60507)*

Hayes, Stephanie, R.D. and Barbara Maynard, R.D. Rotational Bon Appetite! Dallas, TX: WJR and Associates, P.A. dba Environmental Health Center-Dallas, 1986. *Especially for information on rotation. (Environmental Health Center–Dallas, 8345 Walnut Hill Lane, Suite 205, Dallas, TX 75231)*

Jones, Marjorie Hurt, R.N. Super Foods. Coeur d'Alene, ID: Mast Enterprises, Inc., 1990. *Especially for specialty grains (Super Foods) recipes. (Mast Enterprises, Inc., 2615 N. Fourth Street #616, Coeur d'Alene, ID 83814)*

Saltzman, Joanne. Amazing Grains. Tiburon, CA: H.J. Kramer, Inc., 1990. Especially for meat-free recipes. *(H.J. Kramer, Inc., P.O. Box 1082, Tiburon, CA 94920)*

Newsletters

The following newsletters are excellent resources and a subscription would be a valuable addition to your personal informational library.

Canary Connect News. Editors: Sondra K. Lewis and Lonnett Dietrich Blakley. Canary Connect Publications, P.O. Box 5317, Coralville, IA 52241-0317. Phone: (319) 351-2371. 4 issues/year—initial issue, Early 1995. Back issues will be available.

Mastering Food Allergies. Editor: Marjorie Hurt Jones, R.N. MAST Enterprises, Inc., 2615 N. Fourth Street #616, Coeur d'Alene, ID 83814. Phone: (208) 772-8213. 6 issues/year. Back issues available. I highly recommend acquiring back issues.

Carbohydrate Level Resources

Rockwell, Sally, Nutritionist. Coping with *Candida* Cookbook (Revised). Seattle, WA: By the author, 1986. *(Sally J. Rockwell, P.O. Box 31065, Seattle, WA 98103)*

U.S. Department of Agriculture. Nutritive Value of Foods. Washington, DC: Government Printing Office, 1981. *May be available at your state's Department of Agriculture Extension Service.*

* * * * *

Use the space below to write in other books or literature which you find helpful or which are recommended to you.

APPENDIX E
COOPERATIVE FOOD WAREHOUSES IN THE UNITED STATES

Northeastern States

Northeast Cooperatives
P.O. Box 8188
Brattleboro, VT 05304
(802) 257-5856

Massachusettes, Maine, Rhode Island, New Hampshire, Vermont, Connecticut, Eastern New York

Southern States

Orange Blossom Warehouse
1601 NW 55th Place
Gainesville, FL 32653
(800) 372-7061

Florida, Georgia, Alabama, South Carolina, North Carolina

Ozark Cooperative Warehouse
P.O. Box 1528
Fayetteville, AR 72702
(501) 521-2667

Alabama, Arkansas, Georgia, Louisiana, Texas, Oklahoma, Mississippi, Western Texas, Part of Florida, Southern Missouri

Midwestern States

Blooming Prairie Warehouse
2340 Heinz Road
Iowa City, IA 52240
(800) 323-2131
(319) 337-6448

Iowa, Nebraska, Illinois, Indiana, Northern Kansas and Missouri, Southwestern Wyoming, Michigan, Southern South Dakota and Wisconsin

Blooming Prairie Natural Foods
510 Kasota Avenue SE
Minneapolis, MN 55414
(800) 322-8324 in MN
(800) 328-8241 outside MN

Southern Minnesota, Western Wisconsin, South Dakota, North Dakota, and Parts of Iowa

Federation of Ohio River Cooperatives
320 Outerbelt, Suite E
Columbus, OH 43213
(614) 861-2446

District of Columbia, Kentucky, Maryland, Michigan, Northern North Carolina, Ohio, Southeast Indiana, Tennessee, Virginia, West Virginia, Western Pennsylvania

North Farm
204 Regas Road
Madison, WI 53714
(608) 241-2667

Illinois, Indiana, Michigan, North Dakota, Wisconsin; Parts of Minnesota, Montana, Ohio, South Dakota, and Wyoming; Small areas of Iowa and Missouri

Southwestern States

Tucson Cooperative Warehouse
350 S. Toole
Tucson, AZ 85701
(602) 884-9951

Arizona, New Mexico, Las Vegas area, Southern California and Colorado, Middle Texas, Some of Utah

Northwestern States

Idaho Organic Producers Association
2260 E. 4300 N.
Filer, ID 83328
(208) 326-4114
FAX: (208) 326-3388

The state of Idaho does not have a cooperative food warehouse. However, the Idaho Organic Producers Association has agreed to act as a resource in providing information on the food-buying cooperatives which are active in the state.

Southern California

Food-Buying Cooperatives

Bonnie Lange Cooperative
379 Rochester
Costa Mesa, CA 92626
(714) 631-7951

Joyce Watt Cooperative
2731 Vista Heights Road
Orange, CA 92667
(714) 637-7216

Portola Cooperative
Attn: Nancy Woldridge
18812 Vista Modesta
Trabuco Canyon, CA 92678
(714) 589-1634

Red Hill Cooperative
Attn: Noel
11862 Red Hill Avenue
Santa Anna, CA 92667
(714) 832-6108

At publication date we have been unable to locate any Cooperative Food Warehouses in California. However, these four food-buying cooperatives located in southern California may be a good resource for you. This is not an exhaustive list of food-buying cooperatives in southern California. Ask around your area for other possible sources.

If you know of other cooperative food warehouses in the United States, please send me the name, address, phone number, and geographical area serviced for each so I may share the information with others through Canary Connect News newsletter (see Appendix G).

APPENDIX F
ORGANIZATIONS PROVIDING INFORMATION ON ORGANIC FOOD PRODUCTION AND AVAILABILITY

At publication date the following organizations have been contacted and have indicated their willingness to act as an informational resource regarding organic food production and availability in their geographical area. You should be aware, however, that the contact person for some of these organizations may change in the future. If a change does occur, the person listed here should be able to direct you to the currect contact person. When you contact these resources, please mention where you found them.

Arkansas

Ozark Organic Growers Association
HC73 Box 42
Jerusalem, AR 72080
(501) 745-5465
FAX: (501) 745-2589

California

California Certified Organic Farmers
1115 Mission Street
Santa Cruz, CA 95060
(408) 423-2263
FAX: (408) 423-4528

Colorado

Colorado Organic Producers Association
1778 S. Clarkson
Denver, CO 80210
(303) 777-6336

Connecticut

Northeast Organic Farming Association—Connecticut
69 Meetinghouse Hill Road
Durham, CT 06422
(203) 349-1417
OR P.O. Box 386
Northford, CT 06472
(203) 484-2445 (message only)

Idaho

Idaho Organic Producers Association
2260 E. 4300 N.
Filer, ID 83328
(208) 326-4114
FAX: (208) 326-3388

Illinois

Organic Crop Improvement Association—Illinois Chapter
R.R. 1 Box 68
Melvin, IL 60952
Phone/FAX: (217) 388-2888

Iowa

Iowa Organic Growers and Buyers Association
P.O. Box 2935
Iowa City, IA 52244-2935
(No phone available at publication date.)

Organic Crop Improvement Association—Chapter 1 of Iowa
6534 220th Street
Arthur, IA 51431
(712) 367-2442

Maine

Maine Organic Farmers and Gardeners Association
P.O. Box 2176
Augusta, ME 04338
(207) 622-3118

Massachusetts

Northeast Organic Farming Association—
Massachusetts
411 Sheldon Road
Barre, MA 01005
(508) 355-2853

Minnesota

Minnesota Grown Program
Minnesota Department of Agriculture
90 W. Plato Boulevard
St. Paul, MN 55107
(612) 297-2301
Request a copy of Minnesota Grown Farmer to Consumer Directory.

Missouri

Missouri Organic Association
2832 Olde Chelsea
St. Charles, MO 63301
(314) 657-4156

Montana

Alternative Energy Resources
Organization
25 South Ewing Street
Suite 214
Helena, MT 59601
(406) 443-7272
FAX: (406) 442-9120

Nebraska

Nebraska Sustainable Agriculture Society
P.O. Box 736
Hartington, NE 68739
(402) 254-2289
FAX: (402) 254-6891

New Hampshire

New Hampshire Department of Agriculture
P.O. Box 2042
Concord, NH 03302-2042
(603) 271-3685
FAX: (603) 271-1109
Ask for the Certified Organic Farm List.

New Jersey

Northeast Organic Farming Association—
New Jersey
31 Titus Mill Road
Pennington, NJ 08534
(609) 737-6848
FAX: (609) 737-3075

New Mexico

New Mexico Organic Commodity
Commission
P.O. Box 3628
Albuquerque, NM 87108
(505) 266-9849
Ask for a growers list.

New York

Northeast Organic Farming Association—
New York
472 Monkey Run Road
Port Crane, NY 13833
(607) 648-5557

North and South Carolina

Carolina Farm Stewardship Association
115 West Main Street
Carrboro, NC 27510
(919) 968-1030

North and South Dakota

Northern Plains Sustainable Agriculture
Society
HC5 Box 104
Langdon, ND 58249
(701) 256-2424

Oklahoma

Kerr Center for Sustainable Agriculture,
Inc.
P.O. Box 588
Poteau, OK 74953
(918) 647-9123
FAX: (918) 647-8712

Oregon

Oregon Tilth Certified Organic
P.O. Box 218
Tualatin, OR 97062
(503) 692-4877
FAX: (503) 691-2514

Rhode Island

Northeast Organic Farming Association—Rhode Island
P.O. Box 83
Peace Dale, RI 02883
(401) 295-1030

Tennessee

Tennessee Land Stewardship Association
450 Davidson Chapel Lane
Bloomington Springs, TN 38545
(615) 653-4402

Vermont

Northeast Organic Farming Association—Vermont
P.O. Box 697
Richmond, VT 05477
(802) 434-4122

Wisconsin

Organic Crop Improvement Association—Wisconsin
Route 1 Box 1198
Soldier's Grove, WI 54655
(608) 734-3273
FAX: (608) 734-3306

If you know of other organizations providing information on organic food production and availability for states not listed in this appendix, please send me the name, address, and phone number for each so I may share the information with others through Canary Connect News newsletter (see Appendix G).

Appendix G
Canary Connect

Thank you for purchasing *Allergy & Candida Cooking—Rotational Style.* We hope you enjoy reading and using it and that the information and recipes it contains will aid you in your journey towards better health.

We would love to hear from you regarding how this book has affected your life. We also look forward to our future projects and to the continuing effort to provide you with the best, most complete information possible to enhance your health and lifestyle.

Please accept our best wishes as you use this book. You will be in our prayers as you continue the adventure of life and learning.

Sondra Lonnett

* * * * * * *

<u>Upcoming projects for Canary Connect</u>

- <u>Canary Connect News</u> newsletter, published quarterly. First issue early 1995.
- Cooking Video Series, beginning with "Tortillas and More" cooking video to be released in Spring 1995.
- Booklet—Traveling with Food Allergies. Projected publication date currently not set.

<u>Projected articles and columns for Canary Connect News newsletter</u>

Our goal is for the newsletter to fit your needs. Send us your opinions regarding this list so we can know of your interests. You may also send us your list of additions.

- Information on current research, alternative treatment programs, and/or supplements investigated by us and/or shared by <u>Canary Connect News</u> readers on:
  - ◊ *Candida* Related Complex
  - ◊ Chronic Fatigue Syndrome
  - ◊ Food Allergies
  - ◊ Multiple Chemical Sensitivities/Environmental Illness (MCS/EI)
- Helpful hints developed by us and from <u>Canary Connect News</u> readers dealing with food preparation, food allergies, chemical sensitivities, etc.
- Current information and research on FOS (Fructo-oligo-saccharides).
- Meal planning ideas—especially Quick & Easy Meals and Meals Away from Home.
- Resources for hard-to-find food products.
- Recipes, recipes, and more recipes—
  - ◊ that follow the *Candida* control and rotational diet set forth in this book.
  - ◊ that follow the *Candida* control diet.
  - ◊ from you, the readers of <u>Canary Connect News</u>.
- Organic gardening—including growing amaranth greens and herbs.
- Sprouting whole grains.
- Traveling tips.

What Does *Canary Connect* Mean?

The name **Canary Connect** was chosen to illustrate the focus of my endeavors and as a symbol of my goal and purpose. Canaries were used in coal mine tunnels to warn miners of dangerous coal gases. Since canaries are more sensitive to coal gases than humans, they would stop singing (or even die) when the dangerous gases were present in the mine shafts. Coal miners would then know to leave immediately.

Those of us who are affected by Multiple Chemical Sensitivities/Environmental Illness (MCS/EI) have come to regard ourselves as warning canaries for today's world. Since we are more sensitive to chemicals and other dangerous substances present in today's world, we, as human "canaries," are singing out the message of danger to any and all who will hear and respond. We "sing" not only to reach those around us, but to connect with other human "canaries" to share information and techniques that may assist us in our daily lives.

Page Mark Labels for Chapters for Days 1, 2, 3, and 4

Would you like to be able to quickly access the chapters for Days 1, 2, 3, and 4 without fumbling through the book pages? A good way to do this is to place a bright-colored, self-adhesive label over the edge of the first page of each Day's chapter (pages, 97, 147, 197, and 237). Please be careful when placing your label that you do not cover any text on either side of the page. It also works best if you stagger the placement down the edge of the pages. With these bright indicators in place, you will be able to turn quickly to each Day's food list or recipes when you are doing meal planning or preparation.

Foods for Day 1

Animal Protein

88	catfish
98	tuna
103	halibut, sole
124	chicken, chicken egg, Cornish hen, pheasant, quail

Vegetables

6	bamboo shoots
7	Chinese water chestnut
28	beets, chard
36	broccoli, cabbage, radish, turnip, collards
65	celery, parsley*

Grains, Flours, & Baking Foods

6	Kamut®, rice, spelt, teff, wheat

Fruit

40a	pear
40b	apricot, peach, nectarine
40c	raspberry

Sweeteners

6	rice syrup
40a	pear

Oils

40b	almond oil
75	sesame oil

Herbs & Spices

34	cinnamon*
36	dill, dry mustard
65	cumin

Seeds & Nuts

22	pecan
40b	almond
75	sesame seeds

Foods for Day 2

Animal Protein

82	shrimp, crab, prawn, lobster
87	cod (scrod), pollack
129	rabbit
137	beef, buffalo, plain yogurt
n/a	red snapper

Vegetables

11	onion
41	garbanzo (chickpea), lima beans
54	okra
74	potato, tomato, green pepper, eggplant
79	cucumber, pumpkin, spaghetti and zucchini squash
80	lettuce

Grains, Flours, & Baking Foods

19	arrowroot starch
30	amaranth
41	garbanzo bean flour (chickpea)
74	potato starch

Fruit

16	banana, plantain
45	grapefruit, lemon
56	kiwi
79	melons

Sweeteners

Currently recipes for Day 2 are developed using stevia or honey floated from Day 4

Oils

69	olive oil
80	sunflower oil
137	butter, ghee (clarified butter)

Herbs & Spices

11	garlic**
63	allspice, clove
73	basil, marjoram, oregano**, rosemary, sage, savory, thyme
74	cayenne (red) pepper, chili powder**

Seeds & Nuts

79	pumpkin seeds
80	sunflower seeds

Unassigned "Fun Foods" (See explanation on pages 30–31.)

10	pineapple
17	ginger
20	vanilla
26	macadamia nut
33	nutmeg
44	flaxseed and flaxseed oil
50	maple
62	Brazil nut

*Foods that float between Days 1 and 3
**Foods that float between Days 2 and 4

Foods for Day 3

Animal Protein

103	flounder, turbot
106	salmon, trout
121	duck, goose
126	turkey, turkey, egg

Vegetables

28	spinach
36	cauliflower, Brussels sprouts, rutabaga, kale
65	carrots, parsnips, parsley*

Grains, Flours, & Baking Foods

6	barley, corn, millet, oat, rye, wild rice
28	quinoa
47	tapioca starch
52	cream of tartar

Fruit

34	avocado
40a	apple
40b	plum, prune, cherry
52	raisin, grape

Sweeteners

40a	apple
28	FOS—NutriFlora™

Oils

22	walnut oil
36	canola oil

Herbs & Spices

34	bay leaf
34	cinnamon*
65	caraway, fennel

Seeds & Nuts

22	walnut
23	filbert (hazelnut)

Foods for Day 4

Animal Protein

87	haddock	130	squirrel
91	sea bass	134	pork
95	mahi mahi	135	venison
100	swordfish	137	lamb, goat
102	ocean perch	n/a	orange roughy

Vegetables

11	asparagus, leeks
27	sorrel
41	greenbeans, peas, lentils, soybeans, & all beans not on Day 2
70	sweet potato
74	squash—acorn, butternut, & other squash not on Day 2
80	artichoke

Grains, Flours, & Baking Foods

1	agar agar, kombu
27	buckwheat
41	carob powder, kudzu (kuzu) and lentil, soy, navy, & pinto bean flours
80	Jerusalem artichoke flour

Fruit

27	rhurbarb
45	orange, tangerine, tangelo
93	blueberry, cranberry

Sweeteners

27	buckwheat honey
41	clover honey
80	stevia

Oils

41	soy oil
80	safflower oil

Herbs & Spices

11	garlic**
73	oregano**
74	chili powder**
80	tarragon

Seeds & Nuts

41	roasted soy beans
48	cashew

Unassigned "Fun Foods" (See explanation on pages 30–31.)

10 pineapple	26 macadamia nut	50 maple
17 ginger	33 nutmeg	62 Brazil nut
20 vanilla	44 flaxseed and flaxseed oil	

*Foods that float between Days 1 and 3
**Foods that float between Days 2 and 4

Guidelines for writing to authors of

Allergy & Candida Cooking—Rotational Style

We would love to hear from you with comments, questions, and/or miscellaneous information to share with others in Canary Connect News newsletter. However, please follow these simple guidelines when writing so that we can handle the flood of mail effectively and efficiently.

First, please organize your comments, helpful hints, and information to share in Canary Connect News newsletter separate from personal questions.

To submit information to share in Canary Connect News, use page 345 or a photocopy of the page. However, if you desire you may use a separate sheet of paper and format your submission appropriately. If you refer to a published source in your submission, please include the complete bibliographical information. Possible subject areas for which you may desire to make submissions include:

- A question that you would like to submit to CCN readers for their input
- Current information relating to food allergies
- Helpful hints dealing with food preparation and food allergies as well as chemical sensitivities
- Information on available treatment programs and/or supplements for:
  - ◊ *Candida* Related Complex
  - ◊ Chronic Fatigue Syndrome
  - ◊ Food Allergies
  - ◊ Multiple Chemical Sensitivities/Environmental Illness (MCS/EI)
- Meal planning ideas—especially Quick & Easy Meals and Meals Away from Home
- Recipes that follow the *Candida* control diet
- Resources for hard-to-find food products
- Traveling tips

Guidelines to follow when submitting a question for a personal response are:

1. We prefer that you submit only one question per page or half page so that we may respond to each question separately.
2. Questions requiring research may require a longer time to answer, so if you submit only one question per page it may help us respond more quickly to the less-time-consumng questions.
3. Keep questions concise but detailed enough for us to understand the situation and to give you an accurate response.
4. Please put your name, address, and phone number on each page that you send.
5. A personal response to questions requires a self-addressed, stamped envelope.
6. Realize that some questions may be beyond our knowledge, but we will try to at least direct you to someone else. Also, we may rephrase your question and include it in Canary Connect News newsletter for others to respond.
7. Do realize that some questions may take some research time and that a fee may be involved. If a fee is involved, we will inform you of the estimated cost for your approval prior to undertaking the research.

Send to: **Sondra K. Lewis**
c/o Canary Connect Publications, P.O. Box 5317, Coralville, IA 52241-0317

Thank You

Use this half page or a photocopy of it to submit information to be shared in

Canary Connect News

(If you desire, you may use a separate sheet of paper and include the information indicated below.)

Sondra and Lonnett, my submission for Canary Connect News is:

____

____

____

____

____

If needed, continue on back side of this half sheet and/or on a separate sheet of paper.

Please check one:
____ Please sign my first name, last initial, and state
____ Please sign my submission as an anonymous CCN reader

Name ______________________________

Address ______________________________

City/State/Zip ______________________________

Phone number: (day) ________________ (evening) ________________

We prefer at least one number in case we desire more information by phone.

Send your submissions to: Canary Connect News, P.O. Box 5317, Coralville, IA 52241-0317

\- - - - - - - - - - - - - - - - - - - -

Use this half page or a photocopy of it to submit information to be shared in

Canary Connect News

(If you desire, you may use a separate sheet of paper and include the information indicated below.)

Sondra and Lonnett, my submission for Canary Connect News is:

____

____

____

____

____

If needed, continue on back side of this half sheet and/or on a separate sheet of paper.

Please check one:
____ Please sign my first name, last initial, and state
____ Please sign my submission as an anonymous CCN reader

Name ______________________________

Address ______________________________

City/State/Zip ______________________________

Phone number: (day) ________________ (evening) ________________

We prefer at least one number in case we desire more information by phone.

Send your submissions to: Canary Connect News, P.O. Box 5317, Coralville, IA 52241-0317

Use this page or a photocopy of it to order general information from

CANARY CONNECT

However, if you desire you may use a separate sheet of paper, order by the code number in the left column, enclose the appropriate fee listed in the right column, and provide requested mailing address information. See reverse side of this form for FOS scientific articles and abstracts.

SEND REQUESTED INFORMATION TO:

Name
Address
City/State/Zip

CIRCLE THE CODE NUMBER IN THE LEFT COLUMN TO REQUEST THE FOLLOWING INFORMATION:

#	INFORMATION DESCRIPTION	PRICE*
1	Basic FOS information packet including Sondra's success story with *Candida* and food allergies, order form, and the following article: Perna, Peter J., Ph.D., Manager. "Fructooligosaccharides (FOS): An All Natural Food which Promotes *Bifidobacteria* and *Lactobacillus*." Broomfield, CO: Center for Applied Nutrition, ZeaGen, Inc., 530 Interlocken Boulevard, 80021.	NO CHARGE
2	Brochure & Order Form for Chuck's Seafood—Tuna and Salmon (Packed in glass jars)	NO CHARGE
3	Information on how to receive Sondra's personalized assistance regarding specialized recipes and meal planning to fit a personalized rotation	NO CHARGE
4	Information regarding Video Cooking Series or other publications by Canary Connect Publications as it becomes available.	NO CHARGE
5	Brochure & order form for Granny's Old Fashioned Products (See below for low-cost trial sizes available for purchase.)	NO CHARGE
6	Granny's 2oz. Trial Size Circle choice(s) below. $1.50 each or all 7 for $7 (price includes shipping)	
	Subtotal to be Carried Over to Reverse Side of This Page $	

Granny's Old Fashioned Household & Personal Care Products.

Granny's products are specially formulated for the chemically sensitive and are economical, effective, environmentally friendly, and free of fragrance, phosphate, formaldehyde, and dye. All Granny's products are in liquid form.

Please circle your choice(s) of trial sizes ordered above:

Laundry Liquid   Dish/All Purpose Cleaner   Hand & Body Liquid Soap

Protein Shampoo   Tearless Shampoo   Creme Rinse

Hand & Body Moisturizing Lotion

*Prices subject to change without notice.

Order Form for General Information from Canary Connect (continued)

<table>
<tr><th>#</th><th>INFORMATION DESCRIPTION</th><th>PRICE*</th></tr>
<tr><td colspan="2">Subtotal Carried Over from Reverse Side of This Page $</td><td></td></tr>
<tr><td>7</td><td>The items found in code numbers 7 and 8 are more scientific articles on FOS, its uses, and the available research on its effects. They may be more appropriate reading for persons in the health-care professions.
The following three (3) scientific articles and abstracts on FOS:
Modler, H.W., R.C. McKellar, and M. Yaguchi. "Bifidobacteria and Bifidogenic Factors," <u>Journal of Canadian Institute of Food Science and Technology</u>, 21, no. 1 (1990): 29-41.
Hosoya, N., D. Dhorranintra, and H. Hidaka. "Utilization of [U-^{14}C] Fructooligosaccharides in Man as Energy Resources," <u>Journal of Clinical Biochemical Nutrition</u>, 5 (1988): 67-74. Abstract.
Hidaka, H., T. Eida, T. Takizawa, T. Tokunaga, and Y. Tahiro. "Effects of Fructooligosaccharides on Intestinal Flora and Human Health," <u>Bifidobacteria Microflora</u>, 5, no. 1 (1986): 37-50. Abstract.</td><td>Shipping and Handling Charge of $3.00</td></tr>
<tr><td>8</td><td>The three (3) articles and abstracts listed above plus the following twelve (12) scientific articles and abstracts on FOS:
Fukuyasu, T., T. Oshida, and K. Ashida. "Effect of Oligosaccharides on Growth of Piglets and on Bacterial Flora, Putrefactive Substances and Volatile Fatty Acids in Their Feces," <u>Bulletin of Animal Hygiene</u>, 26 (1987): 15-22. Abstract
McKellar, R.C. and H.W. Modler. "Metabolism of Fructooligosaccharides by Bifidobacterium sp.," <u>Applied Microbiology Biotechnology</u>, 31 (1989): 537-541. Abstract.
Mitsuoka, T. "Bifidobacteria and Their Role in Human Health," <u>Journal of Industrial Microbiology</u>, 6 (1990): 263-268.
Mitsuoka, T. "Effects of Long-term Intake of Neosugar (Fructooligosaccharides) on Intestinal Flora and Serum Lipids," <u>Proceedings of the 3rd Neosugar Conference</u>, Tokyo (1986). Abstract.
Mitsuoka, T.; H. Hidaka, and T. Eida. "Effect of Fructooligosaccharides on Intestinal Microflora," <u>Die Nahrung</u>, 31, no. 5-6 (1987): 427-436. Abstract.
Oku, T, T. Tkunaga, and N. Hosoya. "Nondigestibility of a New Sweetener, 'Neosugar', in the Rat," <u>Journal of Nutrition</u>, 114 (1984): 1574-1581. Abstract.
Sano, T. "Effect of Neosugar (Fructooligosaccharides) on Constipation, Intestinal Microflora and Gallbladder Contraction in Diabetics," <u>Proceedings of the 3rd Neosugar Conference</u>, Tokyo (1986). Abstract.
Spiegel, J.E., R. Rose, P. Karabell, V.H. Frankos, and D.F. Schmitt. "Safety and Benefits of Fructooligosaccharides as Food Ingredients," <u>Food Technology</u> (January 1994): 85-89.
Takahashi, Y. "Effects of Neosugar (Fructooligoaccharides) in the Chronic Renal-Failure Patient," <u>Proceedings of the 3rd Neosugar Conference</u>, Tokyo (1986). Abstract.
Tokunaga, T, T. Oku, and N. Hosoya. "Utilization and Excretion of a New Sweetener, Fructooligosaccharides (Neosugar), in Rats," <u>Journal of Nutrition</u>, 119 (1989): 553-559. Abstract
Williams, C.H., S.W. Witherly, and R.K. Buddington. "Influence of Dietary Neosugar on Selected Bacterial Groups of the Human Faecal Flora," <u>Microbial Ecology in Health and Disease</u>, 7 (1994): (accepted for publication).
Yamashita, K., K. Kawai, and M. Itakura. "Effects of Fructo-oligosaccharides on Blood Glucose and Serum Lipids in Diabetic Subjects," <u>Nutrition Research</u>, 4 (1984): 961-966.9.</td><td>Shipping and Handling Charge of $8.00</td></tr>
<tr><td colspan="2">Please send order with payment to:
CANARY CONNECT PUBLICATIONS
P.O. Box 5317
Coralville, IA 52241-0317

TOTAL ENCLOSED $
Check or money order
(US Funds Only)</td><td></td></tr>
</table>

*Prices subject to change without notice.

THANK YOU FOR REQUESTING THE ABOVE ITEMS.
BE SURE TO COMPLETE MAILING INFORMATION ON REVERSE SIDE OF THIS FORM.

RETURN THIS PAGE OR A PHOTOCOPY OF IT TO ORDER

Allergy & Candida Cooking—Rotational Style
by Sondra K. Lewis
with Lonnett Dietrich Blakley

and/or to order your subscription for

Canary Connect News
A quarterly newsletter edited by
Sondra K. Lewis and
Lonnett Dietrich Blakley

Did you enjoy Sondra's recipes, meal planning ideas, helpful hints, general information, and ideas in this book? Do you desire on-going support from Sondra and others regarding *Candida* Related Complex, food allergies, rotational diet, Multiple Chemical Sensitivities/Environmental Illness (MCS/EI), and Chronic Fatigue Syndrome?

Then Canary Connect News newsletter is your answer. Subscribe today for this exciting quarterly newsletter.

For more information regarding subjects and columns to be included in Canary Connect News, see page 340 of this cookbook. Back issues are also available. More information available upon request.

Number of copies of **Allergy & *Candida* Cooking—Rotational Style** ________

Price per copy X $19.95

Subtotal ________

Iowa residents add 5% sales tax ($1 per copy) ________

Shipping & Handling Charge Per Book ________

US Book Rate $2.50
US Priority Rate $5.00
Canada $7.00

Enter my 1 year subscription (4 issues) to **Canary Connect News** ________

US & Canada @ $15 per year
Other countries @ $20 per year

Thank you for your order **TOTAL ENCLOSED $** ________

Send your order with payment (check or money order—US Funds only) to:

CANARY CONNECT PUBLICATIONS
P.O. Box 5317
Coralville, IA 52241-0317

Ship book(s) and/or newsletter to:

NAME ________________________

ADDRESS ________________________

CITY/STATE/ZIP ________________________

RETURN THIS PAGE OR A PHOTOCOPY OF IT TO ORDER

Allergy & Candida Cooking—Rotational Style
by Sondra K. Lewis
with Lonnett Dietrich Blakley

and/or to order your subscription for

Canary Connect News
A quarterly newsletter edited by
Sondra K. Lewis and
Lonnett Dietrich Blakley

Did you enjoy Sondra's recipes, meal planning ideas, helpful hints, general information, and ideas in this book? Do you desire on-going support from Sondra and others regarding *Candida* Related Complex, food allergies, rotational diet, Multiple Chemical Sensitivities/Environmental Illness (MCS/EI), and Chronic Fatigue Syndrome?

Then Canary Connect News newsletter is your answer. Subscribe today for this exciting quarterly newsletter.

For more information regarding subjects and columns to be included in Canary Connect News, see page 340 of this cookbook. Back issues are also available. More information available upon request.

Number of copies of **Allergy & *Candida* Cooking—Rotational Style** ________

Price per copy X $19.95

Subtotal ________

Iowa residents add 5% sales tax ($1 per copy) ________

Shipping & Handling Charge Per Book ________

US Book Rate	$2.50
US Priority Rate	$5.00
Canada	$7.00

Enter my 1 year subscription (4 issues) to **Canary Connect News** ________

US & Canada @ $15 per year
Other countries @ $20 per year

Thank you for your order

TOTAL ENCLOSED $ ________

Send your order with payment (check or money order—US Funds only) to:

CANARY CONNECT PUBLICATIONS
P.O. Box 5317
Coralville, IA 52241-0317

Ship book(s) and/or newsletter to:

NAME ________

ADDRESS ________

CITY/STATE/ZIP ________

Evaluation Form for Allergy & *Candida* Cooking—Rotational Style

Please use this form or a photocopy of it to report any errors such as typos, grammar, or spelling that you see in the cookbook (no matter how small or insignificant). We will use your comments to correct the text before future printings and/or editions, and in future works by the authors in the form of book, video, or newsletter.

We developed this book to be clear and concise, while detailed especially for the inexperienced cook. All efforts have been made to make this book informative, readable, and understandable by people at all levels of experience or expertise in the areas of subject matter and cooking skills.

I prefer that you sign your evaluation form only so that I may contact you if we have a question regarding your comments.

If you want a personal answer to any question (rather than a response printed in Canary Connect News newsletter), you must send a self-addressed stamped envelope. Also, see page 344 for guidelines regarding writing to the authors. Please allow up to several weeks for your answer.

For each category listed below please evaluate clarity, information, and useability with a ranking of 1 to 10 (10 being the highest),

Book Section	Clarity	Information	Useability
Table of Contents			
How to Use This Book			
1. Candida Related Complex (CRC)			
2. Treatments for CRC			
3. Rotational Diet			
4. Specialty Foods			
5. Basic Equipment			
6. Helpful Hints			
7. Meal Planning			
8. Foods, Meal Planning, & Recipes for Day 1			
9. Foods, Meal Planning, & Recipes for Day 2			
10. Foods, Meal Planning, & Recipes for Day 3			
11. Foods, Meal Planning, & Recipes for Day 4			
12. Organics—The Only Way to Go!			
Bibliography			
Appendix A: Food Families			
Appendix B: *Candida* Questionnaire			
Appendix C: Resources			
Appendix D: Recommended Reading			
Appendix E: Cooperative Warehouses			
Appendix F: Availablity of Organic Food			
Appendix G: Canary Connect			
Subject Index			
Recipe Index			
Graphics/Tables/Charts			
Special Sayings			
Book Covers			
Spiral Binding			

Please continue evaluation on reverse side. Thank you!

Cookbook Evaluation Form
(continued)

Did you appreciate that the book was printed with soy bean ink and on nontoxic recycled paper?		Yes		No	No Opinion
How much of the book have you read and begun to apply?	all	most	about half	very little	none
How many of the recipes have you prepared?	up to 10	11–30		31–50	over 50
Would you recommend this book to friends/family/health-care professionals, etc?		Yes		No	Maybe
Would you recommend that your local health-food store carry this book?		Yes		No	Maybe

Other Comments:

____

Evaluation Date: ____________________

Name: ____________________

Address: ____________________

City/State/Zip: ____________________

Phone: ____________________

Please send evaluation form to:

Sondra K. Lewis
c/o Canary Connect Publications
P. O. Box 5317
Coralville, IA 52241-0317

Thank you for taking the time to inform us of your opinions!
They are important to us.

Subject INDEX

(continued)

(continued)

RECIPE INDEX

Never give in—
in nothing great or small,
large or petty—
never give in.
—Winston Churchill

Hold fast to dreams; for if dreams die, life
is a broken-winged bird that cannot fly.
—Lanston Hughes

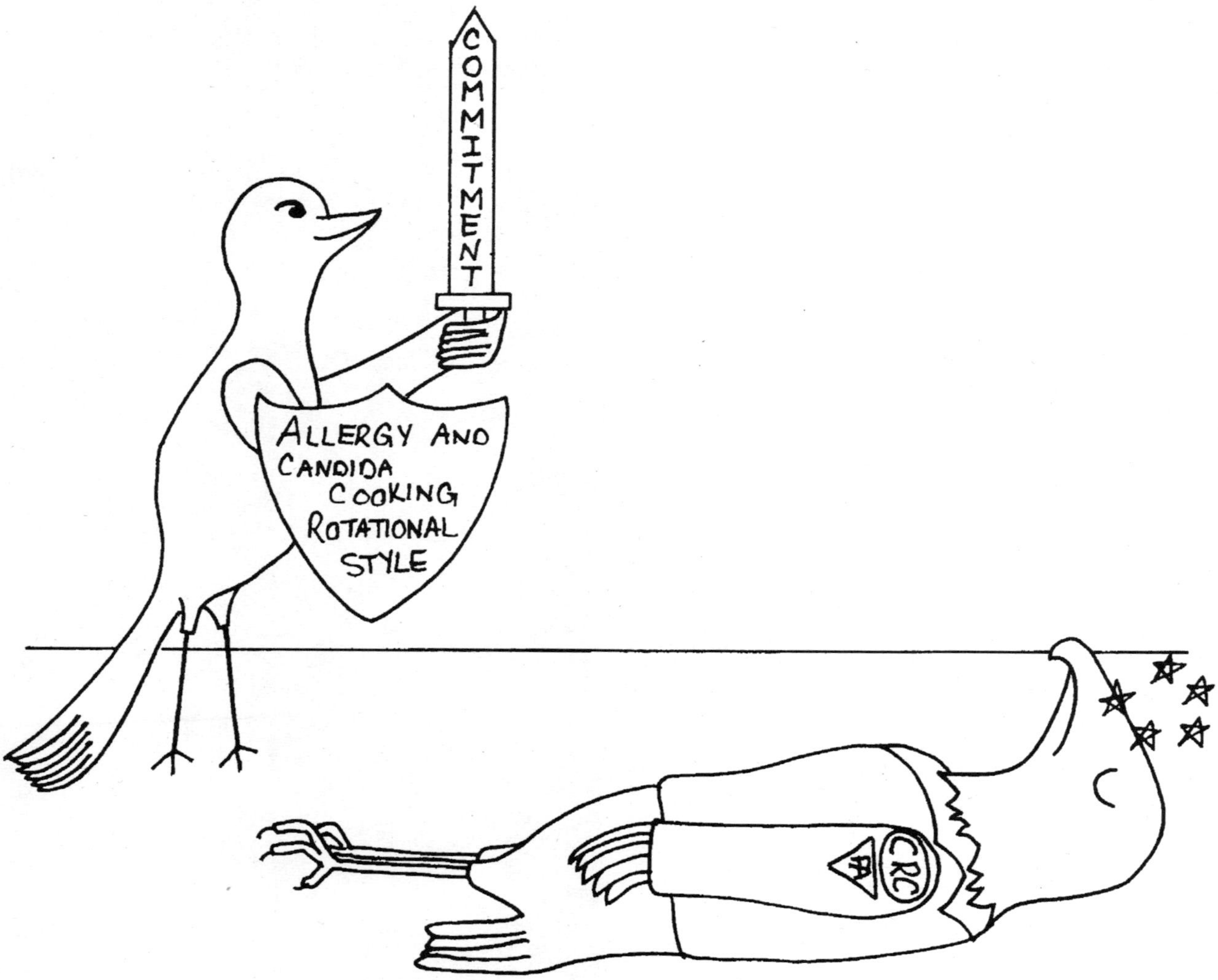